AF342252

A Handbook
of Kidney
Nomenclature
and Nosology

Supported in part by grants from the
Josiah Macy, Jr. Foundation and the
National Library of Medicine, U.S.
Public Health Service (LM 00619)

A Handbook of Kidney Nomenclature and Nosology

Criteria for Diagnosis, Including Laboratory Procedures

Prepared by
The International
Committee for Nomenclature
and Nosology of
Renal Disease

Little, Brown and Company
Boston

Contents

Preface

Every scientific discipline must define its terms, and from time to time redefine, delete, augment, or in other ways change its vocabulary and ways of ordering its subject matter. The rapid developments in research techniques and clinical developments in nephrology over the past twenty-five years have made such a look at nosology and nomenclature mandatory and, some would say, long overdue.

As early as 1966 a number of nephrologists recognized the need for a standard nomenclature, and several groups of physicians had organized to investigate the problem. In the United States the Kidney Foundation of Illinois supported a committee headed by Dr. Robert Kark, and in New York, Eaton Laboratories, Inc. supported a group headed by Dr. Kurt Lange. The Armed Forces Institute of Pathology, represented by Dr. F. K. Mostofi, the Renal Section of the American Heart Association, and the National Kidney Foundation were also early involved in nomenclature discussions.

An informal meeting of representatives of these groups met at the time of the Third International Congress of Nephrology in Washington in September 1966. Those present at the meeting, sponsored by the National Kidney Foundation, included Drs. Kurt Lange, Robert Kark, David P. Earle, E. Lovell Becker, Paul Kimmelstiel,* Louis G. Welt,* President of the NKF, and Neal S. Bricker, President of the American Society of Nephrology.

The result of that meeting was a merger of the Illinois and New York groups into a single committee which became the International Committee for Nomenclature and Nosology of Renal Disease. Dr. Earle, representing the Renal Section of the AHA, was named Chairman, Drs. Kark and Lange, Vice-Chairmen, and Dr. Becker, Secretary-General. The Executive Committee, augmented by Dr. Robert T. McCluskey to represent pathology, agreed that the most efficient way to proceed would be to set up working subcommittees, each charged with a particular field of interest: anatomy, pathology, physiology, clinical medicine, and so on. The sub-

* Deceased

committees were requested to seek outside experts to advise, review, or write particular entries for this volume.

Initial financing for the work of the Committee was provided by Eaton Laboratories and the Kidney Foundation of Illinois. This was augmented by a five-year grant from the Josiah Macy, Jr. Foundation to Cornell University Medical College and, subsequently, by a grant from the National Library of Medicine, U.S. Public Health Service (LM 00619), administered through the Federation of American Societies for Experimental Biology.

From the outset the make-up of the various subcommittees and the roster of advisors has been international. This is in keeping with the Committee's stated goal of producing standard nomenclature and nosology that would have worldwide acceptance. To facilitate communication between countries, several international meetings have been held, and at the time of the Stockholm meeting of the Fourth International Congress of Nephrology in 1969, official representatives were chosen from countries most active in nephrology.

The Stockholm meeting was also the occasion for formal endorsement of the Committee's nomenclature and nosology work by the International Society of Nephrology. Since that time members of the Executive Committee have also explored the future association with the World Health Organization in testing the new vocabulary and classification.

The production of a nomenclature and classification that will be accepted by experts throughout the world is an ambitious undertaking. The Committee acknowledges that disagreements and controversies are inevitable, especially in areas in which new techniques have resulted in new information about kidney structure, function, or pathology derangements. As knowledge proceeds, concomitant modifications in terminology will be essential. Thus, this first attempt at establishing a nomenclature and nosology of renal disease is in no sense the last word. The Committee will feel amply rewarded for its efforts if this volume produces the basis for future discussions among nephrologists throughout the world.

The Executive Committee

Committee Members, Advisors, and Contributors

Theodore Ehrenreich, M.D.

Professor of Pathology, New York Medical
College, New York

Robert B. Jennings, M.D.

Professor of Pathology, Northwestern
University Medical School, Chicago

Renée Habib, M.D.

Director of Research, Hôpital des Enfants
Malades, Paris, France

Robert H. Heptinstall, M.D.

Baxley Professor of Pathology, The Johns
Hopkins University School of Medicine,
Baltimore

Anders Bergstrand, M.D.

Karolinska Institutet, Stockholm, Sweden

Robert T. McCluskey, M.D.

Conrad L. Pirani, M.D.

Professor of Pathology, Columbia
University College of Physicians and
Surgeons, New York

Victor E. Pollak, M.D.

Professor of Internal Medicine, University
of Cincinnati College of Medicine,
Cincinnati

Sheldon C. Sommers, M.D.

Director of Laboratories, Lenox Hill
Hospital, New York

Subcommittee for Anatomy

Chairman

Johannes A. G. Rhodin, M.D.

Chairman, Department of Anatomy, New
York Medical College, New York

Harrison Latta, M.D.

Professor of Pathology, University of
California, Los Angeles (UCLA) School
of Medicine

Jacob Churg, M.D.

Anders Bergstrand, M.D.

Subcommittee for Physiology

Chairman
Theodore N. Pullman, M.D.
Professor of Medicine, The Pritzker School
of Medicine of The University of Chicago

Norman Bank, M.D.
Professor of Medicine, Albert Einstein
College of Medicine, Bronx, New York

Neal S. Bricker, M.D.
Professor and Chairman, Department of
Medicine, Albert Einstein College of
Medicine, Bronx, New York

Norman W. Carter, M.D.
Professor of Internal Medicine, University
of Texas Southwestern Medical School,
Dallas

Marvin Forland, M.D.
Professor of Medicine, The University of
Texas Southwestern Medical School, Dallas

Richard E. Rieselbach, M.D.
Professor of Medicine, University of
Wisconsin Medical School, Madison

Subcommittee for Immunology

Robert T. McCluskey, M.D.

Kurt Lange, M.D.

Subcommittee for Clinical Medicine

Robert M. Kark, M.D., Chairman

E. Lovell Becker, M.D.

J. Denys Blainey, M.D.
Queen Elizabeth Hospital, Birmingham,
England

David P. Earle, Jr., M.D.

Robert H. Heptinstall, M.D.

Howard G. Worthen, M.D.
Professor of Pediatrics, The University
of Texas Southwestern Medical School,
Dallas

George E. Schreiner, M.D.
Professor of Medicine, Georgetown
University School of Medicine,
Washington, D.C.

Herman Villarreal, M.D.
Professor of Medicine, Universidad
Nacional de Mexico, Mexico City

Subcommittee for Radiology

Milton Elkin, M.D.
Chairman, Department of Radiology,
Albert Einstein College of Medicine,
Bronx, New York

Harold A. Baltaxe, M.D.
Associate Professor of Radiology, Cornell
University Medical College, New York

E. Lovell Becker, M.D.

Subcommittee on a Morphological Classification of Renal Diseases

Conrad L. Pirani, M.D., Chairman

Victor E. Pollak, M.D.

Robert B. Jennings, M.D.

Robert T. McCluskey, M.D.

Subcommittee on an Etiological
Classification of Renal Diseases

Robert M. Kark, M.D.

and members of the Subcommittee
for Clinical Medicine

WORLD REPRESENTATIVES OF THE INTERNATIONAL COMMITTEE FOR NOMENCLATURE AND NOSOLOGY OF RENAL DISEASE

Argentina
Dr. Manuel L. Arce
Instituto de Investigaciones Medicas,
Buenos Aires

Australia
Dr. Priscilla Kincaid-Smith
Royal Melbourne Hospital, Victoria

Belgium
Dr. P. Lambert
Hôpital Universitaire Brugmann, Brussels

Brazil
Dr. Heonir Rocha
Universidade Federal da Bahia
Faculdade de Medicina, Bahia

Canada
Dr. Z. F. Jaworski
University of Ottawa, Ottawa, Ontario

Czechoslovakia
Prof. J. Brod
(Previously Prague, Czechoslovakia)
I. Medizinische Klinik und Poliklinik der
Johannes Gutenberg-Universität,
Langenbeckstrasse, West Germany

Denmark

Dr. C. Brun

Centrallaboratoriet Kommunehospitalet,
Copenhagen

East Germany

Dr. R. Natüsch

II. Medizinische Klinik, Charité, Berlin

France

Dr. J. Berger

Hôpital Necker, Paris

India

Dr. Phillipose Koshy

Christian Medical College Hospital,
Vellore, Madras

Ireland

Dr. Michael Carmody

Jervis St. Hospital, Dublin

Italy

Prof. E. Fiaschi

Instituto Patologia Medica Universitá
Policlinica, Padova

Japan

Dr. Kenzo Oshima

Nihon University School of Medicine,
Tokyo

Mexico

Dr. Herman Villarreal

National Institute of Cardiology,
Mexico City

New Zealand

Dr. Robin O. Irvine

Otago Medical School, Dunedin

Peru

Dr. Alfredo Piazza

Miraflores, Lima

Poland

Prof. T. Orlowski

I. Klinika Chorob Wewnetrznych,
Warszawa ul. Nowogrodska

Spain

Prof. L. Hernando

Fundación Jimenez Diaz, Clinica de
Nuestra Sra. de la Concepción, Madrid

Sweden

Prof. A. Bergstrand

Sabbatsberg Sjukhus, Stockholm

Switzerland

Prof. F. Reubi

Berne

Thailand

Dr. Visith Sitprija

Yanava, Bangkok

United Kingdom

Dr. A. W. Asscher

The Royal Infirmary, Cardiff, Wales

U.S.S.R.

Prof. E. M. Tareeva

Academy of Medical Sciences, Moscow

West Germany

Prof. E. Wollheim

Medizinische Universitätsklinik,
Luitpoldkrankenhaus

CONTRIBUTORS

Herbert L. Abrams, M.D.

Harvard Medical School, Boston

Dr. G. A. O. Alleyne

University of the West Indies,
Kingston, Jamaica

Dr. A. W. Asscher

Welsh National School of Medicine,
Royal Infirmary, Cardiff, Wales

Harold A. Baltaxe, M.D.
Cornell University Medical College,
New York

Dr. Frederic C. Bartter
National Heart Institute,
National Institutes of Health,
Bethesda, Maryland

Carl G. Becker, M.D.
Cornell University Medical College,
New York

Dr. Anders Bergstrand
Sabbatsbergs Sjukhus,
Stockholm, Sweden

Dr. Dora Bialestock
Royal Children's Hospital Research
Foundation, Parkville, Victoria, Australia

J. D. Blainey, M.D.
Queen Elizabeth Hospital,
Birmingham, England

Saul Boyarsky, M.D.
Duke University Medical Center,
Durham, North Carolina

Emmanuel L. Bravo, M.D.
Cleveland Clinic Foundation, Cleveland

Jan Brod, M.D., F.R.C.P.
Medizinische Klinik der Medizinischen
Hochscule Hannover Im Krankenhaus
Oststadt der Landeshauptstadt Hannover,
Hannover, West Germany

Claus Brun, M.D.
Kommunehospitalet,
Copenhagen, Denmark

Dr. Harje Bucht
St. Erik's Hospital, Stockholm, Sweden

Charles L. Christian, M.D.
The Hospital for Special Surgery, New York

Jacob Churg, M.D.
Mount Sinai Hospital, New York

B. G. Clarke, M.D.
Peoria, Illinois

Diane W. Crocker, M.D.
Temple University School of Medicine,
Philadelphia

E. M. Darmady, M.D.
General Hospital,
Southampton, England

F. del Greco, M.D.
Northwestern University Medical School,
Chicago

C. E. Dent, M.D.
University College Hospital Medical School,
London, England

Harriet P. Dustan, M.D.
Cleveland Clinic Research Division,
Cleveland

David P. Earle, Jr., M.D.
Northwestern University Medical School,
Chicago

Theodore Ehrenreich, M.D.
New York Medical College, New York

J. Clint Elwood, Ph.D.
State University of New York Upstate
Medical Center, Syracuse

Prof. G. Fanconi
Zurich, Switzerland

Robert Flinn, M.D.
Northwestern University Medical School,
Chicago

Richard Friedenberg, M.D.
Flower and Fifth Avenue Hospital,
New York

J. L. Funck-Brentano, M.D.
Hôpital Necker, Paris, France

H. J. Goldsmith, M.D.
Liverpool Regional Urological Centre–
Sefton General Hospital,
Liverpool, England

Burgess L. Gordon, M.D.
American Medical Association, Chicago

John B. Graham, M.D.
Northwestern University Medical School,
Chicago

Ira Greifer, M.D.
Albert Einstein College of Medicine,
Bronx, New York

Renée Habib, M.D.
Hôpital des Enfants Malades,
Paris, France

Professeur Jean Hamburger
Hôpital Necker, Paris, France

Laurence S. Harris, M.D.
New York Medical College, New York

Robert H. Heptinstall, M.D.
The Johns Hopkins University
School of Medicine, Baltimore

Dr. James M. Holland
Northwestern University Medical School,
Chicago

Melvin Horwith, M.D.
Cornell University Medical College,
New York

Robert Jennings, M.D.
Northwestern University Medical School,
Chicago

Robert E. Johnson, M.D.
University of Illinois College of Medicine
at Urbana

Robert M. Kark, M.D.
Rush Medical College of Rush University,
Chicago

Richard Kessler, M.D.
Northwestern University Medical School,
Chicago

Philip A. Khairallah, M.D.
Cleveland Clinic Foundation, Cleveland

Paul Kimmelstiel, M.D.
University of Oklahoma
College of Medicine, Oklahoma City

Priscilla Kincaid-Smith, M.D.
University of Melbourne
Department of Medicine,
Parkville, Victoria, Australia

Lowell R. King, M.D.
Northwestern University Medical School,
Chicago

John M. Kissane, M.D.
Washington University School of Medicine,
St. Louis

Calvin M. Kunin, M.D.
University of Virginia School of Medicine,
Charlottesville

Kurt Lange, M.D.
New York Medical College, New York

John K. Lattimer, M.D.
Columbia University College of Physicians
and Surgeons, New York

Nathan W. Levin, M.D.
Henry Ford Hospital, Detroit

Charles U. Lowe, M.D.
National Institute of Child Health
and Human Development,
Bethesda, Maryland

Dr. R. W. Luxton
Manchester, England

John F. Maher, M.D.
Georgetown University Hospital,
Washington, D.C.

Dr. Enno Mandema
Department of Medicine, State University of
Groningen, The Netherlands

Dr. Emanuel E. Mandel
Kingsbrook Jewish Medical Center,
Brooklyn, New York

Dr. Victor F. Marshall
Cornell University Medical College,
New York

Robert T. McCluskey, M.D.
Harvard Medical School, Boston

Eugene McKelsey, M.D.
Northwestern University Medical School,
Chicago

John P. Merrill, M.D.
Peter Bent Brigham Hospital, Boston

Robert C. Muehrcke, M.D.
West Suburban Hospital, Oak Park, Illinois

Maria I. New, M.D.
Cornell University Medical College,
New York

Donald E. Oken, M.D.
The Medical College of Virginia,
Richmond

Gerald T. Perkoff, M.D.
Washington University School of Medicine,
St. Louis

Conrad L. Pirani, M.D.
Columbia University College of
Physicians and Surgeons, New York

Victor E. Pollak, M.D.
University of Cincinnati College of
Medicine, Cincinnati

E. V. Potter, M.D.
Northwestern University Medical School,
Chicago

Theodore N. Pullman, M.D.
University of Chicago Pritzker School
of Medicine, Chicago

Arnold S. Relman, M.D.
University of Pennsylvania
School of Medicine, Philadelphia

I. Drummond Rennie, M.D.
Presbyterian–St. Luke's Hospital, Chicago

Johannes A. G. Rhodin, M.D.
New York Medical College, New York

Professor Heonir Rocha
Universidade Federal da Bahia
Faculdade de Medicina, Salvador, Brazil

Theodore Sall, Ph.D.
New York Medical College, New York

I. Herbert Scheinberg, M.D.
Albert Einstein College of Medicine,
Bronx, New York

Norman M. Simon, M.D.
Northwestern University Medical School,
Chicago

Ethan A. H. Sims, M.D.
The University of Vermont College of
Medicine, Burlington

Wesley W. Spink, M.D.
University of Minnesota–Minneapolis
Medical School, Minneapolis

Kurt H. Stenzel, M.D.
Cornell University Medical College,
New York

Maurice B. Strauss, M.D.*
Tufts University School of Medicine,
Boston

Myron Susin, M.D.
Cornell University Medical College,
New York

* Deceased

David M. Wilson, M.D.
Mayo Clinic, Rochester, Minnesota

Max A. Woodbury, M.D.
Duke University School of Medicine,
Durham, North Carolina

Howard G. Worthen, M.D.
University of Texas Southwestern
Medical School, Dallas

Acknowledgments

Glossary photographs reproduced by permission from:

1. Becker, E. L. (Ed.). *Structural Basis of Renal Disease.* Hagerstown, Md., Harper & Row, 1968.
2. Becker, E. L., and Churg, J. *Famous Teachings in Modern Medicine.* New York: MEDCOM, Inc., 1972.

Examination of the Urine: Photographs courtesy of R. Kark.

The Diagnosis of Urinary Tract Infection: Photographs courtesy of T. Sall.

Ophthalmic Diagnosis of Renal Disease: Photographs courtesy of L. Harris.

Radiologic Diagnosis of Renal Disease:
Figures 1, 3, 6, 12, 15, 16, 20, 21, 22, 23, 24, and 35 from *Kidney and Urinary Tract Infections.* Eli Lilly and Company, 1971.
Figures 2, 4, 5, 7, 8, 9, 10, 11, 13, 14, 19, and 28 courtesy of E. L. Becker.
Figures 17, 18, 25, 26, 27, 29, 30, 31, 32, 38, and 39 courtesy of H. Baltaxe.

A Handbook of Kidney Nomenclature and Nosology

I

The Glossaries

Anatomy

afferent arteriole The small artery that enters the glomerulus (Fig. 12, p. 25). See also EFFERENT ARTERIOLE; GLOMERULUS.

afibrillar cell See LACIS CELL, under CELLS.

agranular cell See LACIS CELL, under CELLS.

arcade See ARCHED COLLECTING DUCT, under DUCTS.

arched collecting duct (also *arcade*) See under DUCTS.

arcuate arteries See under ARTERIES.

area cribrosa An area under the top of each papilla, pierced by the openings of the ducts of Bellini (large collecting ducts), from which urine drains into a minor calyx (Fig. 1).

arteries

arcuate arteries Arteries formed by division of the interlobar arteries at the junction of the cortex and the medulla of the kidney. The arcuate arteries course over the base of the pyramid of medullary tissue, giving rise to the interlobular arteries. **capsular arteries** Arteries arising from the perirenal fat and penetrating the renal capsule to the cortex. They may contribute significantly to the renal arterial blood supply. **interlobar arteries** Branches of the renal arteries which course between the renal columns and the border of the medullary pyramids to the corticomedullary junction. There each one divides to form many arcuate arteries. In a unilobar kidney interlobar arteries course between hypothetical lobes (pyramids). **interlobular arteries** Branches of the arcuate arteries. They run radially toward the renal capsule between adjacent medullary rays and give rise to afferent arterioles. **renal arteries** Branches of the abdominal aorta arising at about the first lumbar vertebra. Usually a single branch supplies each kidney, but two or more branches are sometimes seen. Each artery enters its corresponding kidney through the renal hilus, at which point it branches into two vessels to supply the anterior and posterior portions of the renal parenchyma. The two vessels divide further giving rise to the interlobar vessels. Before reaching the hilus each renal artery sends branches to the suprarenal gland, ureter, and fat tissue. **ureteral arteries** Arteries supplying the ureter. Ureteral arteries may be branches of the main renal artery or separate arteries from the aortic branches (Fig. 1).

arteriola recta spuria; arteriola recta vera   See VASA RECTA.

arteriole   See AFFERENT ARTERIOLE; EFFERENT ARTERIOLE.

ascending thick limb   See LOOP OF HENLE; also under TUBULE, RENAL.

axial cell   See MESANGIAL CELL, under CELLS.

axial tissue   See MESANGIUM.

basal lamina branches; basal lamina-like material   See MESANGIAL MATRIX.

basement membrane   See CAPILLARY WALL OF THE GLOMERULUS.

basement membrane-like material   See MESANGIAL MATRIX.

Bellini, duct of   PAPILLARY DUCT, under DUCTS.

Bertin, column of   See COLUMN, RENAL; also under CORTEX, RENAL.

Bowman's capsule; Bowman's space   See GLOMERULAR CAPSULE, under CAPSULE; GLOMERULAR CAPSULAR SPACE.

brush border   A zone of densely packed microvilli which covers the apical surface of the proximal tubular cells (Fig. 17).

calyx   A cup-shaped conduit of the extrarenal collecting system.
major calyx   A large conduit formed by the confluence of several minor calyces and draining into the renal pelvis.   **minor calyx**   A small conduit which terminates around the base of one or more papillae and actively propels urine from the tip of a medullary pyramid into a major calyx (Fig. 1).

capillary, peritubular   See PERITUBULAR CAPILLARY.

capillary tuft   See TUFT, GLOMERULAR.

capillary wall of the glomerulus   A wall consisting of three layers: the inner layer, or endothelium; the middle layer, or basement membrane; and an outer layer of visceral epithelial cells, or podocytes.
endothelium   The endothelium is very thin except where cell nuclei are located. The thin portion (**lamina fenestrata**) is perforated by pores 500 to 1000 Å (50 to 100 nm) in diameter (the **fenestra**), which are believed to be closed by an osmophilic diaphragm thinner than the endothelial cell membrane.
basement membrane   The basement membrane is a continuous structure separating the capillary lumen from the glomerular capsular space. It appears to be composed of three not always clearly discernible layers. The center layer (**lamina densa**) is the thickest one and is electron dense; the inner layer (**lamina rara interna**) and the outer layer (**lamina rara externa**) are electron lucid. The lamina densa contains filaments chemically related to collagen; the laminae rarae are probably composed of glycoproteins and mucopolysaccharides. The filaments appear to be arranged much more compactly than in the mesangial matrix and to lie parallel to the surface.
epithelial cells   The **epithelial cells (podocytes)** of the glomerulus are

attached to the basement membrane by fine cytoplasmic projections called **pedicels**. The cytoplasmic ultrastructure of the epithelial cells includes very fine filaments and microtubules coursing in many directions. The cytoplasm also contains a moderate amount of endoplasmic reticulum, ribosomes, mitochondria, lysosomes, and vacuoles (vesicles). At their periphery the epithelial cells give rise to broad cytoplasmic trabeculae from which most **foot processes** originate. The cytoplasm of the foot processes appears generally denser than that of the cell body and of the trabeculae, particularly in the area where the processes are attached to the basement membrane (**foot process material** or **contractile material**). The space between the foot processes, the **slit pore**, is separated from the basement membrane by a fine diaphragm-like layer called the **filtration slit membrane**. This membrane is covered by a layer of material which is continuous with the surface coat of the foot processes and stains like a polysaccharide. Epithelial cells, in conjunction with endothelial cells and mesangial cells, probably produce and maintain the basement membrane (Figs. 7, 8, 10, and 11).

capsular arteries   See under ARTERIES.

capsular space, glomerular   See GLOMERULAR CAPSULAR SPACE.

capsular veins   See under VEINS.

capsule

glomerular capsule (also *Bowman's capsule*)   The double-layered sac surrounding the glomerular tuft. It consists of a thick basement membrane supporting a layer of parietal epithelial cells. The capsule is surrounded by a layer of connective tissue which is part of the interstitial connective tissue of the kidney. In general, the parietal epithelial cells are low cuboidal or flat, although they may be slightly taller at the tubular pole of the glomerulus, where they are continuous with the cells of the proximal tubules. At the vascular pole of the glomerulus the capsular basement membrane is reflected onto the afferent and efferent arterioles and is continuous with the basement membrane of the glomerular tuft. The parietal epithelial cells of the glomerular capsule are continuous with the visceral epithelial cells or podocytes of the capillary wall. See POLE, VASCULAR.   **renal capsule** (also *external capsule*)   The fibrous tunic enveloping the kidney (Figs. 7 and 8).

cells

afibrillar cell (or Goormaghtigh)   See LACIS CELL.   **agranular cell** See LACIS CELL.   **axial cell**   See MESANGIAL CELL.   **central lobular cell** See MESANGIAL CELL.   **dark cell**   See INTERCALATED CELL.   **deep cell** (also *deep endothelial cell*) See MESANGIAL CELL.   **endothelial cell**   A cell of the inner layer of the capillary wall of the glomerulus, characterized by a large ellipsodial nucleus usually located near the mesangial region and a thinner cytoplasm perforated by fine pores and believed to be closed by a diaphragm. See also CAPILLARY WALL OF THE GLOMERULUS.   **epithelial cell** (also **visceral epithelial cell, podocyte**)   The large octopus-shaped cell of the outer layer of the glomerular capillary wall. See also CAPILLARY WALL OF THE GLOMERULUS. **epithelioid cell** See GRANULAR CELL. **glomerular capsular cell** See PARIETAL (EPITHELIAL) CELL. **granular cell** (also *granular epithelioid cell, epithelioid cell, myoepithelial cell*) A densely granulated cell with characteristic morphology and staining properties found in the walls of afferent and efferent arterioles around the vascular pole of the glomerulus. Granular cells constitute part of the juxtaglomerular apparatus (Fig. 14). See also JUXTAGLOMERULAR APPARATUS. **intercalated cell** (also *dark cell*) A cell found among the principal cells of the collecting duct and also in the distal convoluted tubule. Intercalated cells are characterized by abundant mitochondria and distinguished from the principal cell type by having more basally placed nuclei, many apical vesicles, more numerous apical microvilli, and, in some cases, an increased cytoplasmic density (Fig. 21). **intercapillary cell** See MESANGIAL CELL. **interluminal cell** See MESANGIAL CELL. **interstitial cell** See MEDULLARY INTERSTITIAL CELL. **juxtaglomerular cell** One of several functionally related cell types constituting the juxtaglomerular apparatus at the glomerular hilus. They include the granular cells of the afferent and efferent arterioles, the lacis cells situated in the wedge formed by the arterioles at the vascular pole of the glomerulus, and the cells of the macula densa of the distal tubule (Figs. 13 and 14). **lacis cell** (also *afibrillar cell* [*of Goormaghtigh*], *agranular cell, pseudo-Meissnerian cell*) One of the interstitial cells between the afferent and efferent arterioles at the vascular pole of the glomerulus. Together with granular cells they constitute the polar cushion (Polkissen, lacis celluloconjunctif) or juxtaglomerular body or cell mass. Polar cushion cells are in intimate contact with cells of the mesangium and of the macula densa (Fig. 12). **lacis celluloconjunctif cells** See POLAR CUSHION CELL. **light cell** (also *principal cell*) The major cell type forming the simple cuboidal epithelium that lines the collecting duct. Light cells are characterized by a zone of basal interdigitations and infoldings, with small ovoid mitochondria lying above it. **medullary interstitial cell** One of a population of elongated cells with processes and containing abundant lipid droplets. They are found in the medullary interstitium oriented with their long axes perpendicular to those of adjacent tubules and vessels. **mesangial cell** (also *axial cell, central lobular cell, deep cell, deep endothelial cell, intercapillary cell, interluminal cell, stalk cell, third cell*) An irregularly shaped cell with twisted elongated processes, situated in the stalk region of the capillary tuft. It contains peripherally arranged fibrils, some of which are arranged perpendicular to the cell membrane. Mesangial cells are separated almost completely from the capillary lumen by mesangial matrix and endothelial cytoplasm, although finger-like or balloon-like projections of mesangial cells may extend through the endothelial cells into the capillary lumen

(Figs. 4, 5, 7, 9, and 11). **myoepithelial cell** See GRANULAR CELL. **parietal (epithelial) cell** (also *glomerular capsular cell*) A cell of the parietal layer of the glomerular capsule (see under CAPSULE). It is typically squamous, bulging at the level of the nucleus (Fig. 7). **podocyte** See EPITHELIAL CELL. **polar cushion cell** (also *Polkissen cell, cell of the lacis celluloconjunctif, juxtaglomerular body cell*). A granular or a lacis cell. **principal cell** See LIGHT CELL. **pseudo-Meissnerian cell** See LACIS CELL. **stalk cell** See MESANGIAL CELL. **third cell** See MESANGIAL CELL.

central lobular cell See MESANGIAL CELL, under CELLS.

collecting duct See under DUCTS.

column of Bertin See COLUMN, RENAL; also CORTEX, RENAL.

column, renal Cortical substance found between adjacent medullary pyramids of a multilobar kidney. See also CORTEX, RENAL.

connecting segment See ARCHED COLLECTING DUCT, under DUCTS.

connective tissue fibers See MESANGIAL MATRIX.

corpuscle, renal See GLOMERULUS.

cortex, renal The outer part of the kidney parenchyma extending from the external capsule over the base of the pyramids and dipping down into the space between adjacent pyramids. In general it is dark reddish-brown in color, contrasting with the lighter cone-shaped areas of medulla. In thickness the ratio of cortex to medulla is approximately 1:3. The partitions of cortical substance between adjacent pyramids are called renal columns (also columns of Bertin). The cortex contains glomeruli, proximal convoluted tubules, distal convoluted tubules, and medullary rays (Fig. 1).

cortical nephron See under NEPHRON.

dark cell See CELLS, INTERCALATED.

deep cell or **deep endothelial cell** See CELLS, MESANGIAL.

deep nephron See JUXTAMEDULLARY NEPHRON, under NEPHRON.

descending thick limb See LOOP OF HENLE; also under TUBULE, RENAL.

distal segment (or *distal tubule*) See under TUBULE, RENAL.

ducts

arched collecting duct (also *arcade*) The form taken by the initial segment (sometimes called **connecting segment**) of the collecting tubule for some nephrons. The arcade begins in the deeper region of the cortex, ascends, and passes down into a medullary ray. Such an arcade apparently develops in embryo when the terminal segment of a collecting duct ceases to divide but still induces the formation of new nephrons. The additional nephrons then become attached to the connecting segment of the nephron formed earlier and pass by way of the arcade into the medullary ray. **collecting duct** (also *collecting tubule*) A system of channels draining a group of nephrons. Individual nephrons are connected to collecting tubules. These converge to form ducts of larger diameter, which eventually discharge their contents into the calyces. **duct of Bellini** See PAPILLARY DUCT. **mesonephric ducts** (also *wolffian ducts*) The ducts into which the mesonephric tubules empty after the pronephric tubules degenerate. The mesonephric ducts carry the urine of the embryo from the mesonephros to the bladder or cloaca. **papillary duct** (also *duct of Bellini*) A large collecting duct in the medulla of the kidney, formed by convergence of smaller collecting tubules. Papillary ducts drain into the minor calyces at the area cribrosa. The epithelium lining these ducts is higher than that of collecting tubules in the cortex. In man the cells are all columnar in shape (Fig. 20). **pronephric duct** A duct that grows caudal to the hindgut until it unites with it and converts it into the cloaca. **wolffian duct** See MESONEPHRIC DUCTS.

efferent arteriole The small artery that drains the glomerulus (Figs. 12 and 22). See also AFFERENT ARTERIOLE; GLOMERULUS.

endocytic apparatus A system of cellular organelles specialized for the uptake of macromolecular substances such as proteins. It is well developed in the proximal renal tubule, where it consists of tubular invaginations at the base of the brush border, vesicles, and larger vacuoles. The vacuoles presumably condense and fuse with lysosomes. Hydrolases from the lysosomes then digest the sequestered material (Fig. 18).

endothelial cell See under CELLS.

epithelial cell See under CELLS.

epithelioid cell See GRANULAR CELL, under CELLS.

external capsule See RENAL CAPSULE, under CAPSULE.

fenestra See under CAPILLARY WALL OF THE GLOMERULUS.

filtration slit membrane See under CAPILLARY WALL OF THE GLOMERULUS.

foot process, foot process material See under CAPILLARY WALL OF THE GLOMERULUS.

glomerular capillary wall See CAPILLARY WALL OF THE GLOMERULUS.

glomerular capsular space (also *Bowman's space, urinary space*) The interior space between the glomerular capsule and the glomerular tuft. The glomerular filtrate drains into this space (Figs. 7 to 11).

glomerular capsule (also *Bowman's capsule*) See under CAPSULE.

glomerular hilus See HILUS, GLOMERULAR.

glomerular stalk See MESANGIUM.

glomerular tuft See TUFT, GLOMERULAR.

glomerulus (also *renal corpuscle*) An almost spherical structure at the beginning of a nephron, composed of a double-layered sac (the glomerular or Bowman's capsule) and an enclosed network of branching and anastomosing capillaries (the tuft) and associated mesangium. The glomerulus has a vascular pole (the glomerular hilus), where the afferent arteriole enters and the efferent arteriole leaves, and a tubular pole, where the space between the double-layered sac and the capillary tuft becomes confluent with the lumen of the tubule. The term glomerulus is sometimes used to denote the capillary tuft alone, or all the renal corpuscle except the parietal layer of the glomerular capsule (Figs. 2, 3, 7, 10 to 12). **primitive glomerulus** The glomerulus at about 8 weeks' gestation. An S-shaped cavity forms in a cluster of nephrogenic cells in the metanephros. The end of the upper limb, closest to the surface of the kidney, communicates with the ampulla of a ureteral branch. The lower limb branches into a double-layered structure. The outer layer, lined by flattened cells, forms the glomerular (Bowman's) capsule. The inner layer, lined by columnar cells, will become the epithelial cells. A capillary penetrates the cavity, splits into six to eight loops, and with the epithelial cells forms the glomerular tuft. See also CAPILLARY WALL OF THE GLOMERULUS.

granular cell   See under CELLS.

Henle, loop of   See LOOP OF HENLE.

hilus

glomerular hilus   See POLE, VASCULAR; also GLOMERULUS. **renal hilus** A vertical slit on the medial concave surface of the kidney through which pass the renal artery, renal vein, pelvis or ureter, renal nerves, and some of the renal lymphatics (Fig. 1).

intercalated cell   See under CELLS.
intercapillary cell   See MESANGIAL CELL, under CELLS.
intercapillary tissue   See MESANGIUM.
interlobar arteries   See under ARTERIES.
interlobular arteries   See under ARTERIES.
interluminal cell   See MESANGIAL CELL, under CELLS.
interstitial cell   See MEDULLARY INTERSTITIAL CELL, under CELLS.

juxtaglomerular apparatus   A cushion of cells (the **juxtaglomerular body** or **mass**) at the hilus of the glomerulus, together with the macula of the distal renal tubule, thought to be functionally related. The cells of the juxtaglomerular body consist of (1) granular epithelioid or myoepithelial cells found mainly in the wall of the terminal part of the afferent and efferent arterioles, where they replace smooth muscle cells. These cells contain dense granules bounded by a membrane and are relatively homogeneous in the mature state, and (2) a group of cells with relatively less dense granules (agranular or lacis cells, afibrillar cells of Goormaghtigh, pseudo-Meissnerian cells) situated in the wedge formed by the afferent and efferent arterioles at the vascular pole of the glomerulus. Lacis cells are in intimate contact with the granular cells of the mesangium and macula densa (Figs. 12 to 14).

juxtaglomerular cell See under CELLS. See also JUXTAGLOMERULAR APPA-
RATUS.

juxtamedullary nephron See under NEPHRON.

lacis cells See under CELLS.

lacis celluloconjunctif cell See POLAR CUSHION CELL, under CELLS.

lamina densa See under CAPILLARY WALL OF THE GLOMERULUS.

lamina fenestrata See under CAPILLARY WALL OF THE GLOMERULUS.

lamina rara externa See under CAPILLARY WALL OF THE GLOMERULUS.

lamina rara interna See under CAPILLARY WALL OF THE GLOMERULUS.

light cell See under CELLS.

lobe A morphologic unit of the kidney consisting of a pyramid of medulla
and the cup-shaped cap of the cortex surrounding it along its base and
sides. In some animals the kidney has only one lobe (unilobar) while
in others several lobes are found (multilobar) (Fig. 1).

lobular stalk See MESANGIUM.

lobule

    glomerular lobule One of the capillary loops of the glomerular tuft
(Fig. 5). It is wound around a terminal portion of the stalk. See also
TUFT, GLOMERULAR. **renal lobule** A structural unit of kidney parenchyma consisting of a central medullary ray surrounded by nephrons
which drain into the collecting ducts of the ray. Interlobular arteries,
parallel to the medullary ray, are situated between lobules (Fig. 1).

loop of Henle A portion of the tubule of a nephron extending from the
cortex into the medulla and/or papillae and returning to the cortex.
As originally described by Henle it is composed of the following parts
of the renal tubule: (1) proximal segment, straight portion (**thick
descending limb**), (2) **thin limb**, and (3) distal segment, straight
portion (**thick ascending limb**) (Fig. 6). See also under TUBULE,
RENAL.

lymphatics, renal The renal lymph vessels running along the large blood
vessels in the hilus or through the capsule. Some of them are said to
empty into the renal pelvis and may be a source of proteinuria in patho-
logical conditions.

lysosome A membrane-bounded cellular organelle which contains a variety
of hydrolytic enzymes used for the digestion of material sequestered
by the cell. The sequestered material can be derived from an external
source (**heterophagy**) or from part of the cell itself (**autophagy**). Cells
of all parts of the uriniferous tubule contain lysosomes, but they are
particularly abundant in cells of the proximal convoluted segment
(Fig. 18).

macula densa (also *pars maculata*) See under TUBULE, RENAL.

major calyx See under CALYX.

matrix See MESANGIAL MATRIX.

medulla   The inner part of the kidney, which in man is composed of 6 to
18 conical structures (pyramids). In gross specimens these appear
lighter in color than cortical tissue and have a striated appearance
caused by the parallel arrangement of nephron segments and blood
vessels. A pyramid begins at the level of the arcuate arteries and is
composed of tubular elements, portions of the collecting ducts, the
vasa recta, and capillaries.

medullary ray   Radially directed bundles of longitudinally oriented tubules
and vessels extending from the base of the medullary pyramid into the
cortex. They form the center of a renal lobule and are considered to be
part of the cortex.

medullary zones   In some species, such as the rat, gross divisions (inner
and outer) of the medullary pyramid according to which segments of
the nephrons are contained within each. The inner zone contains thin
limbs of the loops of Henle as well as large collecting ducts, capillaries,
interstitium, and interstitial cells. In man, the nephron segments are
less precisely arranged (Figs. 1 and 6).

mesangial cells   See under CELLS.

mesangial matrix   (also *basal lamina branches, basal lamina-like material,
basement membrane-like material, connective tissue fibers, sponge
fibers*)   A continuous meshwork of extracellular material which fills
the space between the mesangial cells. The material is similar to that
of the capillary basement membrane and other basement membranes
but is less compact. The matrix consists of filaments, chemically related to collagen, and of a homogeneous ground substance which is
probably composed of mucopolysaccharides and glycoproteins. The
mesangial matrix is permeable to various substances of large molecular
size and to aggregates; such material may also become localized in the
matrix. Mature collagen filaments are rarely present (Fig. 4).

mesangium   (also *axial tissue, glomerular* or *lobular stalk, intercapillary
tissue*)   The tissue of the glomerulus, which extends from the vascular
pole, runs between the capillaries, and forms the centers of the individual lobules. It is composed of mesangial cells and intercellular substance or matrix and is covered by a continuous layer of basement
membrane and epithelial cells. (Figs. 7, 8, and 11).

mesonephric duct   See under DUCTS.

mesonephros   (also *mesonephric kidney*)   In man, the temporary excretory organ during embryonic life. Nephrogenic mesoderm at the level
of somites 14 to 26 forms glomerular tubules that are longer and more
complicated than those of the pronephros. The tubules drain into the
duct formed in relation to the pronephros, thus converting it into the
mesonephric duct.

metanephrogenic blastema   In the embryo, a condensed mass of tissue, at
the caudal end of the nephrogenic mesoderm, which forms the nephrons of the metanephros.

metanephros (also *metanephric kidney*) The functional permanent kidney of mammals, birds, and reptiles. Glomerular nephrons develop from the caudal region of the nephrogenic mesoderm and fuse with branches of the ureteric bud (**metanephric duct**) to form uriniferous tubules.

microbody, peroxisome A cellular organelle found in the proximal renal tubule. It is surrounded by a single membrane, has a moderately dense matrix, and frequently contains a dense core-like structure called a **nucleoid**. Microbodies contain catalase and oxidase enzymes and appear to play a role in the metabolism of hydrogen peroxide. They also may be involved in gluconeogenesis.

microvillus A small finger-like process of a cell. Microvilli may be abundant and regular, as in the brush border of the proximal tubule, or less abundant and irregular, as in the distal tubule (Fig. 17).

minor calyx See under CALYX.

multilobar kidney A kidney having more than one lobe (6 to 18 lobes have been reported in man) (Fig. 1).

myoepithelial cell See GRANULAR CELL, under CELLS.

neck, tubular In certain species, a short segment with low epithelium connecting the tubular pole of the glomerulus to the proximal convoluted tubule (Fig. 8).

nephron The functional unit of the renal parenchyma, consisting of the glomerulus and the attached tubule (Fig. 6).
  cortical nephron (also *superficial nephron*) A nephron whose glomerulus lies in the outer portion of the cortex near the external capsule of the kidney. Cortical nephrons are usually characterized by short loops of Henle. **juxtamedullary nephron** (also *deep nephron*) A nephron whose glomerulus lies in the cortex near the medullary border. Juxtamedullary nephrons are generally characterized by loops of Henle which penetrate deeply into the medulla, unlike the loops of superficial or cortical nephrons, which are generally shorter. Deep nephrons do not have prominent juxtaglomerular granular cells, whereas superficial nephrons do. The efferent glomerular arterioles of deep nephrons are surrounded by prominent smooth muscle cells before dividing into vasa recta spuria in the renal pyramid. No such prominent smooth muscle cells are seen in the efferent arterioles of the superficial glomeruli. It has been claimed that these structural differences are an expression of functional differences (Fig. 6).

papilla The apex of the medullary pyramid (Fig 1). See also AREA CRIBROSA; CALYX.

papillary duct (also *duct of Bellini*) See under DUCTS.

parietal cell See under CELLS.

parietal epithelium   See GLOMERULAR CAPSULE, under CAPSULE.

pars convoluta   See TUBULE, RENAL.

pars maculata   See under TUBULE, RENAL.

pars recta   See under TUBULE, RENAL.

pedicel   See under CAPILLARY WALL OF THE GLOMERULUS.

pelvis, renal   The funnel-shaped area of the extrarenal collecting system draining the calyces proximally and narrowing to form the ureter distally. It is covered by transitional epithelium (Fig. 1).

peritubular capillary   Part of a capillary network surrounding a renal tubule, formed predominantly by the branching of efferent arterioles (Figs. 23 and 24).

peroxisome microbody   See MICROBODY, PEROXISOME.

podocyte   See EPITHELIAL CELL, under CELLS; see also under CAPILLARY WALL OF THE GLOMERULUS.

polar cushion   (also *Polkissen lacis celluloconjunctif*)   See under JUXTA-GLOMERULAR APPARATUS; see also LACIS CELL, under CELLS.

pole, tubular   (also *urinary pole*)   The side in the glomerulus where the proximal convoluted segment of the renal tubule originates and where the glomerular capsular space is continuous with the tubular lumen. The tubular pole is opposite the vascular pole (Fig. 8). See also GLO-MERULUS.

pole, vascular   (also *glomerular hilus*)   The site where the afferent arteriole penetrates the glomerulus and the efferent arteriole leaves it. Between the two arterioles, cells of the polar cushion are continuous with the mesangium (Fig. 12). See also GLOMERULUS; JUXTAGLOMERULAR APPARATUS.

Polkissen   See under JUXTAGLOMERULAR APPARATUS; see also LACIS CELL, under CELLS.

pore, slit   See under CAPILLARY WALL OF THE GLOMERULUS.

principal cell   See LIGHT CELL, under CELLS.

pronephric duct   See under DUCTS.

pronephros   (also *pronephric kidney*)   The earliest form of excretory system, developing at the end of the third week of an embryo. It is formed of sets of pronephric tubules which arise from the nephrogenic mesoderm at the level of somites 7 to 13. In man these tubules appear to be nonfunctional and transitory. They empty into a pronephric duct on each side. The ducts grow caudal to the hindgut until they unite with it and convert it into the cloaca.

proximal convoluted segment   See under TUBULE, RENAL.

proximal segment   See under TUBULE, RENAL.

pseudo-Meissnerian cell   See MESANGIAL CELL, under CELLS; also JUXTA-GLOMERULAR APPARATUS.

pyramid, renal   A conical division of medullary tissue. The bases of renal pyramids are adjacent to the cortex, and their apices, or papillae, project into the lumen of the minor calyces (Fig 1).

ray, medullary   See MEDULLARY RAY.
renal arteries   See under ARTERIES.
renal capsule   See under CAPSULE.
renal column   See COLUMN, RENAL.
renal corpuscle   See GLOMERULUS.
renal sinus   See SINUS, RENAL.
renal tubule   See TUBULE, RENAL.
renal veins   See under VEINS.

sinus, renal   A narrow, crescent-shaped cavity which indents the renal parenchyma on its medial aspect. The ureter, blood vessels, lymphatics, and nerves enter and exit from the kidney through the renal hilus, which is continuous with the sinus. The small reservoir formed by the sinus is the **intrarenal pelvis,** which drains urine from all parts of the kidney (Fig. 1).

slit pore   See under CAPILLARY WALL OF THE GLOMERULUS.
sponge fibers   See MESANGIAL MATRIX.
stalk cell   See MESANGIAL CELL, under CELLS.
stalk, glomerular   See MESANGIUM.
superficial nephron   See CORTICAL NEPHRON, under NEPHRON.

thick ascending limb   See under LOOP OF HENLE; TUBULE, RENAL.
thick descending limb   See under LOOP OF HENLE; TUBULE, RENAL.
thin limb   See under LOOP OF HENLE; TUBULE, RENAL.
third cell   See MESANGIAL CELL, under CELLS.
tubule, collecting   See COLLECTING DUCT, under DUCTS.
tubule, renal (also *uriniferous tubule*)   For descriptive purposes the renal tubule is divided into a proximal segment originating at the glomerular capsule, a thin intermediate portion, and a distal segment emptying into a collecting tubule. Each segment is further subdivided anatomically.

proximal segment   The initial part of the proximal segment is extremely tortuous and for this reason is called the **proximal convoluted segment** (*pars convoluta*). It comprises much of the cortex. In mammalian species it is characterized by epithelial cells of complex shape whose basal infoldings and lateral processes interdigitate extensively with those of adjacent epithelial cells. The cells also have an extensive luminal border of microvilli (the brush border), a well-developed endocytic apparatus, abundant elongated mitochondria in the lateral interdigitating processes, and numerous microbodies (Figs. 16 to 19). The latter part of the proximal segment, the **straight portion** (*pars recta*), or **thick descending limb,** is located in the medullary ray and the outer stripe of the outer zone of the medulla. As compared with the convoluted portion the cells comprising this region are less complex in shape and are characterized by a well-developed microvillous border (brush border), a less well developed endocytic apparatus, rounder mitochondrial profiles, fewer lysosomes, and more numerous microbodies (Fig. 6).

thin segment (also **thin limb**) The thin segment constitutes part of or, in some cases, the entire loop of Henle. It descends from the pars recta of the proximal segment, turns, and ascends to the pars recta of the distal segment. The descending portion is generally longer than the ascending portion. Thin limbs can be found in the inner stripe of the outer zone (descending segments) and in the inner zone (ascending and descending segments), and in man they may sometimes be located in the outer zone and even in the medullary ray. The epithelium comprising the wall of the thin segment is characterized by low height and extremely irregular shape, with well-developed lateral interdigitating processes. The more proximal cells of the descending limb are usually more irregular in shape and have more microvilli than the distal cells, which are more simplified in shape (Fig. 20).

distal segment This portion of the tubule is composed of an initial **straight portion** (*pars recta*), an **intermediate** section (*pars maculata*), and a convoluted terminal portion (*pars convoluta*). The initial straight section ascends in the outer zone of the medulla and in the medullary ray, where it forms the **thick ascending limb** of the loop of Henle. The epithelial cells lining this portion of the distal segment are of greater height than those of the thin segment and are characterized by their elaborate shape and their many lateral interdigitating processes containing numerous elongated mitochondria. They are somewhat lower than those of the distal convoluted portion but are similar to them (Fig. 15). **intermediate portion** (*pars maculata; macula densa*) When the straight portion of the distal segment returns to the cortex, it passes between the afferent and efferent arterioles of its originating glomerulus. The nuclei of the epithelial cells on one side of the wall of the distal tubule in this region are especially close together and appear dense with basophilic stains. For this reason the region is called the *macula densa* (dense spot). The bases of the macula densa cells lie adjacent to the granular and agranular juxtaglomerular cells of the polar cushion, suggesting a functional relationship between these two structures. The tubular basement membrane in this area is thin and irregular. **convoluted portion** (*pars convoluta*) The tortuous cortical portion of the distal segment begins at the end of the macula densa. In mammalian species, it is characterized by cells of complex shape with lateral processes which interdigitate extensively with those of adjacent cells. The cells have only a few microvilli on their luminal surfaces, many elongated mitochondria within their cytoplasm, an endocytic apparatus, and a few lysosomes (Figs. 6 and 18).

tubule, uriniferous Sec TUBULE, RENAL.

tuft, glomerular (also *capillary tuft; vascular tuft*) The vascular part of the glomerulus, consisting of a network of capillaries. See also under GLOMERULUS.

unilobar kidney A kidney having only one lobe.

ureter Tube from kidney to the bladder consisting of a *pars abdominalis* and a *pars pelvina*. The ureter is lined with transitional epithelium surrounded by circular and longitudinal smooth muscle.

ureteral arteries See under ARTERIES.

ureteral veins See under VEINS.

ureteric bud In the embryo, a diverticulum of the mesonephric duct which grows into the metanephrogenic tissue and branches to form the extrarenal collecting system as well as the collecting ducts up to the region of the connecting portion.

urinary pole See POLE, TUBULAR.

urinary space See GLOMERULAR CAPSULAR SPACE.

uriniferous tubule See TUBULE, RENAL.

vasa recta (*arteriolae rectae*) Arterioles and capillaries which accompany the nephrons into the medulla and supply the papillae. **Vasa recta spuria** arise from the efferent glomerular arterioles. **Vasa recta vera** arise as arterioles directly from interlobular or arcuate arteries.

vascular pole See POLE, VASCULAR; and under GLOMERULUS.

vascular tuft See TUFT, GLOMERULAR; and under GLOMERULUS.

veins

> **capsular veins** Veins from superficial cortical capillaries passing through the renal capsule to the vessels in the perirenal fat. **renal veins** Veins formed by the union of the three lobar veins (upper, hilar, and lower). The vein on each side is usually single but it is not uncommon to find two or three. Because of its role in the embryo, the left renal vein is longer than the right and has a large drainage area that includes the suprarenal gland, gonad, part of the diaphragm, and part of the body wall. **ureteral veins** Veins draining either directly into the main renal vein or indirectly into the inferior vena cava (Fig. 11).

visceral epithelium See CAPILLARY WALL OF THE GLOMERULUS.

wall, glomerular capillary See CAPILLARY WALL OF THE GLOMERULUS.

wolffian duct See MESONEPHRIC DUCT, under DUCTS.

zone, medullary See MEDULLARY ZONES.

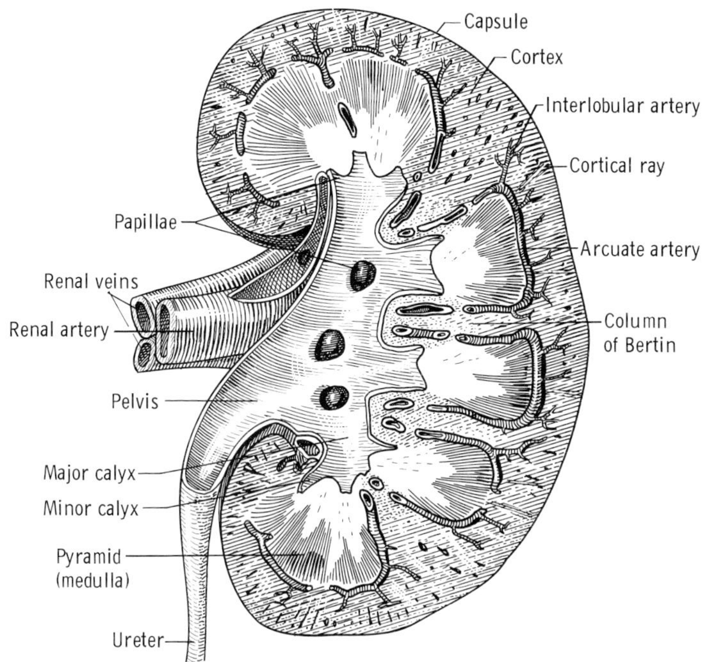

Fig. 1. Human kidney in sagittal section.

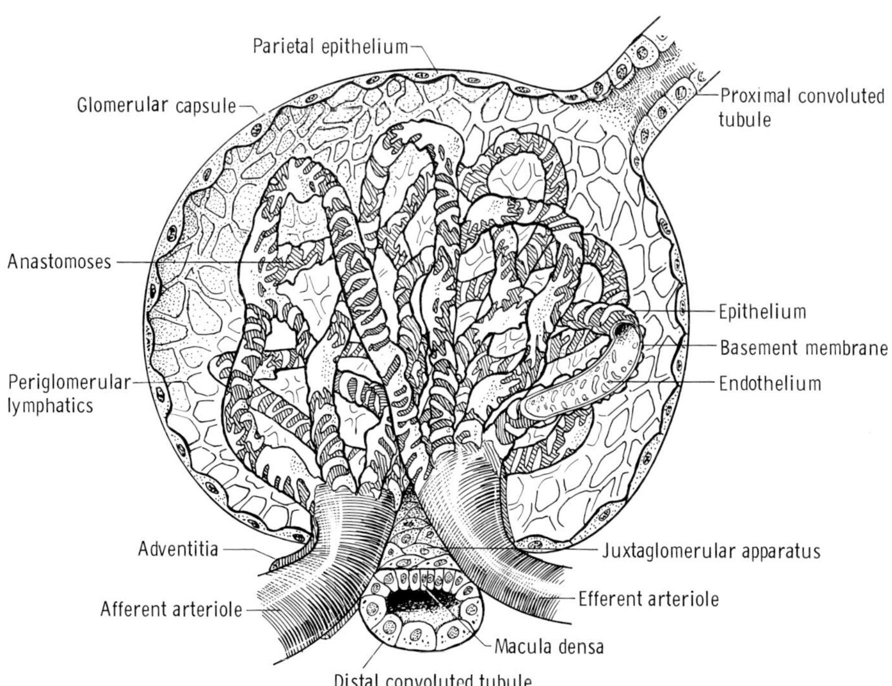

Fig. 2. Three-dimensional drawing of a human glomerulus (mesangium not shown).

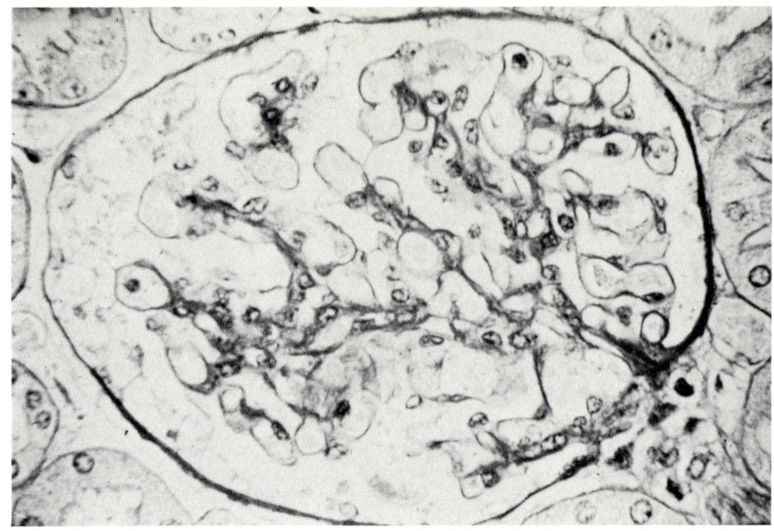

Fig. 3. A normal human glomerulus. (Courtesy of J. Churg.)

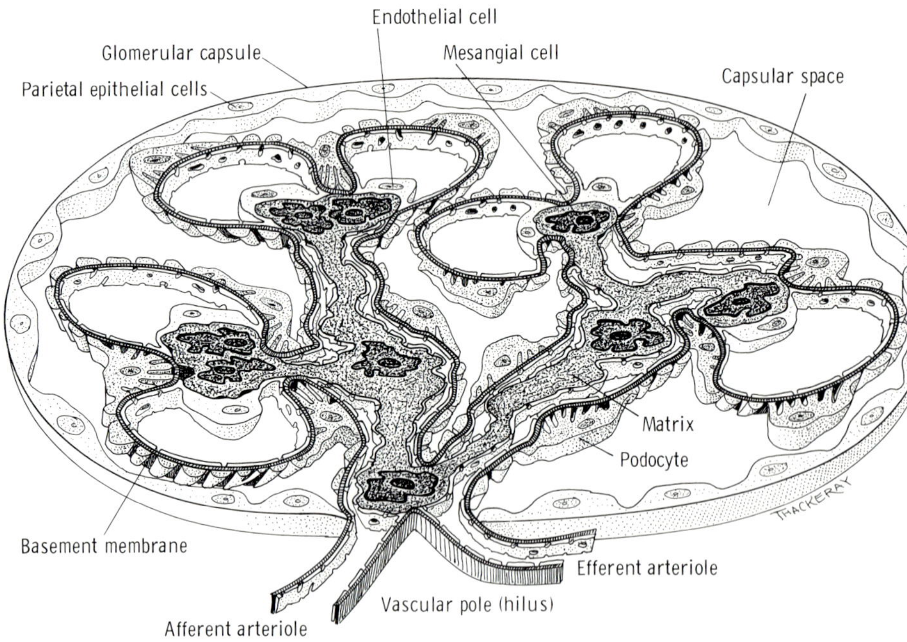

Fig. 4. Glomerulus in cross-section through the vascular pole. Mesangial cells and matrix extend from the vascular pole, run between the capillaries, and form the centers of the individual lobules.

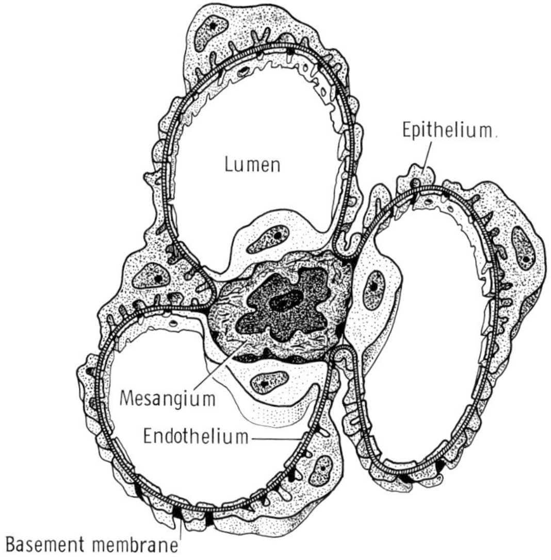

Fig. 5. Single glomerular lobule. The center of the lobule is formed by the mesangial stalk, which is cut across in this section. Note the single mesangial cell.

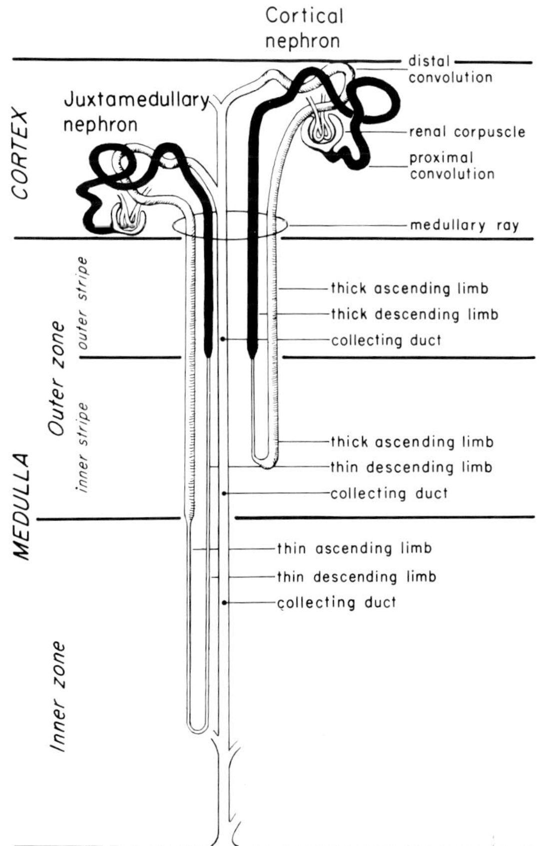

Fig. 6. Schematic diagram of mammalian nephrons showing relationship of segments of the nephron to zones of the kidney. (From B. F. Trump and R. E. Bulger, Morphology of the Kidney, in Becker [1].)

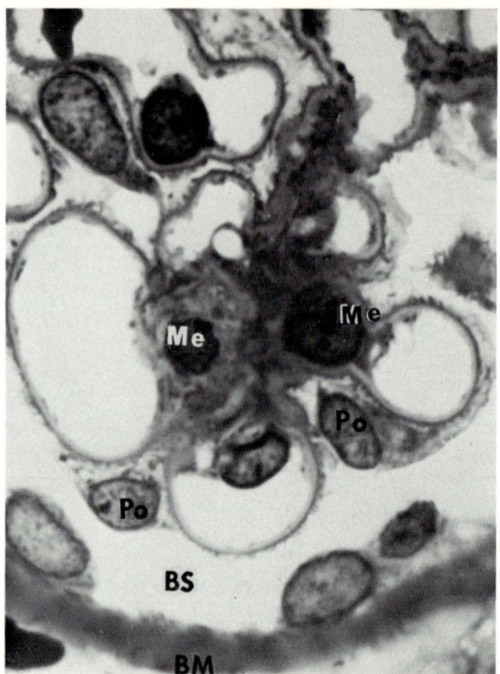

Fig. 7. Light micrograph showing the edge of a human glomerulus. At the edge of the picture a basement membrane (*BM*) can be seen underlying the cells of the parietal layer of the glomerular capsule. Profiles of several capillary loops are visible. The mesangial cells (*Me*) lie in the hilar region near the vascular pole. The podocytes (*Po*) sit in the capsular (Bowman's) space (*BS*) and have long extensions which form a layer over the basement membrane between the podocytes and the capillary. (From B. F. Trump and R. E. Bulger, Morphology of the Kidney, in Becker [1].)

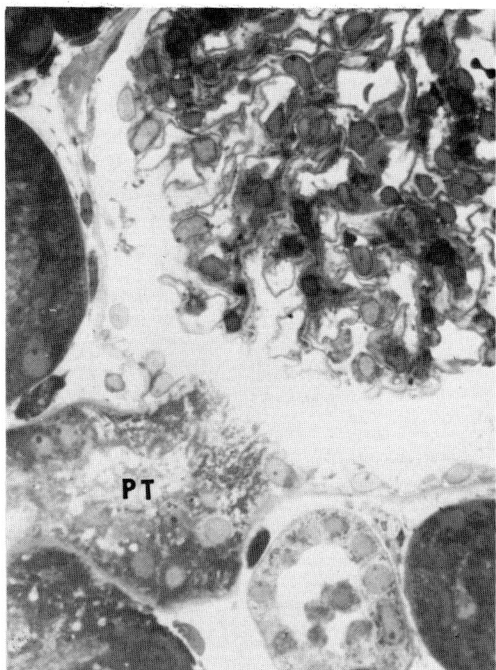

Fig. 8. Light micrograph of a human glomerulus, showing the tubular pole. The flattened cells of the parietal layer of the glomerular capsule end abruptly, and the cells of the proximal convoluted tubule (*PT*) begin at the junction with only a slight constriction in the diameter of the tubule. This constricted area is the only neck segment present in the human. (From B. F. Trump and R. E. Bulger, Morphology of the Kidney, in Becker [1].)

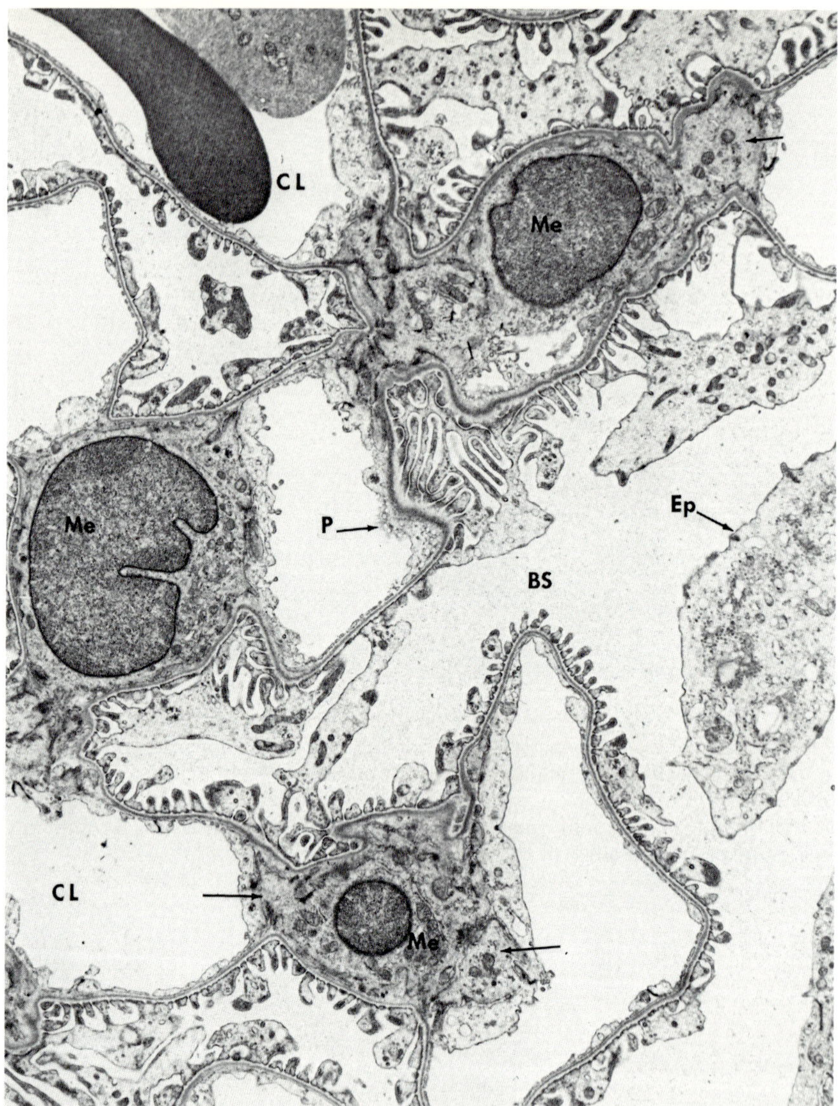

Fig. 9. Electron micrograph showing part of a rat glomerulus. The podocytes (*Ep*) lie in the glomerular capsular (Bowman's) space (*BS*) and have processes (pedicels) which form a layer along the basement membrane. The capillary lumina (*CL*) are lined by endothelium that is attenuated and contains pores (*P*). Mesangial cells (*Me*), seen near the axial region, have processes which extend into, and in some cases through, the endothelium (*arrows*). (From B. F. Trump and R. E. Bulger, Morphology of the Kidney, in Becker [1].)

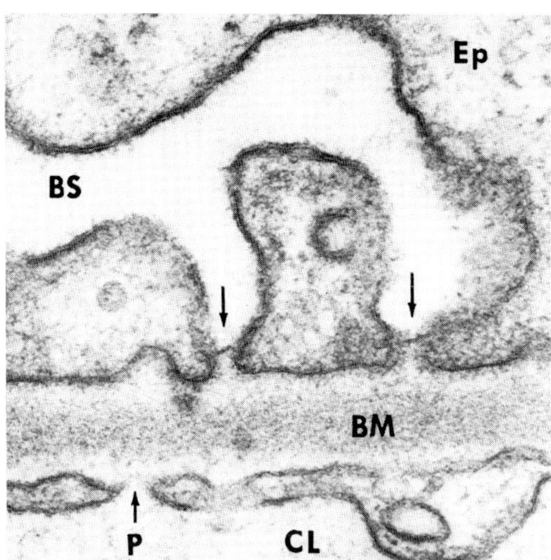

Fig. 10. Electron micrograph of a rat glomerulus, showing the filtration barrier. At the top is the layer of pedicels bridged by the filtration slit membranes (*arrows*). The pedicels rest on the basement membrane (*BM*). The thin layer of endothelium seen beneath that is interrupted by pores (*P*). *CL*, capillary lumen; *BS*, Bowman's space; *Ep*, visceral epithelium. (From B. F. Trump and R. E. Bulger, Morphology of the Kidney, in Becker [1].)

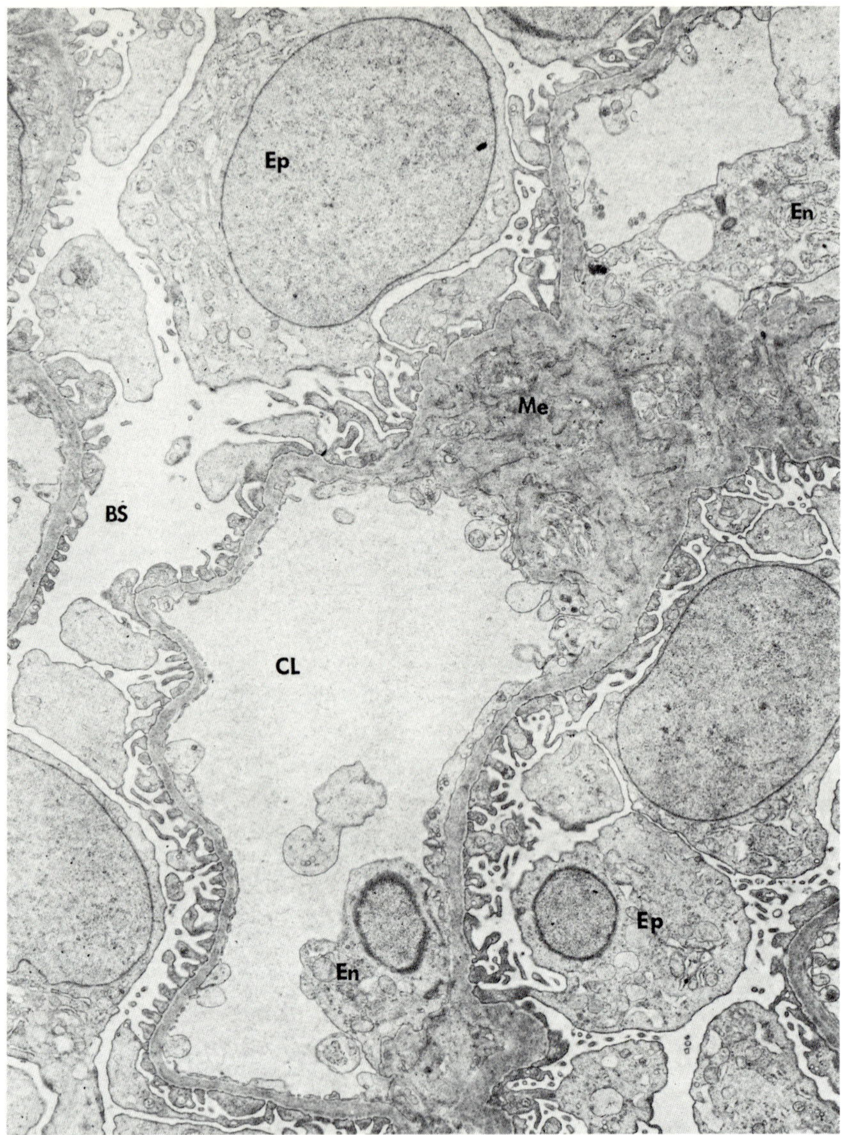

Fig. 11. Electron micrograph of a human glomerulus, showing appearance and relationship of visceral epithelium (*Ep*), mesangium (*Me*), endothelium (*En*), and capillary lumen (*CL*). *BS*, Bowman's space. (From B. F. Trump, and R. E. Bulger, Morphology of the Kidney, in Becker [1].)

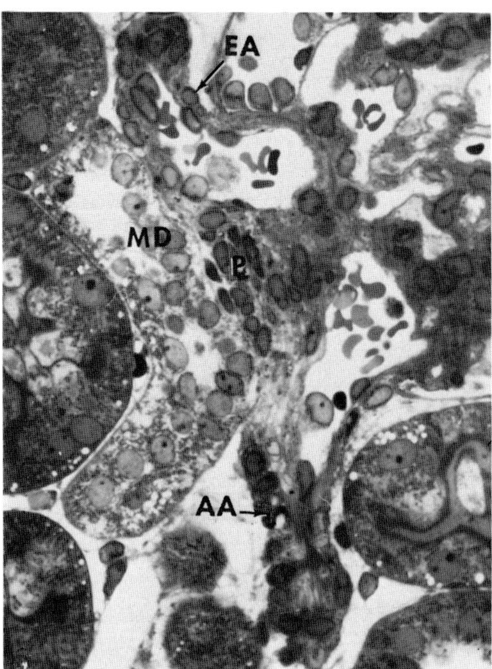

Fig. 12. Light micrograph of a human juxtaglomerular apparatus, showing the afferent (*AA*) and efferent (*EA*) arterioles with a group of cells, the polar cushion (*P*), in the space between. The macula densa (*MD*) of the distal tubules can be seen running between the afferent and efferent arterioles. (From B. F. Trump and R. E. Bulger, Morphology of the Kidney, in Becker [1].)

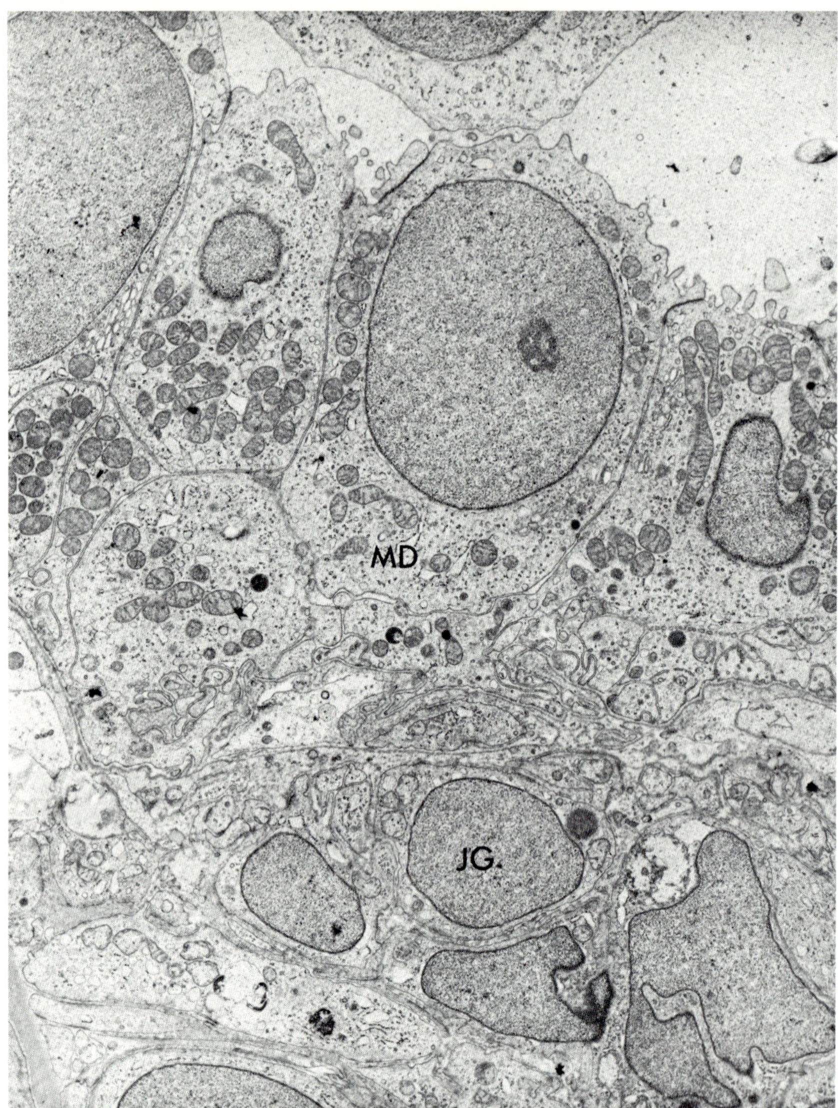

Fig. 13. Electron micrograph showing the macula densa region (*MD*) of a human juxtaglomerular apparatus. The cells of the macula densa are characterized by little cytoplasm and interdigitating processes. Some of the adjacent cells of the polar cushion (*JG*) can be seen. (Courtesy of R. E. Bulger.)

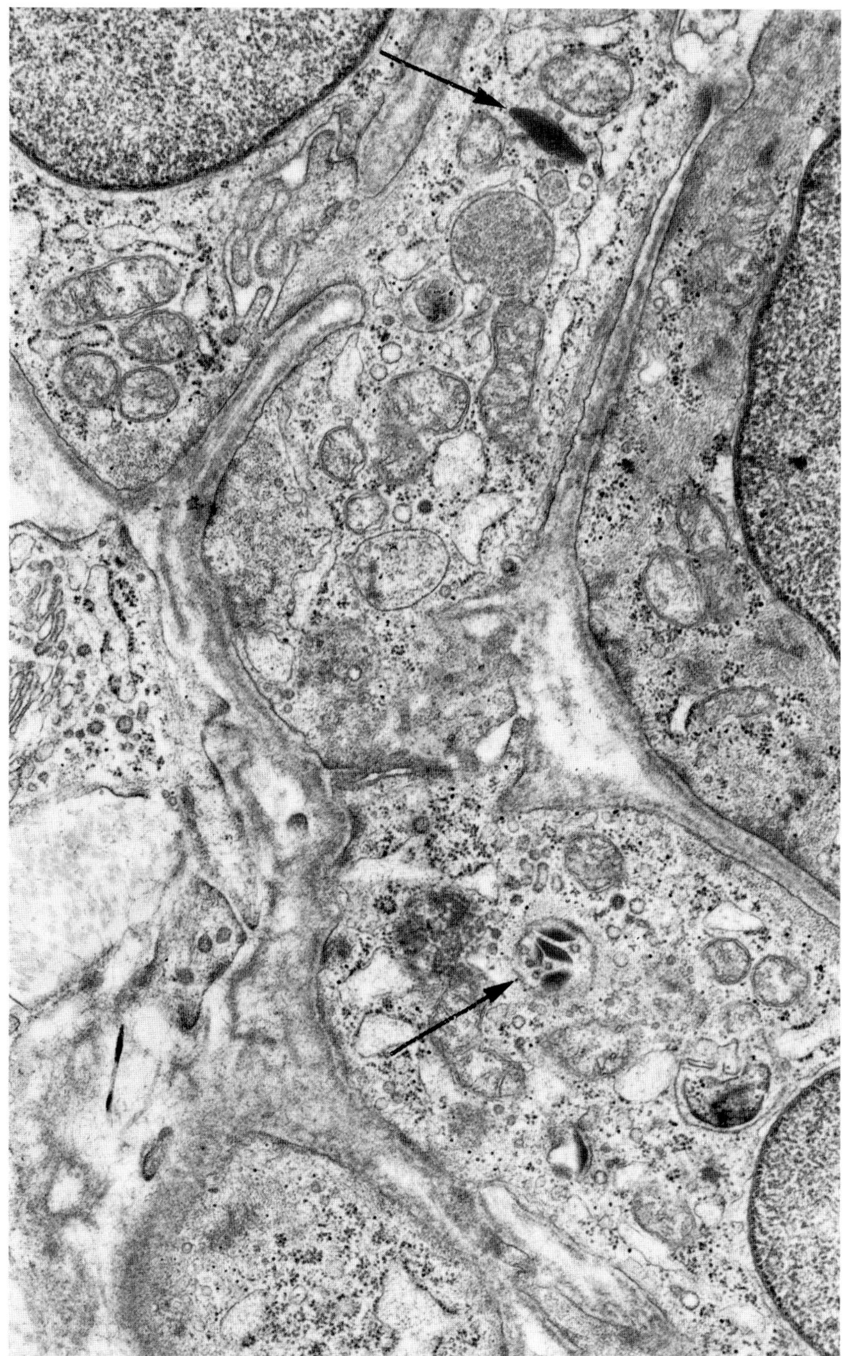

Fig. 14. Electron micrograph showing human juxtaglomerular epithelioid cells which contain characteristic granules (*arrows*). (Courtesy of R. E. Bulger.)

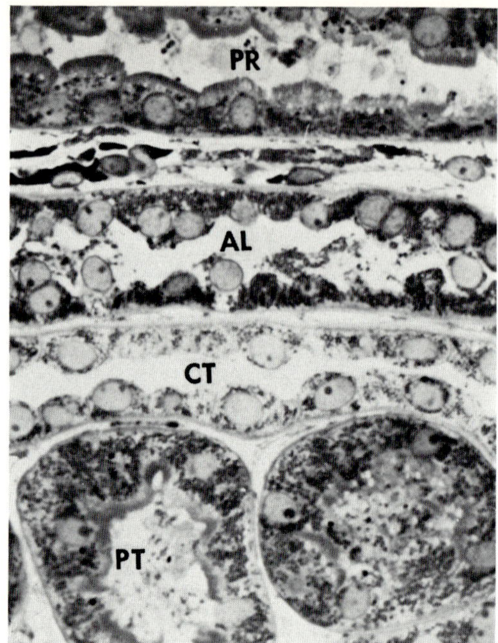

Fig. 15. Light micrograph showing the human pars recta (*PR*) of the proximal tubule, a pars recta of the distal tubule (*AL*), and a collecting duct (*CT*) in the medullary ray. Two profiles of adjacent proximal convoluted tubules (*PT*) can be seen. The cells of the pars recta of the distal tubule (thick ascending portion) project into the lumen in the region of the nucleus; their basal cytoplasm is filled with mitochondria oriented generally perpendicular to the basement membrane. (From B. F. Trump and R. E. Bulger, Morphology of the Kidney, in Becker [1].)

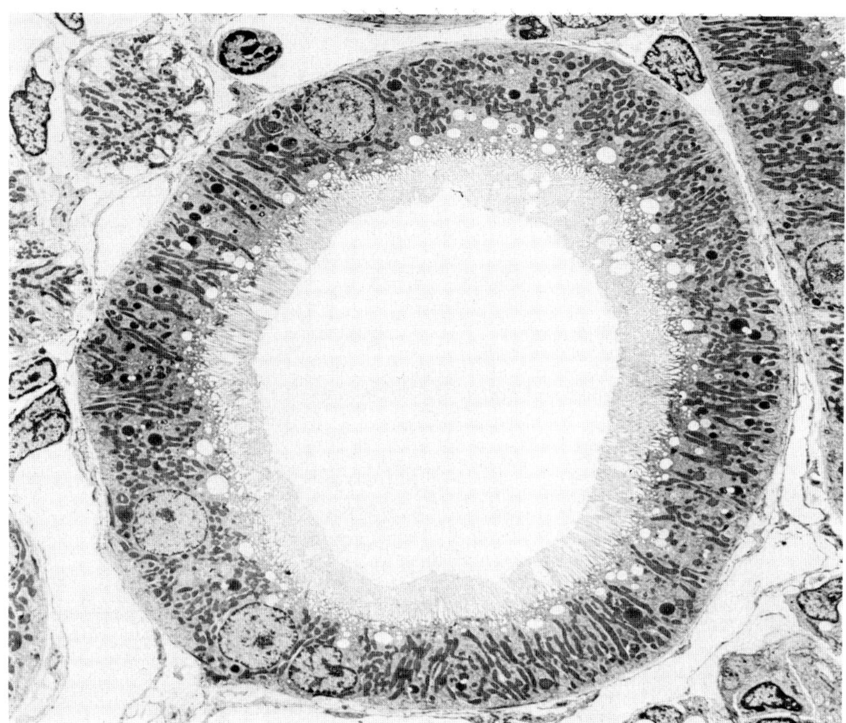

Fig. 16. Electron micrograph of the proximal convoluted tubule of a rat, fixed with glutaraldehyde in a slightly hypotonic tyrode solution. The tubular lumen is round, and the brush border has a regular arrangement. The mitochondria are largely oriented perpendicular to the basement membrane. (Lead citrate stain.) (From A. B. Maunsbach, The influence of different fixatives and fixtation methods on the ultrastructure of rat kidney proximal tubule cells. J. Ultrastruct. Res. 15:283, 1966.)

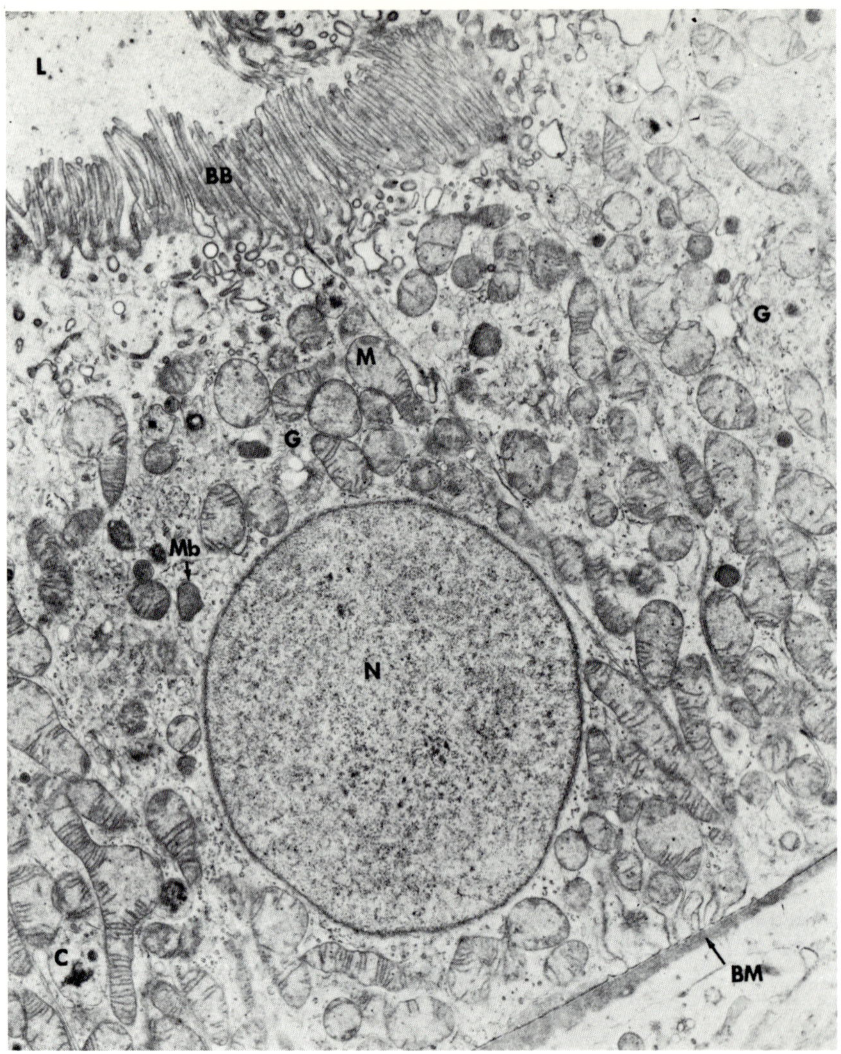

Fig. 17. Electron micrograph of a human proximal convoluted tubule, show-
ing mitochondria (*M*), brush border (*BB*), nucleus (*N*), microbodies (*Mb*),
Golgi apparatus (*G*), cytosomes (*C*), and the other components of the cell.
BM, basement membrane; *L*, tubular lumen. (Courtesy of C. Craig Tisher in
B. F. Trump and R. E. Bulger, Morphology of the Kidney, in Becker [1].)

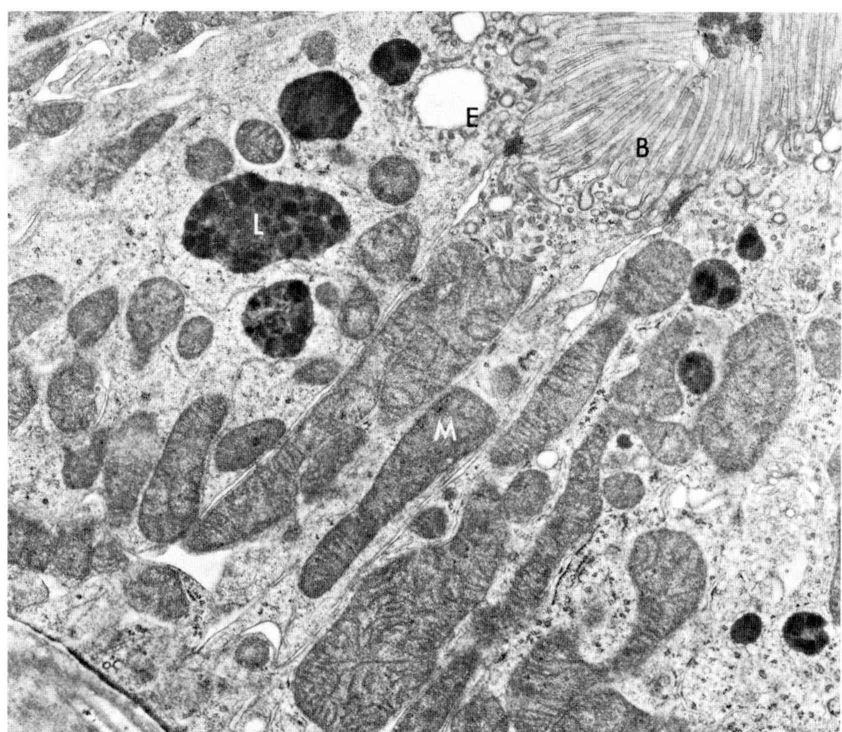

Fig. 18.   Electron micrograph showing a portion of human proximal convoluted tubules. Note the microvillous brush border (B), the apical endocytic apparatus (E), the dense lysosomes (L), and the large mitochondria (M) which characterize this segment (From W. H. Chapman, R. E. Bulger, R. Cutler, and G. Striker, *The Urinary System, an Integrated Approach*. Philadelphia. Saunders, 1973.)

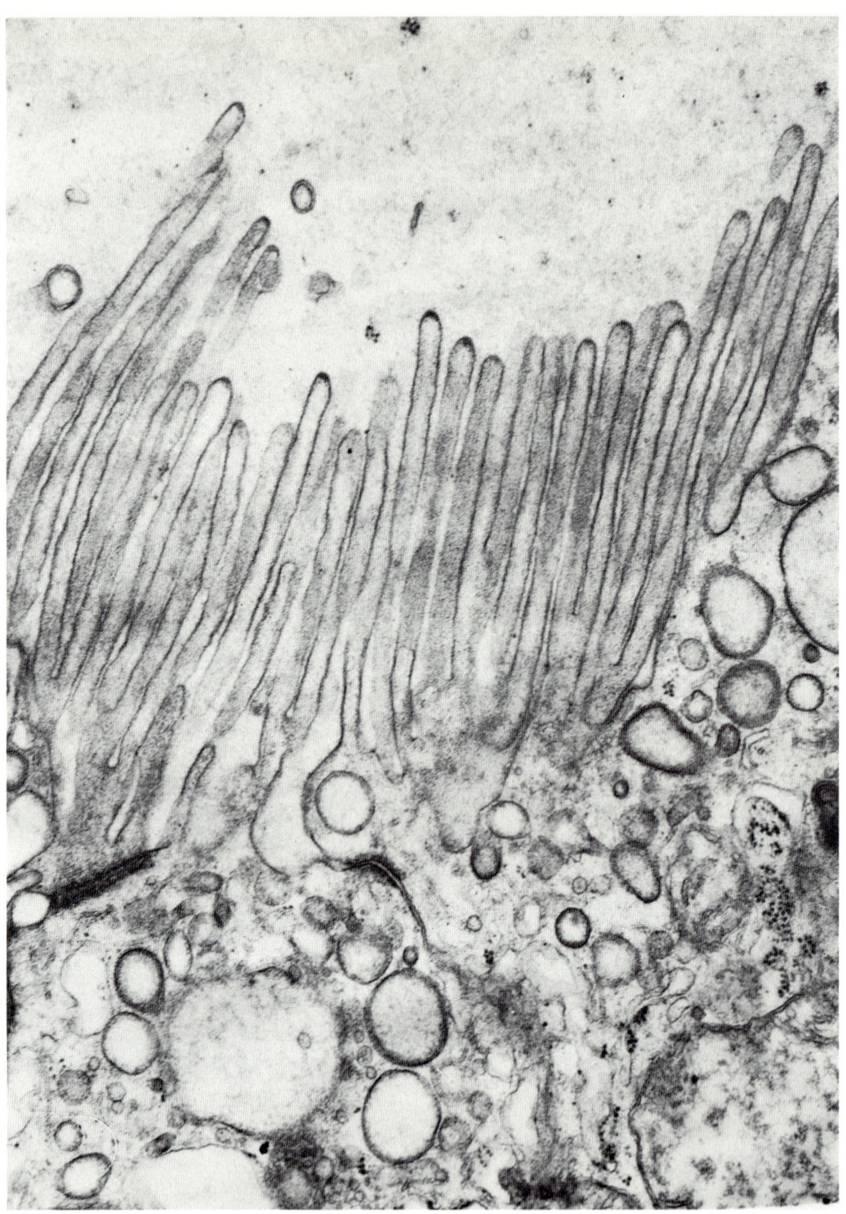

Fig. 19. Portion of proximal tubular cell showing brush border with invaginations and vacuoles. (From *Kidney and Urinary Tract Infections*, Eli Lilly and Company, 1971.)

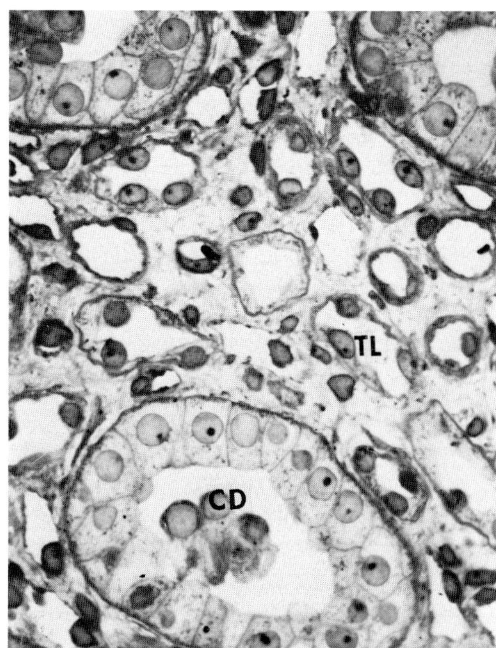

Fig. 20. Light micrograph of a human papilla in which large collecting ducts (*CD*) and thin limbs (*TL*) can be seen. (From B. F. Trump and R. E. Bulger, Morphology of the Kidney, in Becker [1].)

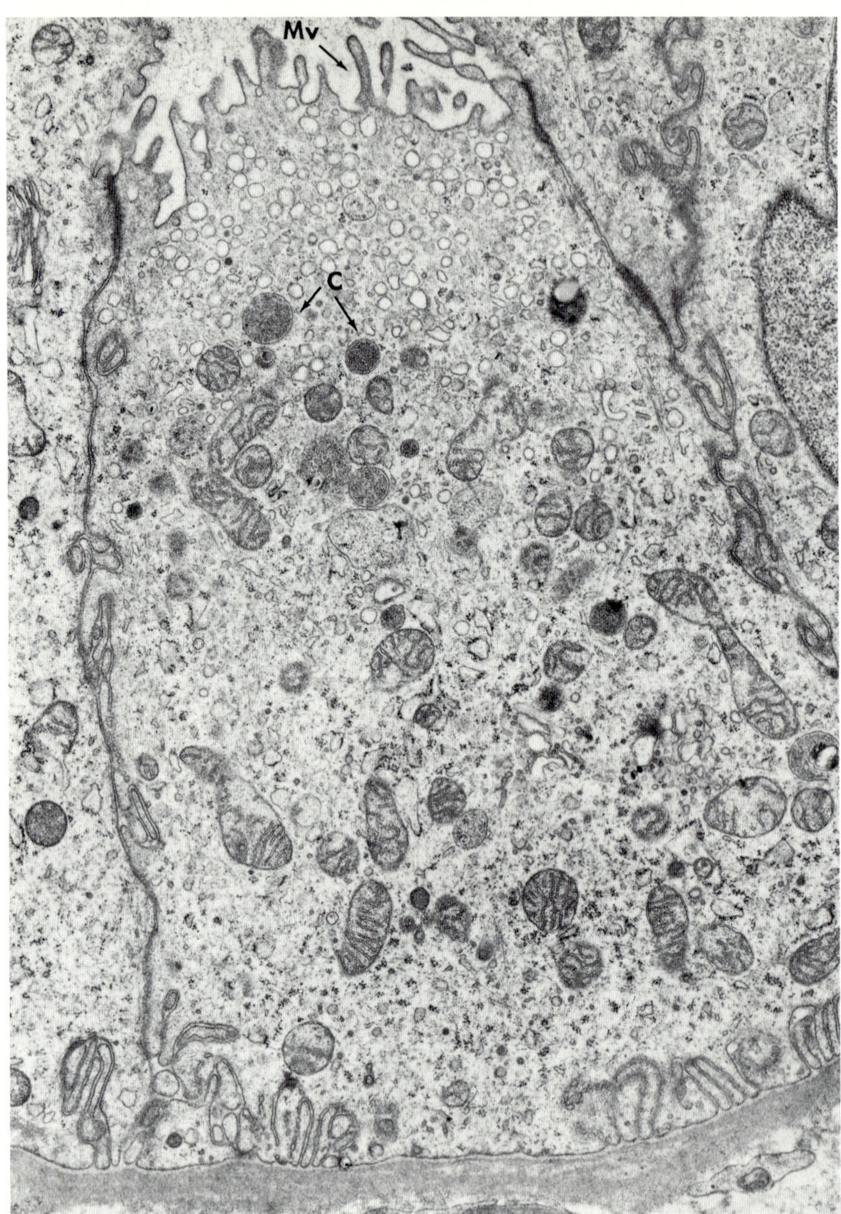

Fig. 21. Electron micrograph of a human cortical collecting tubule, showing a dark cell. The cell exhibits microvilli (*Mv*) along the luminal surface and contains numerous mitochondria and cytosomes (*C*). Several cisternae of rough-surfaced endoplasmic reticulum can be identified, and there are numerous profiles of free ribosomes. The apical region of the cell is filled with a collection of vesicular profiles. (From B. F. Trump and R. E. Bulger, Morphology of the Kidney, in Becker [1].)

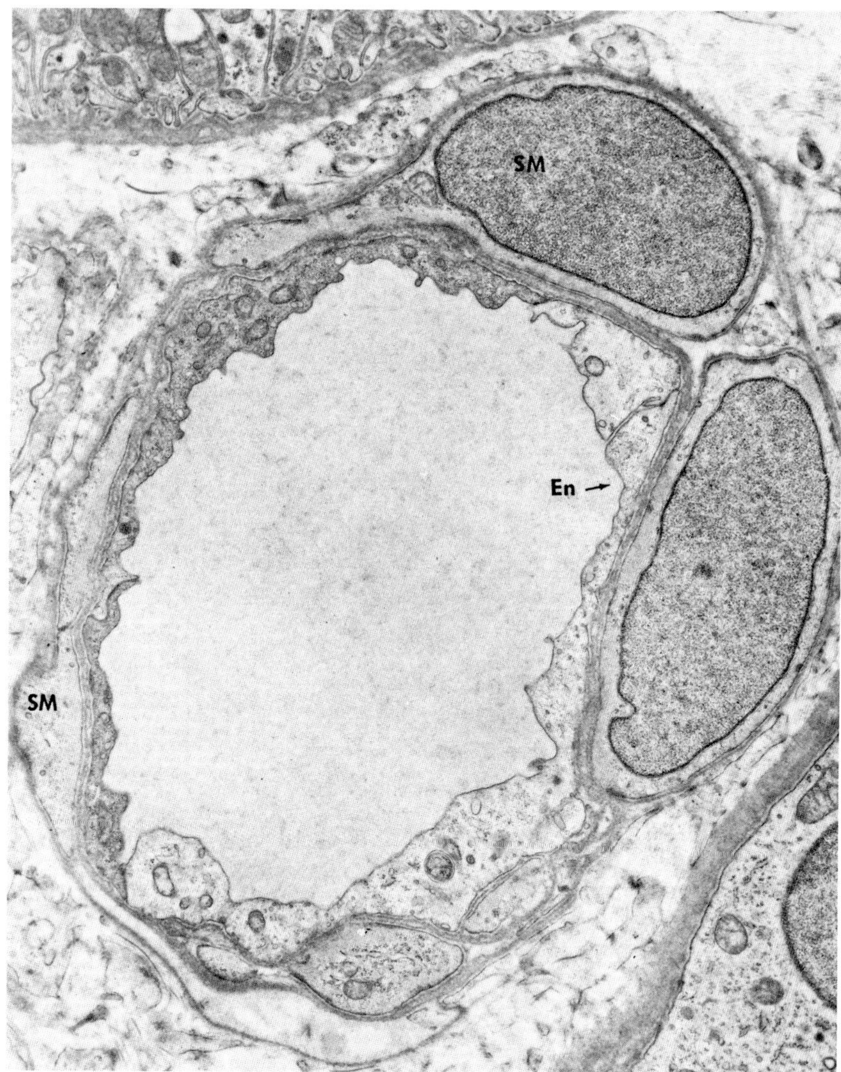

Fig. 22. Electron micrograph of a medullary efferent arteriole from a human kidney, showing an unperforated endothelium (*En*) and a partial covering of smooth muscle (*SM*). (Courtesy of C. Craig Tisher in B. F. Trump and R. E. Bulger, Morphology of the Kidney, in Becker [1].)

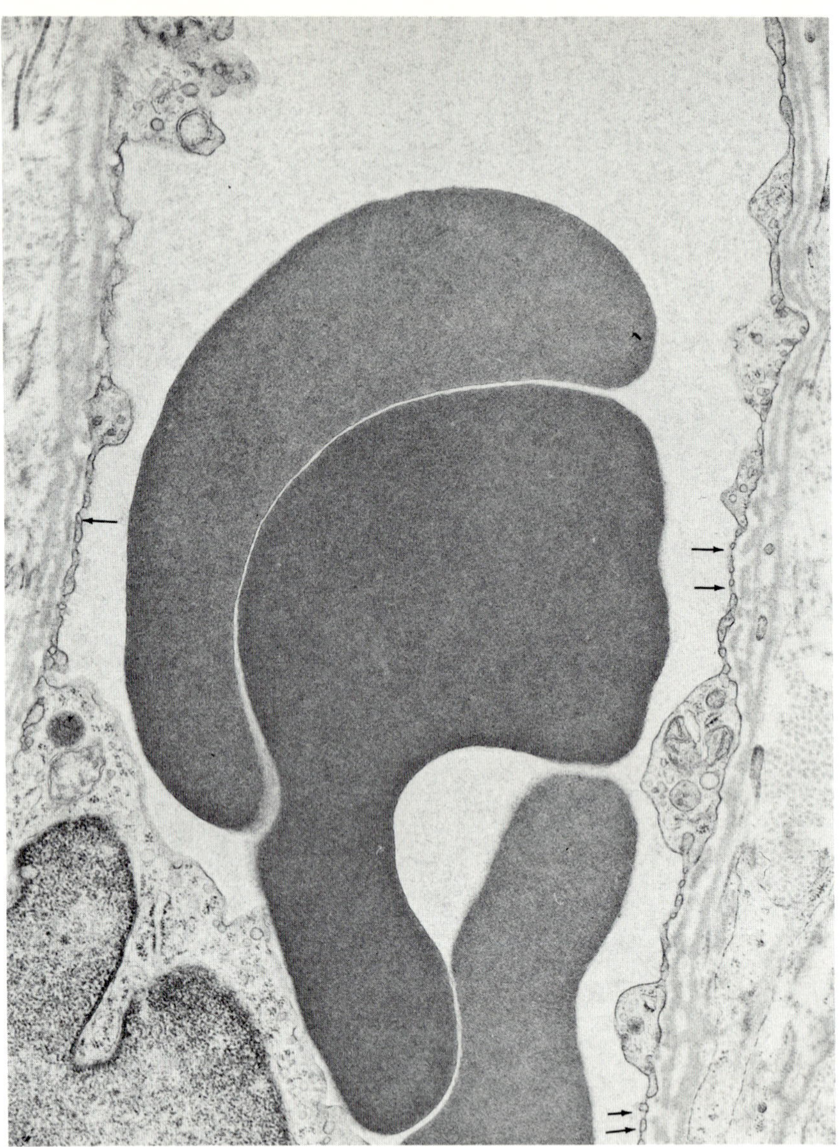

Fig. 23. Electron micrograph of a capillary from the inner medulla of a human kidney, showing an endothelium perforated by pores (*arrows*). The pores are bridged by thin diaphragms. (From B. F. Trump and R. E. Bulger, Morphology of the Kidney, in Becker [1].)

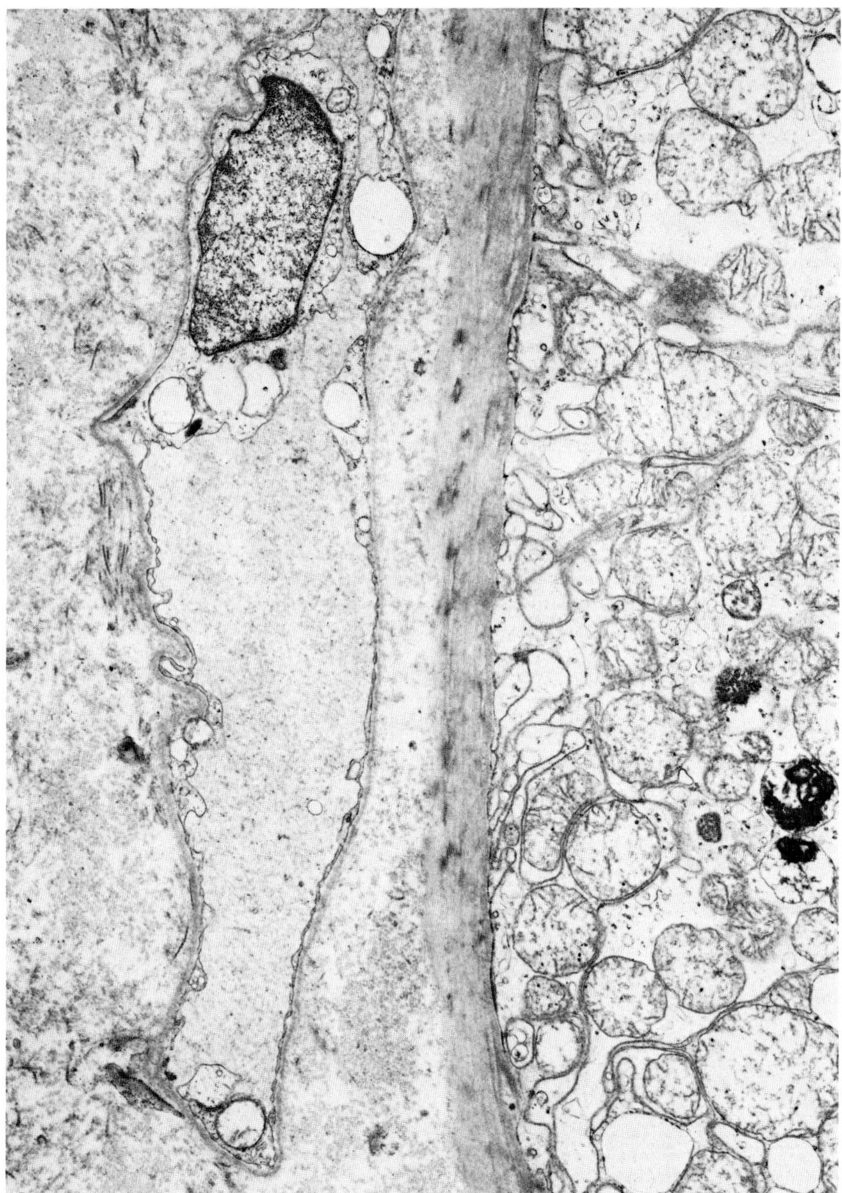

Fig. 24. Electron micrograph of peritubular capillary lying close to the proximal tubule. The wall of the capillary is thin and contains numerous fenestrations; these are present here only in cross section and hence resemble a string of approximately oval beads. Other structures of the capillary visible are the endothelial cell nucleus and the basement membrane. The proximal tubular cell contains numerous mitochondria and is enveloped by a prominent basement membrane. The interstitium contains a collagen-like material. (From *Kidney and Urinary Tract Infections*, Eli Lilly and Company, 1971.)

Immunology

adjuvant A substance which, when added to an antigen, increases antibody production. Some adjuvants act by accelerating the resorption of the antigen into phagocytizing cells (aluminum hydroxide, calcium, and aluminum phosphate). Others supposedly prolong retention of the antigen at the site of deposition. Substances in the latter group contain mineral oils and emulsifiers, whose microdrop composition protects the antigen from rapid destruction. **Freund's adjuvant** Complete: a mixture of killed mycobacteria, mineral oil, and Arlacel A. Incomplete: mineral oil and Arlacel A.

allele One of alternative forms of a gene that have the same locus on homologous chromosomes.

allograft (also *homograft*) A graft of tissue or organ taken from a donor of the same species as the recipient but not from an identical twin. Compare AUTOGRAFT; ISOGRAFT; XENOGRAFT.

alternate pathway (also *amplification loop*) A pathway that parallels the classic route of activation of complement activity (C1, C4, C2) which triggers the terminal attack mechanism and may, but does not necessarily, involve antibody. Properdin factors A and B and euglobulin factor appear to be the constituents by which C3b, the major fragment of the initial step in C3 cleavage, induces the formation of additional C3 cleavage. Factor B in turn acts to split C3, thereby leading to a positive feedback or amplification effect.

antibody A serum globulin synthesized in response to a specific antigen. See also IMMUNOGLOBULIN.

anti-GBM disease See ANTIGLOMERULAR BASEMENT MEMBRANE ANTIBODY DISEASE.

antigen A substance, usually a protein or carbohydrate (polysaccharide) which, when introduced into the body, stimulates the production of an antibody. An antigen possesses immunogenicity and specificity. **autologous antigen** An antigen derived from the body itself.

antigen-antibody complex (also *immune complex*) A complex formed of antigen and antibody and components of complement. When formed in marked antigen excess, complexes are generally soluble. See also IMMUNE COMPLEX DISEASE.

antiglomerular basement membrane antibody disease (also *anti-GBM disease*) Glomerular disease caused by antibodies directed against constituents of the glomerular basement membrane and characterized by a completely continuous ("linear") accumulation of immunoglobulins and complement in the membrane. Experimentally such disease may result from heterologous antibodies against glomerular basement membrane (Masugi nephritis). Autoantibodies to glomerular basement membrane are thought to be the basis for the glomerular changes found in patients with lung purpura (Goodpasture's syndrome) and certain other human glomerular diseases.

antilymphocyte serum An immune serum produced in a heterologous species, which reduced lymphocytes by complement-dependent lysis.

antimetabolite A chemical structurally resembling a particular metabolite but competing with, replacing, or antagonizing it at some points within its metabolic pathway.

autoantibody An antibody produced by either unchanged or altered (e.g., haptenized) autogenous material or by activation of otherwise inactive (tolerant) immunologically competent cells. The cytotoxic damage produced by such autoantibodies is called **autoimmune aggression.**

autograft Any tissue removed from one part of a person's body and applied to another part. Compare ALLOGRAFT; ISOGRAFT; XENOGRAFT.

autoimmune aggression See under AUTOANTIBODY.

autoimmune glomerulonephritis See STEBLAY NEPHRITIS.

autologous antigen See under ANTIGEN.

autologous immune complex disease See under IMMUNE COMPLEX DISEASE.

β_1**C** See under COMPLEMENT.

beta 1C globulin See under COMPLEMENT.

C3 See under COMPLEMENT.

CH$_{50}$ A unit designating the amount of hemolytic complement activity which produces fifty percent hemolysis in an antigen-antibody system, usually sheep erythrocytes and anti-sheep erythrocyte guinea pig antibody.

complement A system of serum factors activated by the allosteric alteration of antigen under the influence of antibody in the presence of most kinds of antigen-antibody complexes. The component most easily demonstrable within tissue by the immunofluorescence staining technique is the third one, **C3** (previously designated β_1C globulin). **Complement activity** is a better term, since complement is not a uniform substance but is characterized and measured by its activity in an antigen-antibody system. The complement activity results from nine components and at least three inhibitors. C1 (subunits C1q, C1r, C1s) is first fixed to IgG or IgM and C1s is activated to become C1 esterase.

C1 esterase acts on C4 and C2 to form the enzyme convertase which cleaves the substrate C3. A histamine liberator (anaphylatoxin, a split product of C3) is formed, and immune adherence and phagocytosis occur. The activation of C5, C6, and C7 results in a complex formation with potent chemotactic activity, and polymorphonuclear leucocytes are attracted to the area of immunoreaction. Finally, the activation of C8 and C9 is responsible for the production of lytic lesions.

complement profile The distribution of the known and determinable components of complement activity in a given serum. This probably varies in the different renal diseases that are based on immunologic reactions.

complex, antigen-antibody See ANTIGEN-ANTIBODY COMPLEX.

complex, immune See ANTIGEN-ANTIBODY COMPLEX.

Coon's technique See IMMUNOHISTOLOGIC METHOD.

enhancement Prolongation of the survival of an allograft as a consequence of the action of humoral antibody against donor histocompatibility antigens which are absent from the host.

Freund's adjuvant See under ADJUVANT.

gene A unit of heredity.

genome A complete set of hereditary factors such as is contained in a haploid set of chromosomes.

glomerulonephritis, autoimmune See STEBLAY NEPHRITIS.

graft See ALLOGRAFT; AUTOGRAFT; ISOGRAFT; XENOGRAFT.

H-2 locus A chromosomal region in mice that houses the genes which control the specificities of a large number of antigens. The role of these genes is preeminent in tissue transplantation.

haploid Posessing a single member of each chromosome pair. A **haploid number** is one-half the total chromosome number of a diploid cell.

haplotype In transplantation, the antigens controlled by one HL-A unit or contained on one chromosome. Since an individual inherits two such HL-A units, one from each parent, each haplotype represents half his full complement.

hapten (also *haptene*) Usually a simple chemical substance but sometimes a more complex derivative of certain bacteria or viruses which determines the immunologic specificity of an antigen. Haptens do not possess immunogenicity themselves but can couple with other nonimmunogenic substances to produce immunogenicity. The antibody which forms in response reacts not only with the haptenized antigen but also with the original nonimmunogenic substance.

heterologous Derived from a different species or from a different part.

Heymann's nephrosis An experimental disease produced in rats by injection of homologous kidney extracts and Freund's adjuvant. The disease has been shown to be due to deposition of circulating complexes composed of autoantibodies and autologous antigens derived from renal tubular epithelial cells.

histocompatibility Tissue compatibility in reference to antigens determining the transplantability of tissue.

HL-A unit The complex genetic unit that controls a large number of antigenic specificities which are the major histocompatibility factors in man. The HL-A system is very similar to the H-2 locus system in mice.

homograft See ALLOGRAFT.

homologous Of a graft, derived from the same species; of chromosomes, possessing the same genes or alleles.

IgA Immunoglobulin of external secretion (saliva, bronchial secretion, intestinal fluid, etc.) Also present in serum. Serum concentration 150–400 mg/100 ml. Molecular weight 160,000. Does not cross placenta, does not fix complement except in presence of lysozyme.

IgD Serum concentration 0.3–40 mg/100 ml. Molecular weight 150,000.

IgE Present in external secretions. Elevated in allergic conditions. Serum concentration 300 ng/ml. Molecular weight 200,000.

IgG The major immunoglobulin in human serum. Serum concentration 800–1600 mg/100 ml. MW 150,000. Fixes complement, crosses human placenta. Subclasses are IgG1, IgG2, IgG3, and IgG4 (IgG4 does not fix complement).

IgM Serum concentration 50–200 mg/100 ml. Molecular weight 900,000. Fixes complement, does not cross placenta.

immune complex See ANTIGEN-ANTIBODY COMPLEX.

immune complex disease A disease in which the lesions (which occur principally in glomeruli, but sometimes also in arteries or heart valves) are due to deposition of antigen-antibody-complement (immune) complexes. The antigens involved may be exogenous (including material of bacterial or viral origin) or autologous. Although a variety of histologic types of glomerular lesions may be produced by immune complexes, they are all characterized by granular, irregular ("lumpy, bumpy") accumulation of immunoglobulins in glomeruli and by corresponding electrondense deposits. Complexes may be demonstrated in aggregates along either side of the basement membrane, or within it, or within mesangial regions, and are seen in several human glomerular diseases, including acute poststreptococcal glomerulonephritis, lupus nephritis, and membranous nephropathy. **autologous immune complex disease** Immune complex disease in which the circulating complexes are composed of autologous antigens and autoantibodies. It is probably the basis for the glomerular lesions in lupus nephritis.

immunofluorescence staining technique   See IMMUNOHISTOLOGIC METHOD.

immunoglobulin   One of several classes of serum proteins which principally include antibodies. There are several major classes of immunoglobulins: IgG (or 7S gamma globulin), IgM (or 19S gamma globulin), IgA, and IgE. (See individual entries.) These are separable on the basis of electrophoretic mobility, molecular weight, and other criteria. The major component is IgG, which is present in most immune complexes responsible for glomerular disease. IgM, IgA, and IgE also are sometimes present in glomerular deposits.

immunohistologic method   (also *Coon's technique; immunofluoresence staining technique*)   A technique consisting of staining kidney biopsy specimens (or other tissues) with previously labeled heterologous antibodies. Fluorescein isothiocyanate, the label most commonly used, causes the area in which the antigen is located to fluoresce an intense apple-green under the ultraviolet microscope. Rhodamine, which may also be used as a label, produces a red-orange fluorescence.

isogenic   Genetically alive.

isograft   A piece of tissue or organ transplanted from one member of an identical twin pair to another or between animals isogenic with respect to histocompatibility genes. Compare ALLOGRAFT; AUTOGRAFT; XENOGRAFT.

nephritis, Steblay   See STEBLAY NEPHRITIS.

nephrosis, Heymann's   See HEYMANN'S NEPHROSIS.

self   The property of the antibody-forming apparatus to recognize a body protein as belonging specifically to its own body. This ability is acquired in the prenatal and perinatal period. Failure to recognize a protein as "self" leads to antibody formation. This is presumably the basis of systemic lupus erythematosus, wherein body-owned nucleoproteins are handled like foreign proteins and antibodies are produced.

serum, antilymphocyte   See ANTILYMPHOCYTE SERUM.

Steblay nephritis   (also *autoimmune glomerulonephritis*)   An experimental disease produced by immunizing sheep with heterologous glomerular basement membrane preparations plus Freund's adjuvant. The glomerular lesions have been shown to be due to autoantibodies directed against constituents of the glomerular basement membrane.

tolerance   A state of specific nonreactivity to an antigen, induced by prior exposure to the antigen under special circumstances.

xenograft   A tissue or organ graft taken from a donor of a species different from that of the recipient. Compare ALLOGRAFT; AUTOGRAFT; ISOGRAFT.

Pathology

abnormalities   See BASEMENT MEMBRANE ABNORMALITIES; EPITHELIAL CELL
ABNORMALITIES.

abscess, kidney   See Clinical Glossary.

adherent capsule   See CAPSULE, ADHERENT.

adhesion, glomerular   Attachment between the capillary loops of the glomerular tuft and the glomerular capsule, or attachment of one capillary
loop to another (Fig. 25). It may be fibrinous or fibrous and may occur
with or without proliferation of epithelial cells (see CRESCENT). Adhesions may be associated with pseudotubules (see PSEUDOTUBULE).

adipose tissue in the interstitium   In atrophic kidneys, increased adipose
tissue that replaces disappearing renal parenchyma without actually
penetrating the interstitial tissue. See MEDULLARY LIPOMATOSIS.

amyloid   See INTERSTITIAL INFILTRATES.

argyrophilic deposit   See under GLOMERULAR DEPOSITS, BASEMENT MEM-
BRANE ABNORMALITIES.

Armanni-Ebstein lesion   See under INCLUSIONS.

atrophy

> **juxtaglomerular cell atrophy**   Shrinkage of the cell and possibly also
> a reduction in number of juxtaglomerular cells. This kind of atrophy is
> believed to be associated with subnormal blood renin levels and is
> characteristic of primary aldosteronism and certain other hypertensive
> conditions. It appears to be reversible.   **renal** or **kidney atrophy** (also
> *contracted kidney*)   A decrease in size and weight of the kidney. See
> also HYPOPLASIA, RENAL and KIDNEY, CONTRACTED in Clinical Glossary.
> **tubular atrophy**   Wasting of the tubules. This is usually the result of
> tubular ischemia or obstruction but may also be caused by severe
> cellular injury. The tubules may be normal in size, collapsed, or
> dilated. On light microscopy the atrophic cells are seen to be cuboidal
> or flattened, with pale, often vacuolated, cytoplasm. The vacuoles
> commonly reflect the presence of lipid concentrated in the subnuclear
> portion of the cells. There may be a marked decrease in the number
> of organelles, and the microvilli of the proximal tubules are short and
> sparse. The basement membranes of atrophic tubules are often con-

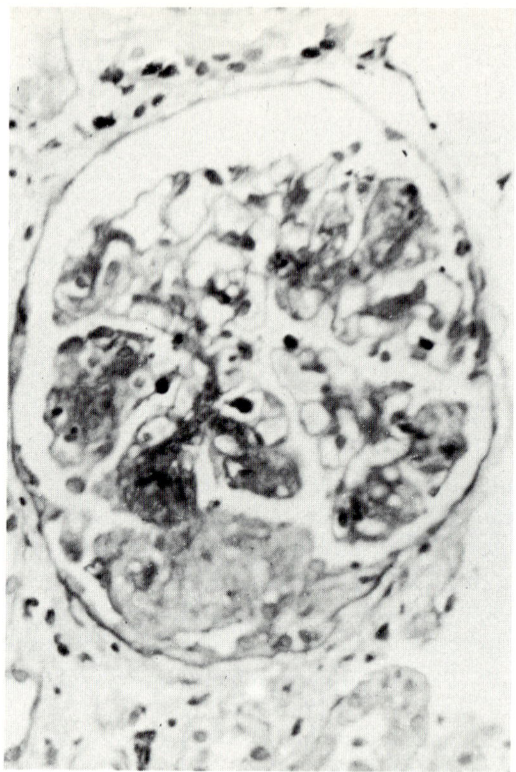

Fig. 25. Glomerular adhesion. The capillary tuft is attached to a small fibrous crescent. (Courtesy of J. Churg.)

siderably thickened. The process that produces atrophy may also lead to the complete disappearance of tubular cells (Figs. 26 and 27).

autophagy See FOCAL CYTOPLASMIC DEGRADATION.

basement membrane abnormalities
   capsular abnormalities See GLOMERULAR CAPSULAR THICKENING. **glomerular capillary basement membrane thickening** Thickening may be caused by formation of additional layers either on the endothelial or, more frequently, on the epithelial side of the membrane, covering part or all of the glomerulus. The extra layers may be less dense and less homogeneous or more dense than the original lamina densa and may have an irregular or wavy luminal border. Projections or **spikes** may form on the epithelial side. Thickening may also be caused by deposits and/or **splitting** of the dense layer into two or more layers, giving the basement membrane a mottled appearance. Subendothelial formation of mesangial matrix (sometimes called **argyrophilic deposit**

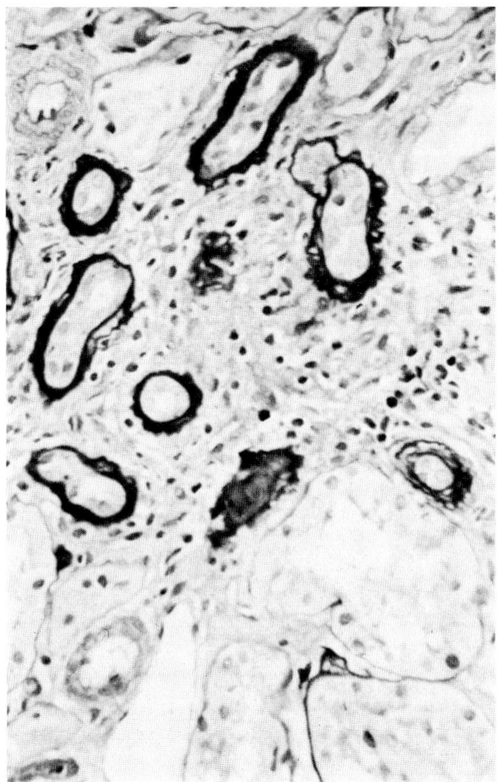

Fig. 26. Tubular atrophy. The atrophic tubules have thick basement membranes and are separated by interstitial fibrous tissue containing inflammatory cells. (Courtesy of J. Churg.)

or **membranoid material**) identifiable by electron microscopy may appear as reduplication or splitting of the basement membrane on light microscopy. Thickening must be distinguished from wrinkling, present normally over the mesangial stalk and pathologically in damaged glomeruli (e.g., ischemia). Thickening may be segmental or diffuse. Changes in density and/or texture of the basement membrane may also be present and may reflect chemical or physical abnormalities (Figs. 28, 29, 30, and 31). **glomerular capillary basement membrane thinning** Thinning may be caused by distention of the lumen or of the whole lobule by blood, by inflammatory cell proliferation, or by cellular edema. **tubular abnormalities** The tubular basement membrane may be thinner or thicker than normal. Thickening may be homogeneous or lamellar, diffuse or segmental, with or without deposits (Fig. 26).

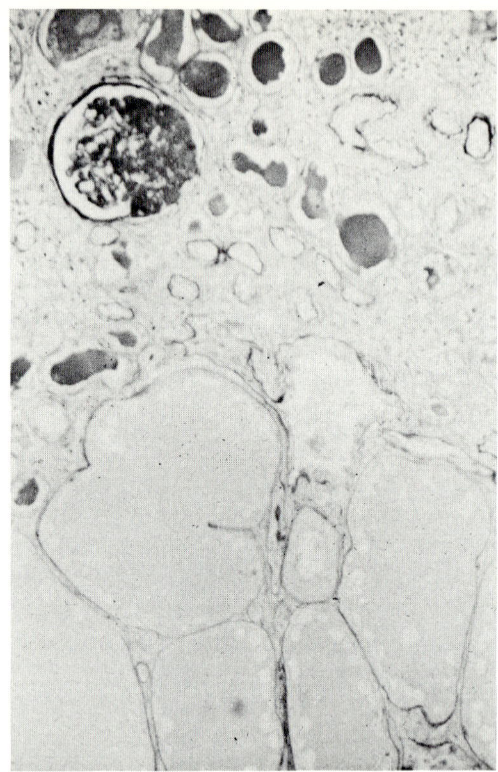

Fig. 27. Tubular atrophy and dilatation. Right, a partly sclerosed glomerulus and small atrophic tubules containing dense casts. Left, markedly dilated tubules filled with pale staining protein precipitate. (Courtesy of J. Churg.)

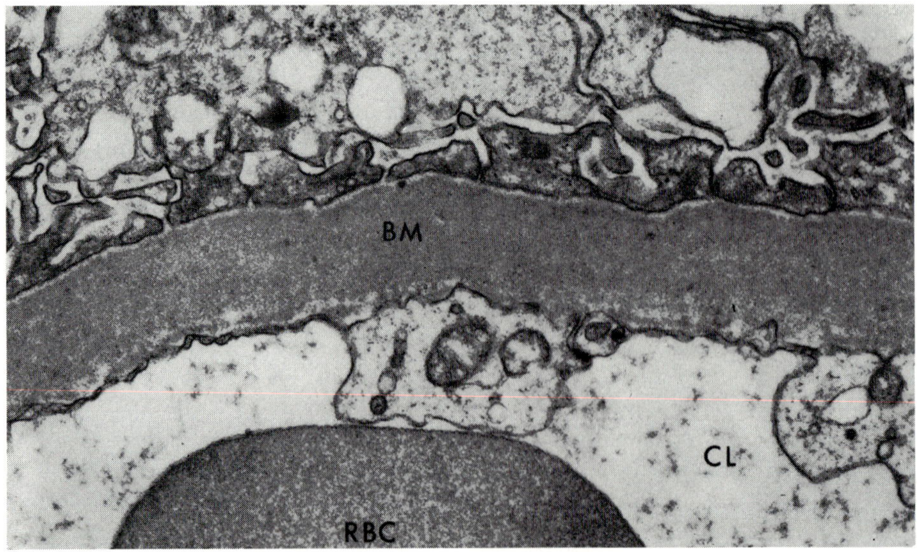

Fig. 28. Basement membrane (*BM*) of the capillary wall diffusely thickened in a case of early diabetic glomerulosclerosis: *RBC*, red blood cell; *CL*, capillary lumen. (From J. Churg, Electron Microscopic Aspects of Renal Pathology, in Becker [1].)

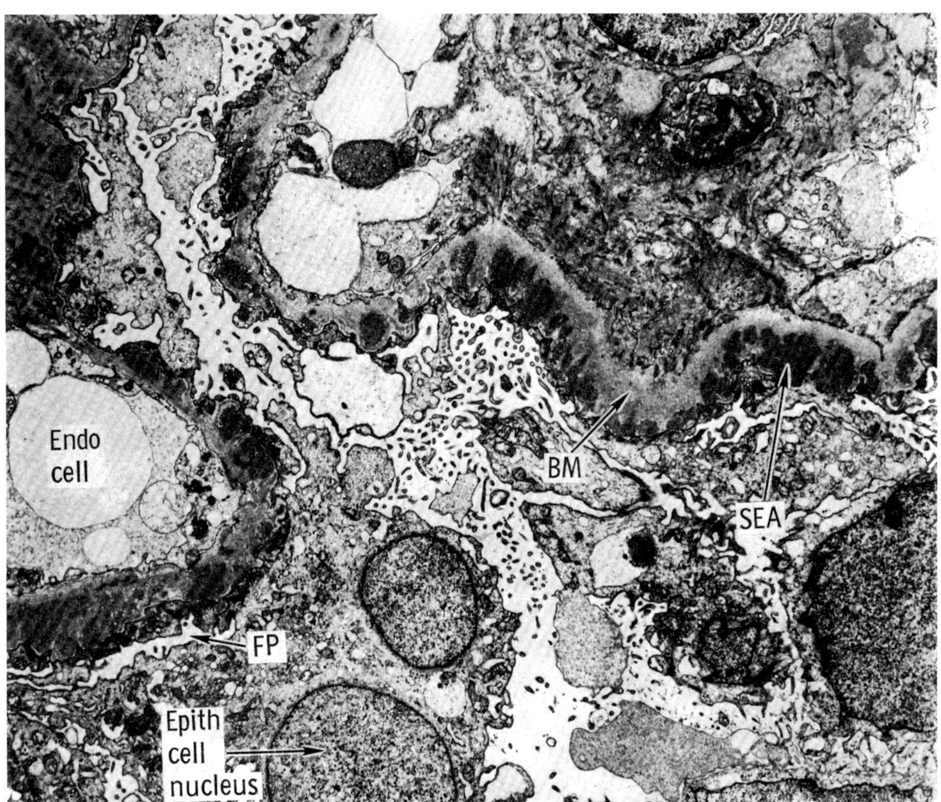

Fig. 29. Electron photomicrograph of kidney biopsy from a patient with membranous nephropathy. The subepithelial accumulation of electron-dense material (*SEA*) is very prominent. There is thickening of the basement membrane (*BM*) and fusion of the foot processes (*EP*). An endothelial cell (*Endo cell*) and an epithelial cell nucleus (*Epith cell nucleus*) are also seen. (Courtesy of J. Churg in E. L. Becker, The Nephrotic Syndrome in Adults with Glomerulonephritis, in Becker [1].)

bleb   A pale, nearly structureless, roughly spherical protrusion of cytoplasm into the capillary lumen. Blebs usually arise from mesangial cells which protrude between or through endothelial cells; they may also arise from endothelial cells. They are observed under normal and pathologic conditions and may result from fixation or other types of artifact (Fig. 32).

Bowman's capsule thickening   See GLOMERULAR CAPSULAR THICKENING.

cake kidney   See KIDNEY, CAKE in Clinical Glossary.

calcification, renal   Deposition of calcium in tubular cells, interstitium (see under INTERSTITIAL INFILTRATES, arteries, and occasionally glo-

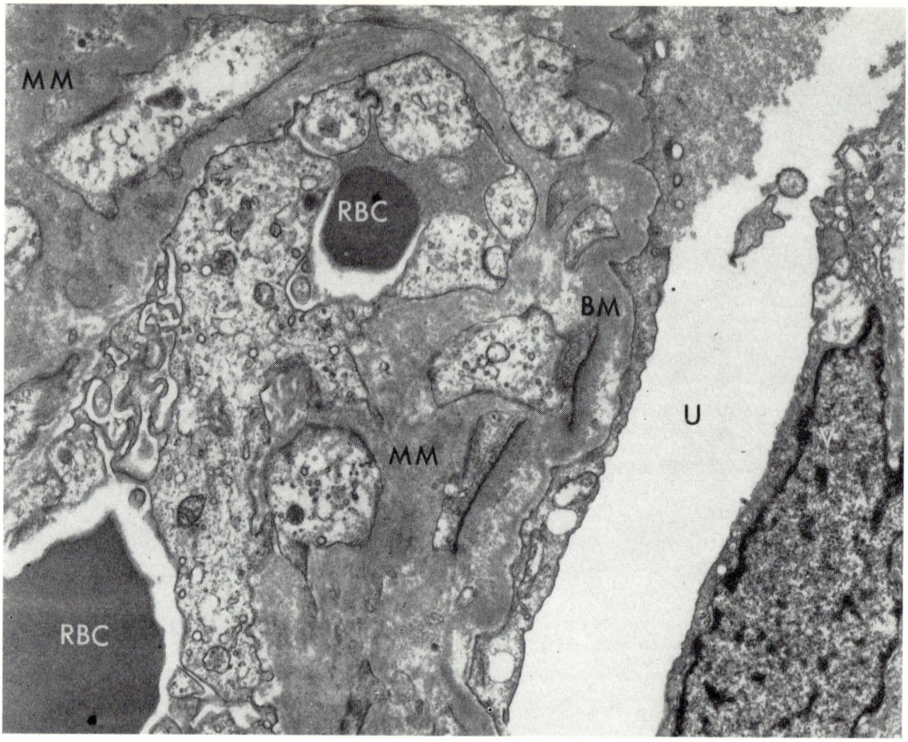

Fig. 30. Membranoproliferative glomerulonephritis with nephrotic syndrome. Part of a glomerulus showing edematous endothelial cells and a narrow lumen containing red blood cells (*RBC*). The foot processes are fused. The basement membrane (*BM*) is slightly irregular and mottled. Between the basement membrane and the endothelium are thick strands of mesangial matrix (*MM*); these surround the lumen and join the expanded mesangium near the top of the picture. *U*, urinary (glomerular capsular) space. (From J. Churg, Electron Microscopic Aspects of Renal Pathology, in Becker [1].)

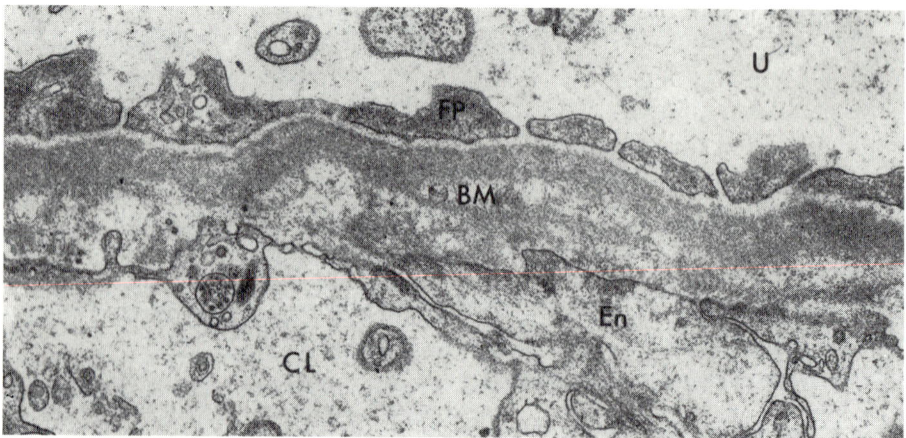

Fig. 31. Splitting and mottling of the basement membrane (*BM*) in a case of subacute glomerulonephritis. *CL*, capillary lumen; *En*, endothelial cell; *FP*, foot process; *U*, urinary (glomerular capsular) space. (From J. Churg, Electron Microscopic Aspects of Renal Pathology, in Becker [1].)

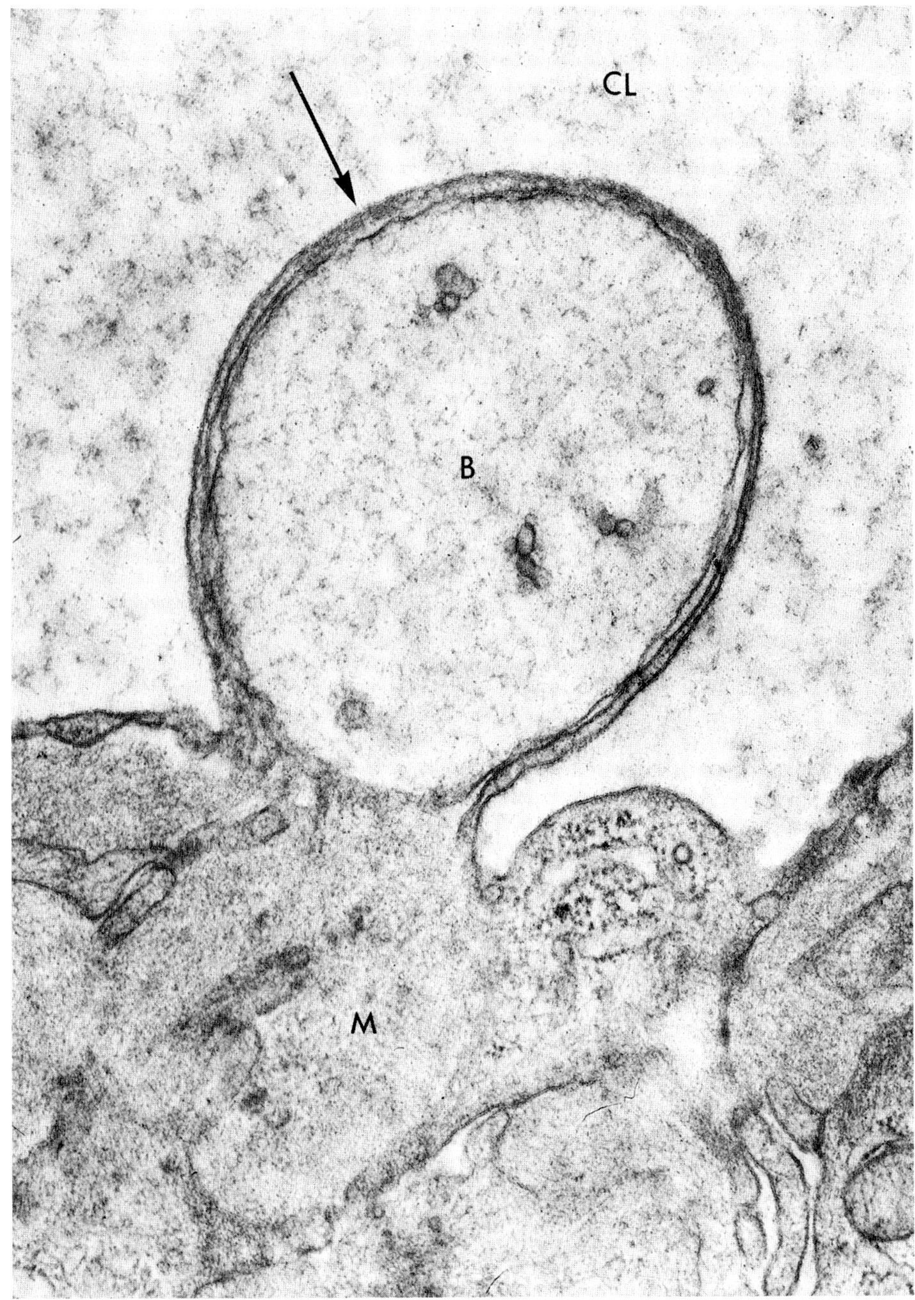

Fig. 32. An intracapillary bleb. This is a portion of mesangial cell cytoplasm filled with fluid (*B*) which protrudes into the capillary lumen (*CL*). It is covered by a thin layer of endothelial cytoplasm (*arrow*). *M*, mesangium. (Courtesy of A. Bergstrand.)

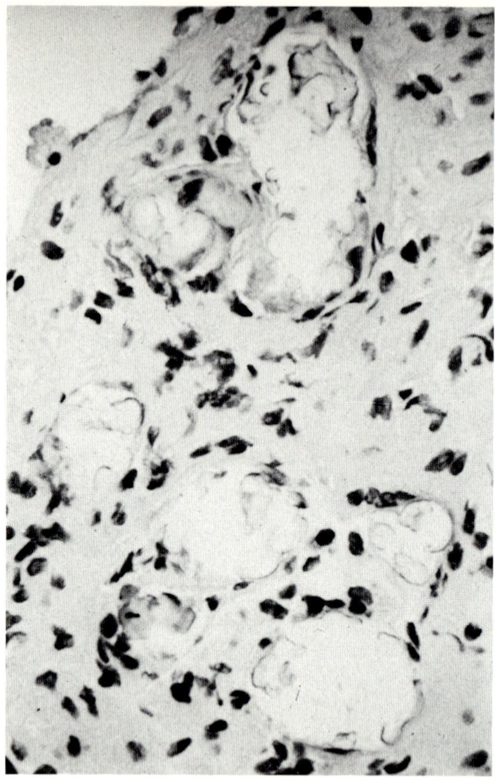

Fig. 33. Calcification of the kidney. Pale-staining rounded and irregular calcium deposits are found in the tubular lumina. (Courtesy of J. Churg.)

meruli. In the proximal tubular cells calcium deposition follows excessive calcium mobilization or hypercalcemia of diverse origin, e.g., hyperparathyroidism and excessive vitamin D intake. It may occur as intracytoplasmic aggregates or as deposits in the mitochondrial matrix, in the subbasilar and extracellular spaces, and along the tubular basement membrane (Fig. 33).

calyceal lesion See PELVIC AND CALYCEAL LESIONS.

capillary collapse, glomerular Wrinkling and thickening of the capillary walls with constriction and obliteration of the capillary lumen (See also SCLEROSIS OF GLOMERULI.)

capillary congestion, glomerular Dilatation of glomerular capillaries by red blood cells. Parts or all of the glomerular tuft may be affected.

capillary dilatation

glomerular See CAPILLARY CONGESTION, GLOMERULAR. **lymphatic** See LYMPHATIC CAPILLARY DILATATION.

capillary wall thickening, glomerular Thickening may be caused by any of the following, singly or in combination: endothelial edema or hyperplasia, thickening of the basement membrane, epithelial hyperplasia or edema, deposits, and mesangial ingrowth between the endothelium and the basement membrane. Thickening may also result from poorly defined layers of basement membrane material (**membranoid**) in a subepithelial location (Figs. 28, 29, 30, and 31). (See also BASEMENT MEMBRANE ABNORMALITIES; EDEMA; GLOMERULAR DEPOSITS.)

capsular drop Accumulation of hyalin in the glomerular capsule. See also HYALINE LESION.

capsule, adherent Adherence to the kidney surface by the renal capsule, which may have become thin or focally or diffusely thickened. Fragments of cortex may be torn off if the capsule is peeled away.

carbohydrate in tubular cells See under INCLUSIONS.

casts Cylindrical, refractile, alkaline-soluble precipitates shaped by development in the renal tubules. Casts are seen usually in the distal segments of the nephron but occasionally appear in the proximal segments (Fig. 40).

Granular casts usually are composed of desquamated and fragmented tubular cells, although some consist of fragmented erythrocytes. They may be brown without containing demonstrable hemoglobin. **Hyaline casts** consist of precipitated protein mixed with Tamm-Horsfall protein of tubular origin. **Leukocyte (polymorph) casts** indicate inflammation in the kidney. **Pigmented casts** are brown in cases of hemoglobinuria and muddy yellow in jaundice. **Red cell casts** as well as single red blood cells in the tubular lumina result usually from glomerular hemorrhage and occasionally from peritubular hemorrhage.

cholesterol granulomata See under INTERSTITIAL INFILTRATES.

cloudy swelling See under EDEMA.

colloid See under INCLUSIONS.

congestion, capillary See CAPILLARY CONGESTION, GLOMERULAR.

contracted kidney See KIDNEY, CONTRACTED in Clinical Glossary.

crescent A buildup of several cell layers in a crescentic shape, caused by proliferation of parietal (glomerular capsule) cells and probably also of the visceral epithelial cells (podocytes) of the glomerulus. The cells rest in a framework of fibrin, basement membrane, and collagen. Crescents are classified as **cellular**, **fibrocellular**, or **fibrous** depending upon the predominant component (Figs. 25, 34, and 50).

crystal formation Phenomena occurring when crystals of protein (in multiple myeloma), calcium oxalate, uric acid, cystine, leucine, and of various poorly soluble sulfonamide drugs, occur mainly in the distal segments of the nephron. Occasionally, crystals of protein and of calcium (hydroxyapatite) occur also in the cell cytoplasm. Rarely, small calculi form in the collecting ducts.

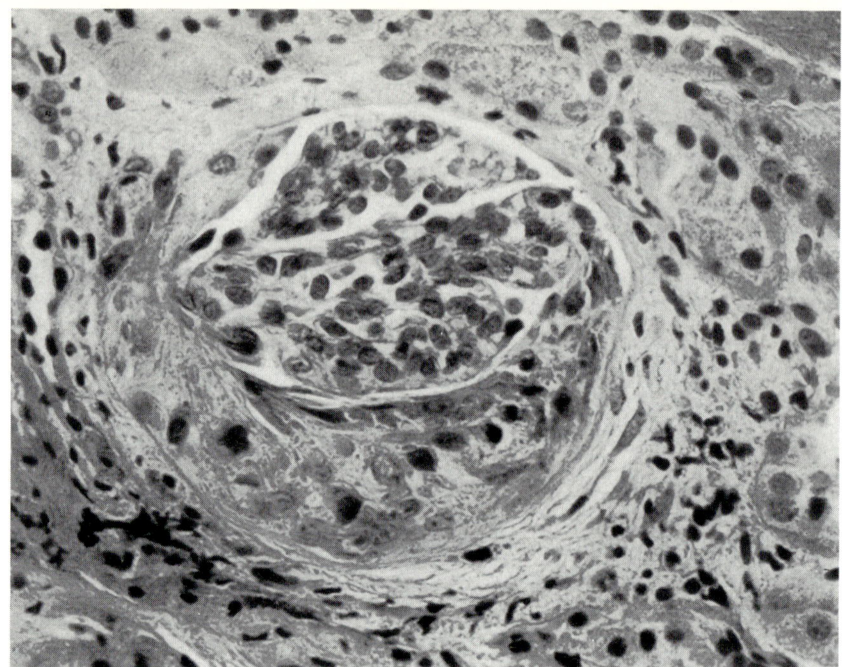

Fig. 34. Crescent in the only diseased glomerulus of six studied in the first biopsy of a patient 30 days after onset of gross hematuria. The hematuria developed 5 days after the onset of acute pharyngitis. At the time of the biopsy the urine contained many erythrocytes but no protein. H&E. (From R. C. Bates, R. B. Jennings, and D. P. Earle, Acute nephritis unrelated to group A hemolytic streptococcus infection: Report of ten cases. *Am. J. Med.* 23:510, 1957.)

degranulation, juxtaglomerular cell   See under HYPERTROPHY.

deposits   See GLOMERULAR DEPOSITS; INTERSTITIAL INFILTRATES.

diffuse glomerular lesion   A lesion involving all or nearly all glomeruli.

diffuse glomerulosclerosis   See SCLEROSIS OF GLOMERULI.

droplets

> **hyaline droplet**   A round, refractile, strongly acidophilic structure, PAS- and silver methenamine–positive, which may very in size from a fraction of a micron to several microns. There are two types: those consisting mainly of protein and those containing lipofuscin (see below).   **lipid droplet**   An accumulation of lipid in a tubular cell as a result of excessive reabsorption of lipid from the tubular fluid or because of an inability of the cell to metabolize normal amounts of lipid. In light microscopic preparations lipid droplets are perceived as vacuoles (in paraffin-embedded tissue) or as sudanophilic droplets (in frozen sections). On electron microscopy they appear either as minute droplets or as larger rounded or irregular bodies surrounded by a single membrane and filled with either black (osmiophilic) or

gray (weakly osmiophilic) material. **lipofuscin granule** A type of hyaline droplet, containing lipofuscin, that is usually the result of cellular damage. Lipofuscin granules are yellowish brown in unstained sections and may be recognized by light microscopy using special stains or by electron microscopy, under which they have the appearance of lysosomes or autophagic vacuoles filled with granular and membranous material (myelin figures). **protein droplet** A type of hyaline droplet, consisting mainly of protein, occurring in proteinurias of various origins. Protein droplets are found mostly in the proximal segments of tubules, sometimes predominantly in the tubular neck at its point of origin from the glomerulus, and represent protein from tubular fluid. There is little quantitative correlation between protein droplets and degree of proteinuria, but there is often some concomitant ischemia (e.g., malignant nephrosclerosis). On electron microscopy protein droplets appear as homogeneous electron-dense structures usually surrounded by a single membrane (**phagosomes** or **phagolysosomes**). **PAS-positive droplet, interstitial** A droplet which stains with periodic–acid Schiff reagent (PAS) and which may appear in interstitial cells in experimental potassium deficiency, in experimental chronic pyelonephritis, and in human xanthogranulomatous pyelonephritis. See also INCLUSIONS.

ectopic glomerulus See GLOMERULUS, ECTOPIC.

edema

    endothelial cell edema Swelling manifested by decreased density of cytoplasm, relative decrease in number of organelles, and decreased density of some organelles (e.g., mitochondria). Endothelial cell edema leads to a loss of pores and the formation of intraluminal blebs (Figs. 30 and 32). **epithelial cell (podocyte) edema** Swelling manifested by pale areas devoid of organelles. The cell organelles, especially of the rough endoplasmic reticulum and Golgi apparatus, may increase, especially when there are basement membrane changes. **interstitial edema** Excess fluid in interstitial tissue resulting in separation of tubules. This may be seen in acute tubular necrosis, acute pyelonephritis, acute glomerulonephritis, preeclampsia, eclampsia, and in the nephrotic syndrome, especially when the latter is associated with renal vein thrombosis. In persistent and long-standing edema, increased numbers of reticulum fibers and collagen may be found in the interstitial space. **tubular edema** (also *cloudy swelling; tubular cloudy swelling; hydropic change*) Severe cellular edema of the renal tubule cells, manifested by dilatation if endoplasmic reticulum, increase in size and number of vacuoles, swelling of mitochondria, decrease in number of ribosomes, and formation of loose cytoplasmic areas devoid of organelles. These changes represent the first stage of acute cellular degeneration or acute cellular injury. Hydropic change due to injury is often difficult to distinguish from that caused by postmortem change, since interruption of blood supply leads to edema within a matter of minutes. See also SWELLING, GLOMERULAR CELL.

endothelial cell edema See under EDEMA.

epithelial cell (podocyte) abnormalities See under EDEMA; INCLUSIONS; FOOT PROCESS LOSS.

extracapillary cell A visceral or a parietal epithelial cell. See under CELLS in Anatomy Glossary.

exudative lesion See HYALINE LESION.

fatty change (also *fatty degeneration*) The accumulation of lipid, usually in the basal portion of the tubular cell. Fatty change is often difficult to distinguish from lipid inclusion (see LIPID DROPLET, under DROPLETS). Fatty change is usually combined with other degenerative changes such as cloudy swelling (see under EDEMA) and vacuolar change. Its presence is taken to mean a severe degree of degeneration.

fibrin cap See HYALINE LESION.

fibrinoid A cellular, finely fibrillar and granular, electron-dense material, seen by light microscopy to be strongly acidophilic. It contains plasma protein, including a large portion of fibrin or fibrinogen or their derivatives.

fibrinoid cap See HYALINE LESION.

fibromuscular hyperplasia of the renal artery See ARTERIES, RENAL, ABNOR-MALITIES OF, in Clinical Glossary.

fibrosis, glomerular See under SCLEROSIS OF GLOMERULI.

foam cells See under INTERSTITIAL INFILTRATES.

focal cytoplasmic degradation (also *autophagy*) A process in which damaged portions of cytoplasm are sequestered within single-membrane-lined vacuoles (**autophagic vacuoles, cytosegresomes**). The sequestered portions are broken down by hydrolytic enzymes into masses of membrane and granular material. The function of the cell is disturbed little, if at all.

focal glomerular lesion A lesion involving some but not all glomeruli (usually less than half the number of glomeruli in a microscopic section).

foot process loss (also *foot process fusion; smudging*) Coalescence of individual epithelial cell foot processes into a continuous layer of cyto-plasm closely apposed to the basement membrane. Loss may be focal or diffuse and may disappear spontaneously or after treatment with steroids. It is often accompanied by formation of villi or pseudovilli (see PSEUDOVILLUS) on the free surfaces of the epithelial cells, and the fused foot processes often contain increased amounts of dense material (foot process material, see Anatomy Glossary). Foot process loss may be associated with proteinuria (see Clinical Glossary) as an isolated finding, accompany proliferative or sclerosing changes, or exist to a small extent in normal individuals (Fig. 35).

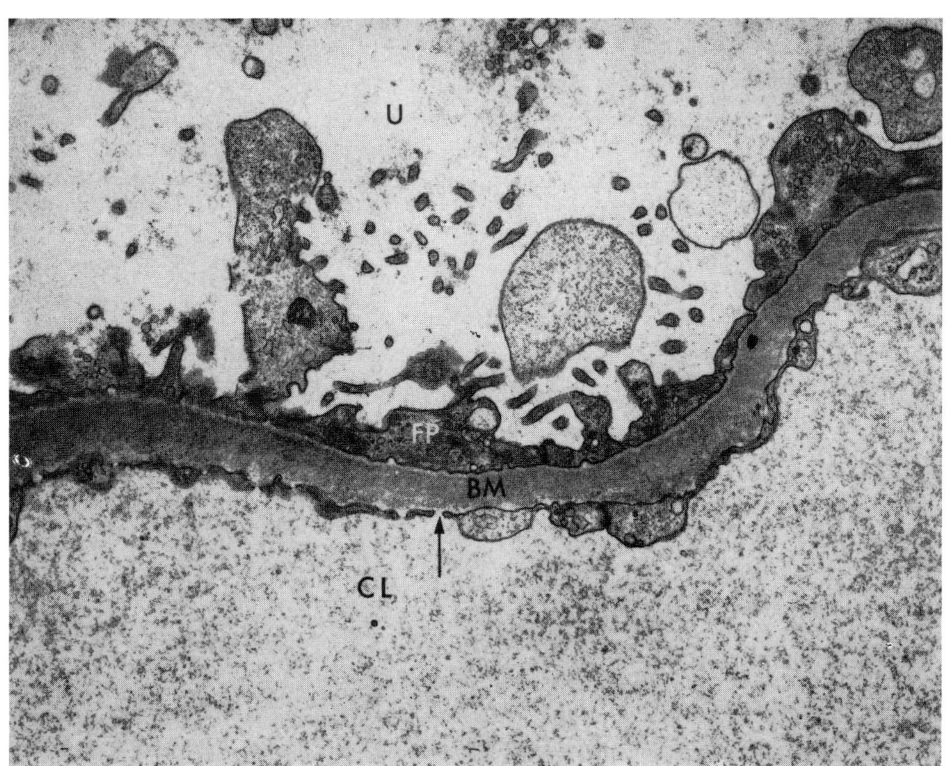

Fig. 35. Extensive fusion of foot processes (*FP*) and development of pseudo-villi projecting into the glomerular capsular space. The basement membrane (*BM*) is slightly irregular but not thickened. The endothelium is unchanged. An endothelial pore (*arrow*) can be seen. From a patient with idiopathic nephrotic syndrome. CL, capillary lumen; U, urinary (glomerular capsular) space. (From J. Churg, Electron Microscopic Aspects of Renal Pathology, in Becker [1].)

glomerular capsular thickening (also *Bowman's capsule thickening*) Thickening, either segmental or covering the entire glomerulus, due to one or more of the following processes: (1) thickening of the outer collagenous layer, (2) thickening and lamination of the basement membrane proper, (3) proliferation of parietal epithelial cells with crescent formation, and (4) accumulation of deposits (Fig. 36) (see CAPSULAR DROP).

glomerular deposits Extracellular accumulation of material not normally present in the glomerulus. (Increase in material normally present, e.g. mesangial matrix, is not a deposit. When mesangial matrix is present between basement membrane and endothelium it is referred to by some as **agryrophilic deposit** or **membranoid material**. See under BASEMENT MEMBRANE ABNORMALITIES.)

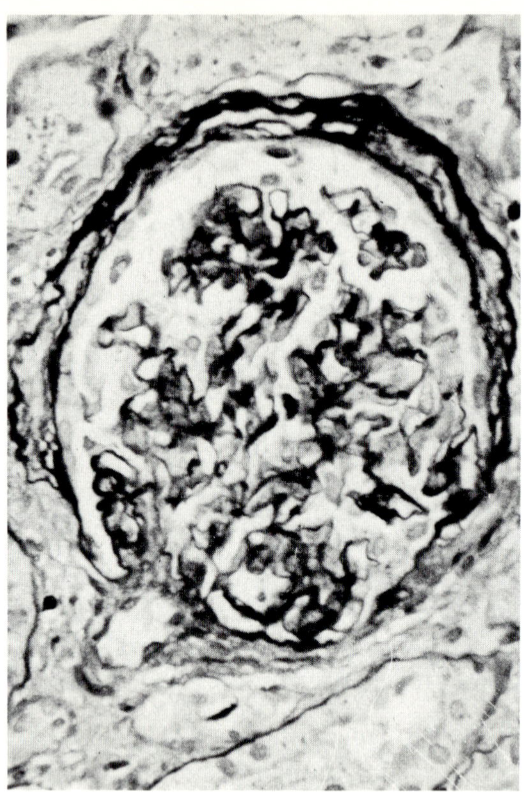

Fig. 36. Marked thickening and splitting of the glomerular (Bowman's) capsule. (Courtesy of J. Churg.)

Nature: The precise composition of most deposits is not known. Usually they are made up of protein, but they may also contain or consist entirely of lipids, DNA, and various metals (such as silver, iron, and calcium). Among the proteins immunoglobulins, complement, and fibrinogen are often found. Some deposits have a specific structure (e.g., amyloid fibrils or fibrin); others can be recognized by their density, staining reactions, or appearance under immunofluorescence. **Fibrinoid deposits** are made up of brightly eosinophilic, smudgy, finely granular or fibrillar material which may contain fibrin and/or other proteins and which stains red rather than blue with the usual trichrome stains. **Hyaline deposits** consist of eosinophilic, homogeneous, glassy material which contains little or no fibrin but may contain lipid.

Localization: Deposits may be found in any part of the glomerulus: the capillary wall, capillary lumen, mesangium, capsule, or capsular space. In the **capillary wall** they may be located in or on either side of the basement membrane. Visualization of deposits in the capillary wall usually requires electron microscopy, but it may be accomplished by using special stains and light microscopy if the deposits are sufficiently large. Some deposits can be visualized by the use of appropriate fluorescinated antibodies and fluorescence microscopy. **Subepithelial deposits** are usually discontinuous and may be separated by attachments of epithelial cells to the basement membrane. They assume various shapes which are referred to as humps, domes, half-domes, flames, and so forth. The epithelial cell foot processes are usually fused over the deposits, and the underlying basement membrane may be indented (Fig. 37). **Subendothelial deposits** form a layer between the basement membrane and the endothelium, occasionally encircling the capillary loop. Their endothelial aspect is often scalloped or irregular. The outer aspect may not be sharply separated from the basement membrane and may extend into it. The density of the deposits varies: it may be greater, similar to, or less than that of the basement membrane. Some deposits may have the appearance of scattered dense granules (Fig. 38). Deposits within the **basement membrane** must differ sugnificantly from the basement membrane to be identified by electron microscopy. They are probably quite common, although usually associated with subepithelial or subendothelial deposits (Fig. 39). Occasionally deposits extend from the endothelium through the entire thickness of the basement membrane to the epithelium (e.g., in amyloidosis). **Mesangial deposits** may appear separately or together with subendothelial and intrabasement membrane deposits and are similar to the latter in structure and density. They may lie within the mesangial matrix or between the matrix and the mesangial cell cytoplasm (Fig. 40).

glomerular lobulation Abnormal prominence of the lobules of the glomerulus, sometimes in association with hyaline deposits. This pattern may occur in a number of disease states, particularly in membranoproliferative and/or hypocomplementemic nephritis and in poststreptococcal glomerulonephritis.

glomerular necrosis See under NECROSIS.

glomerular obsolescence See under SCLEROSIS OF GLOMERULI.

glomerulosclerosis See SCLEROSIS OF GLOMERULI.

glomerulus, ectopic A glomerulus found in the adventitia of the intrarenal vessels and in the peripelvic tissue. It probably represents a nephron that has retained connection with branches of the ureteric bud. Tubules may also be found in the same location.

glycogen in tubular cells (also *Armanni-Ebstein lesion;* Fig. 41) See under INCLUSIONS.

granuloma, granulomata See under INTERSTITIAL INFILTRATES.

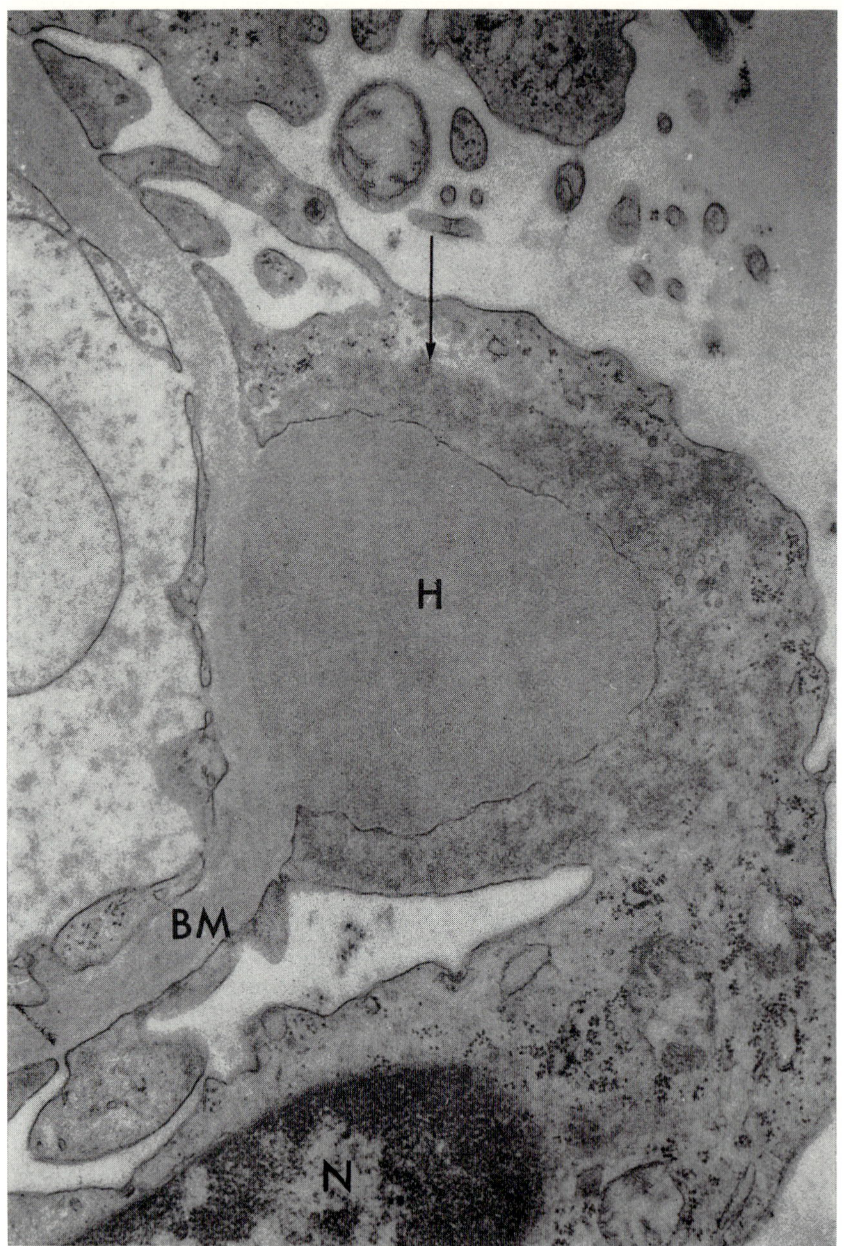

Fig. 37. Biopsy material showing a typical hump (*H*) with a fine granularity, denser than the basement membrane (*BM*). The cytoplasm of the epithelial cell covering the hump contains a zone of greater density (*arrow*). N, epithelial cell nucleus. (From P. B. Herdson, R. B. Jennings and D. P. Earle, Fine structure of post-streptococcal acute glomerulonephritis. *Arch. Path.* 81:117, 1966. © 1966, American Medical Association.)

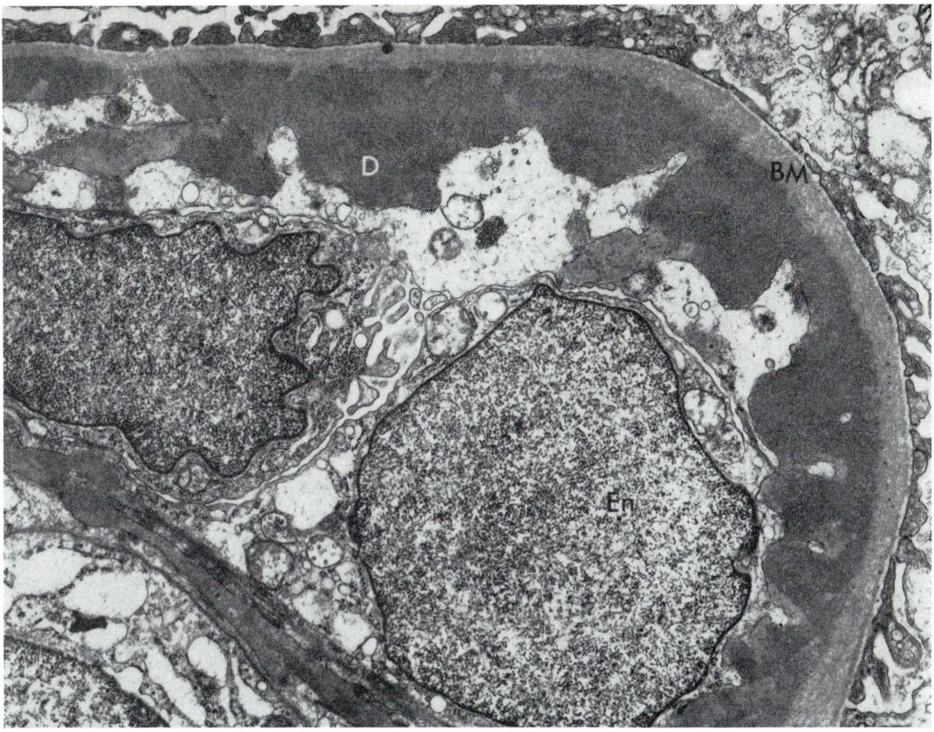

Fig. 38. Lupus nephritis. Part of a glomerular capillary showing dense irregular deposits (*D*) between the basement membrane (*BM*) and the edematous endothelium. This corresponds to the wire loop appearance seen under the light microscopc. (From J. Churg, Electron Microscopic Aspects of Renal Pathology, in Becker [1].)

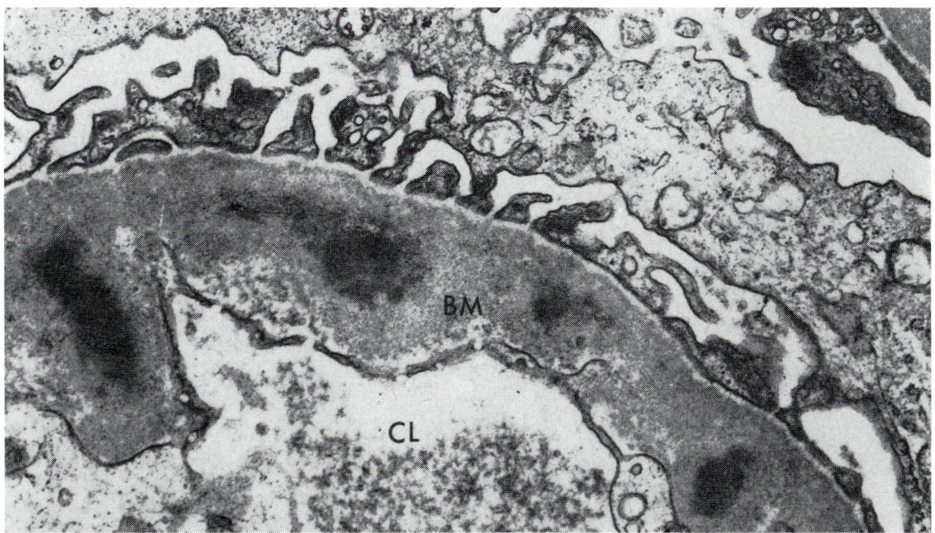

Fig. 39. Dense deposits within a thickened basement membrane (*BM*). From a patient with hepatic (cirrhotic) glomerulosclerosis. *CL*, capillary lumen. (From J. Churg, Electron Microscopic Aspects of Renal Pathology, in Becker [1].)

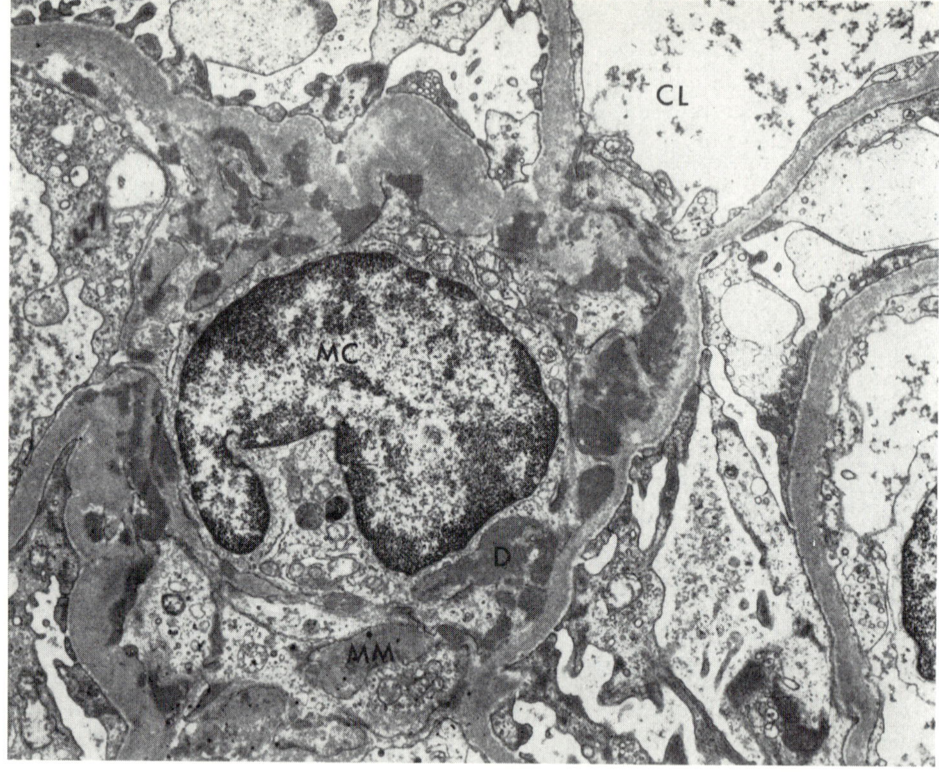

Fig. 40. Lupus nephritis. Mesangial region of a glomerular lobule showing a single cell surrounded by matrix and by electron-dense deposits. *CL*, capillary lumen; *D*, deposits; *MC*, mesangial cell; *MM*, mesangial matrix. (From J. Churg, Electron Microscopic Aspects of Renal Pathology, in Becker [1].)

hemorrhage, glomerular The presence of blood in the glomerular capsular space.

hemorrhage in the interstitium See INTERSTITIAL INFILTRATES.

hyalin Acellular material, glassy and homogeneous (under light microscopy) or very finely granular (under electron microscopy), containing proteins (such as plasma proteins), mucopolysaccharides, and a variety of lipids. Hyaline stains intensely with eosin and periodic acid–Schiff's reagent (PAS), stains red with trichrome stains, and does not stain with periodic acid–silver methenamine (PASM).

hyaline droplet See under DROPLETS.

hyaline lesion (also *exudative lesion, insudative lesion*) Accumulation of hyalin in any of several locations in the glomerulus: (1) in the lumen of one or more capillary loops, often in the periphery of the tuft. It may fill the lumen or form a crescent-shaped subendothelial deposit (Fig. 42). (Obsolete terms: *fibrin cap, fibrinoid cap*); (2) in the glo-

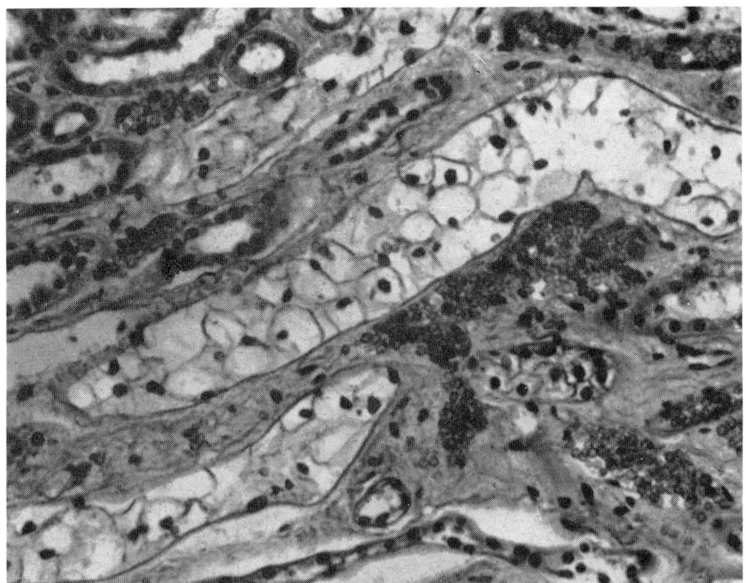

Fig. 41. Armanni-Ebstein cells in a straight portion of a proximal convoluted tubule. The cytoplasm appears empty; the cytoplasmic membrane sharp and stiff. H&E. (From P. Kimmelstiel, Diabetic Nephropathy, in Becker [1].)

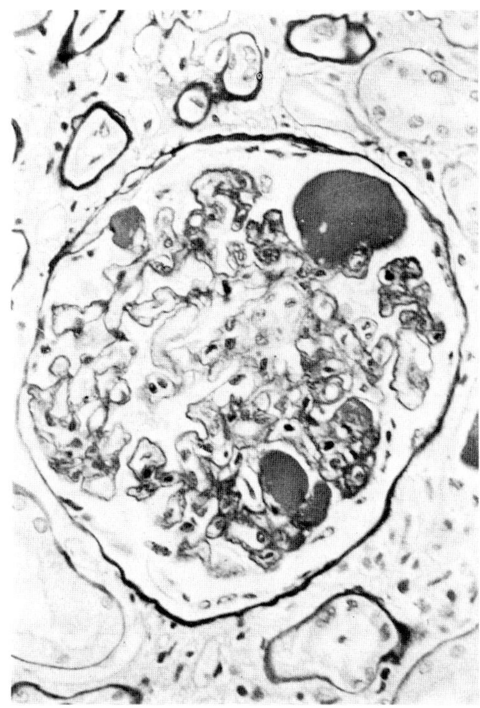

Fig. 42. Hyaline (exudative, insudative) glomerular lesions. Dark-staining nodules along the periphery of the glomerulus represent an accumulation of hyaline material in the capillary lumina. (Courtesy of J. Churg.)

merular (Bowman's) capsule (*capsular drop*); (3) lying free in the glomerular capsular space. See also GLOMERULAR DEPOSITS.

hyaline thrombus   See under THROMBOSIS.

hyalinized glomerulus   See SCLEROSIS OF GLOMERULI.

hydropic change   See under EDEMA.

hypercellularity (*hyperplasia*)   Abnormal increase in the number of cells normally constituting an organ or body tissue.

    extracapillary hypercellularity   Proliferation of visceral and/or parietal epithelial cells.

    glomerular hypercellularity   Proliferation of mesangial, endothelial, or epithelial cells, commonly seen in glomerulonephritis. It may affect a segment or the whole glomerulus and may be focal or diffuse. The number of cells observed in the glomerulus is dependent on the thickness of the section examined. In the glomerular tuft an appearance of hypercellularity may be given by accumulation of polymorphonuclear leukocytes (Fig. 43). See also LEUKOCYTE ACCUMULATION.

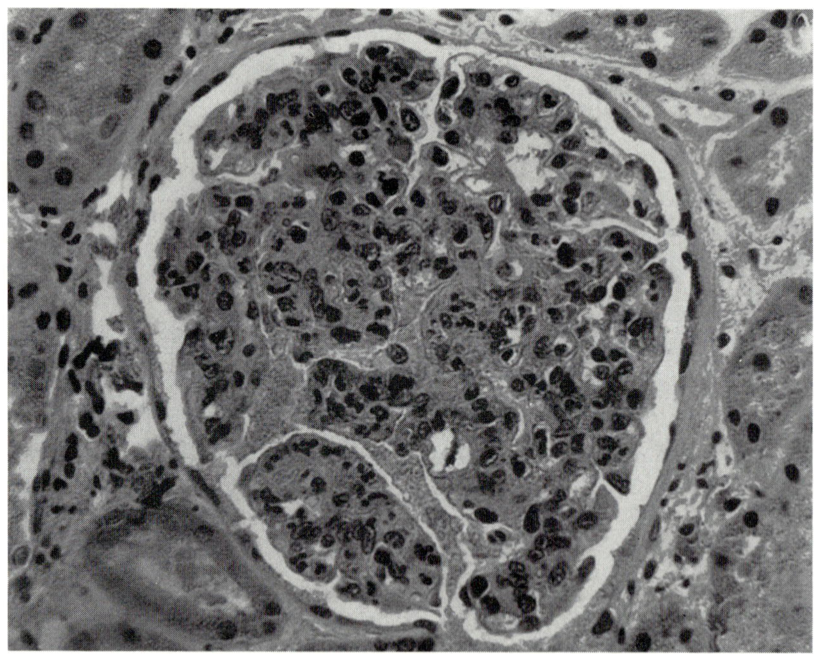

Fig. 43.   Glomerulus obtained at the first biopsy of a patient 13 days after the onset of acute glomerulonephritis. Hypercellularity is due to the presence of more than 40 polymorphonuclear neutrophils per 2-μ section plus proliferation of endothelial cells. At the time of biopsy, urine contained 3+ protein and 10 to 14 erythrocytes; BUN was 30 mg per 100 ml, and blood pressure 140/90 mm Hg. H&E. (From R. B. Jennings and D. P. Earle, Acute Glomerulonephritis, in Becker [1].)

intracapillary or endocapillary hypercellularity Proliferation of mesangial and/or endothelial cells. (It is often difficult to distinguish between the two kinds of cells on light microscopy.)

tubular hypercellularity Proliferation of tubular cells which may be seen around casts, seen particularly in multiple myeloma. The proliferated cells often fuse to form multinucleated giant cells. Excessive proliferation may also occur during cell regeneration.

hypergranulation, juxtaglomerular cell Abnormally large numbers of granules in the juxtaglomerular cell. This condition reflects both renin hypersecretion and renin storage and may be accompanied by hypertrophy and hyperplasia. These changes are associated with large distorted nuclei. Intranuclear invaginations of cytoplasm may simulate inclusions.

tubular cell inclusions Most commonly proteins, lipids, carbohydrates, colloids, and metals may accumulate in the cytoplasm of tubular cells. These substances are either finely dispersed in the cytoplasm or, more often, aggregated within single-membrane-lined vesicles called secondary **lysosomes** or **phagosomes** (digestive vacuoles). The material usually enters the cell from the tubular lumen either by diffusion or via pinocytotic vacuoles but sometimes is derived from the bloodstream through the peritubular capillaries; some of it may also represent breakdown products of the cell's own cytoplasm. Most **carbohydrates** of medium molecular weight (dextran) or of low weight (sucrose, mannitol, glucose, etc.), when absorbed in large amounts, probably accumulate in tubular cells and lead to the formation of vacuoles. This occurs primarily in cells of the proximal convoluted segments of tubules. With the exception of dextran it has not been possible to demonstrate these substances in the vacuoles because of their solubility. Accumulation of **glycogen** (*Armanni-Ebstein lesion*) in the straight portions of the proximal segments of renal tubules produces coarse, poorly defined vacuoles which are seen by light microscopy in specimens stained with hematoxylin and eosin. Glycogen is best seen following fixation with 100% alcohol but is partly preserved with other fixatives and can be demonstrated with the PAS process. On electron microscopy, glycogen appears as an accumulation of dark granules each measuring 200 to 400 Å in diameter. The Armanni-Ebstein lesion occurs in patients with increased renal venous blood renin levels, and often with hypertension, secondary aldosteronism, or both.

hyperplasia   See HYPERCELLULARITY.

hypertrophy

glomerular cell hypertrophy Enlargement of epithelial, endothelial, or mesangial cells of the glomerulus associated with either edema or inclusions. See also under EDEMA.

juxtaglomerular cell hypertrophy Enlargement of the juxtaglomerular cells, associated with a reduction in arterial blood flow and sometimes accompanied by **degranulation.** Degranulation may indicate excessive renin secretion without comparable storage.

nephron hypertrophy Enlargement of the glomerular tuft, proximal tubules, and lining (with normal components), as seen among the residual functioning nephrons in chronic renal disease, or, in compensatory hypertrophy following contralateral nephrectomy, hypertrophy of the whole nephron.

hypoplasia, renal See Clinical Glossary.

inclusions Intracellular accumulation of abnormal substances.

epithelial cell inclusions Large and small vacuoles, lipid and protein inclusions, and hyaline droplets, often present in epithelial cells.

intranuclear cell inclusions Inclusions in the nucleus of tubular cells which may be of viral origin (cytomegalic inclusion disease, see Clinical Glossary), be due to heavy metals (lead, bismuth), or arise from other causes. They are acidophilic, distinct from the nucleolus, and, in the case of heavy metals, acid fast. Cells bearing inclusions may become large and atypical poorly controlled diabetes (Fig. 41). **Iron** in the form of hemosiderin or ferritin accumulates in the tubular cells as tiny particles or larger intravacuolar aggregates which tend to persist. It sometimes appears as a result of breakdown of absorbed hemoglobin. Some of the accumulated material may be discharged back into the tubular lumen. Cells containing large amounts of iron tend to atrophy (Fig. 44).

infarct, kidney surface Necrotic area caused by occlusion of arcuate or larger arteries. A kidney surface infarct is pyramidal with its base at the cortex. In the early stages it is slightly elevated, sharply demarcated, and red or gray-red in color. After several days it beomes gray-yellow, pale, slightly depressed, and poorly demarcated, with a surrounding narrow red zone. Old scars are shrunken, V-shaped, and markedly depressed.

ingrowth See MEMBRANOPROLIFERATIVE LESION.

insudative lesion See HYALINE LESION.

interposition See MEMBRANOPROLIFERATIVE LESION.

interstitial cell edema See under EDEMA.

interstitial infiltrates Substances penetrating the interstitium may include deposits, cells of certain types, or material associated with fibrosis. The pattern and distribution of interstitial tissue infiltrates in response to disease or stimuli varies with the nature of the underlying cause and may be useful in determining that cause.

amyloid deposits in the interstitial tissue are seen predominantly in the medulla (Figs. 45 and 46). The term **para-amyloid** is used by some to designate an acidophilic material similar to amyloid by light microscopy but without its characteristic staining reactions. It may be seen in

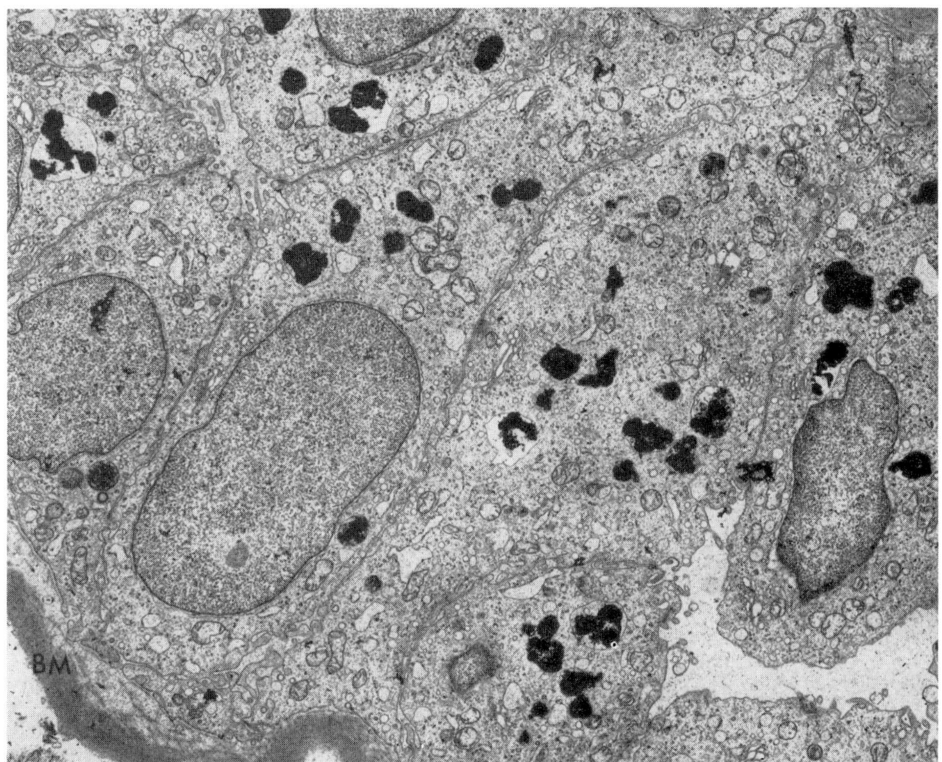

Fig. 44 Dense iron inclusions in the tubular cells of a rabbit with iron ne-
phropathy. Most of the deposits are found in single-membrane-lined vacuoles.
(From J. Churg, Electron Microscopic Aspects of Renal Pathology, in
Becker [1].)

older individuals and in papillary necrosis. **Calcium** may be deposited
in the tubular basement membrane and extend into the peritubular
interstitial tissue, may be deposited directly in interstitial foam cells,
or may be extruded into the interstitium from destroyed tubules. It is
often associated with fibrosis and cellular infiltrates. **Cholesterol
granulomata** are clusters of nucleated giant cells with cholesterol clefts.
Crystals may be found in the interstitial tissue following destruction
of tubules, which are their primary site of deposition (see CRYSTAL
FORMATION). Crystals formed from uric acid or urates, with a cellular
reaction and giant cells are most frequently encountered. **Eosinophils**
may predominate in allergic angiitis and drug sensitivity and in other
interstitial reactions of unknown cause. There may be proliferation of
fibroblasts and formation of **collagen fibers** in long-standing diseases
such as glomerulonephritis, pyelonephritis, potassium deficiency, nephrosclerosis, analgesic abuse, and endemic Balkan nephropathy, and

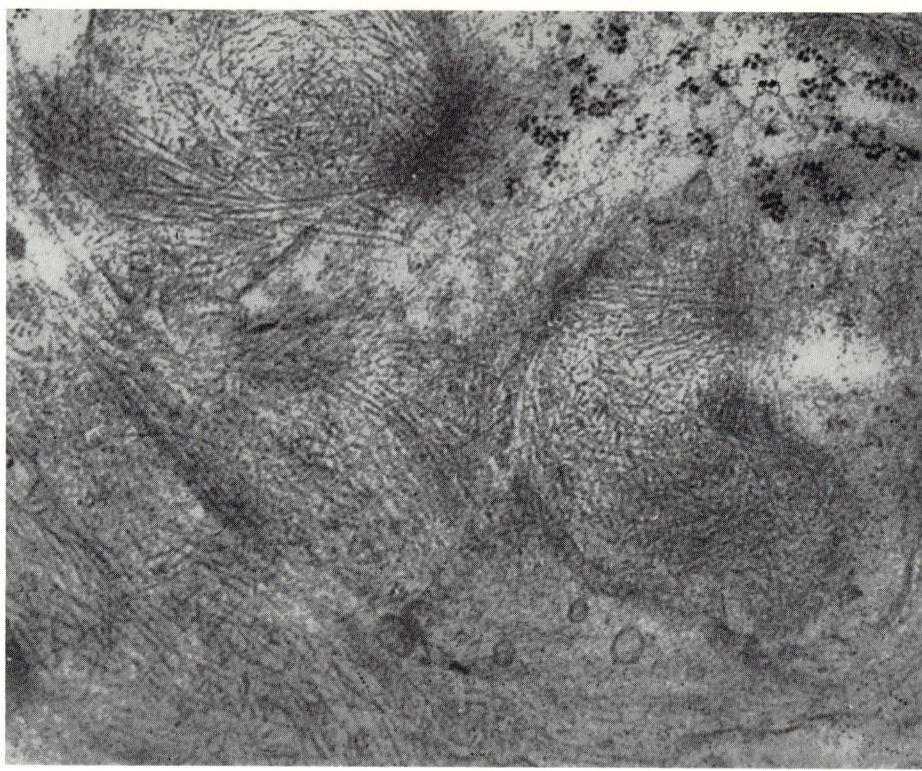

Fig. 45.   Amyloidosis. Part of a glomerulus showing replacement of mesangial matrix by amyloid fibers. (From J. Churg, Electron Microscopic Aspects of Renal Pathology, in Becker [1].)

also in interstitial cell edema. **Foam cells** are large, finely vacuolated macrophages which contain neutral fat, mucopolysaccharides, phospholipids, and cholesterol and may be derived from circulating mononuclear cells, tubular cells, interstitial cells, or lymphatic endothelial cells. They may be seen in the nephrotic syndrome, hereditary nephritis, chronic glomerulonephritis, chronic pyelonephritis, and, in association with giant cells, in xanthogranulomatous pyelonephritis (Fig. 47). **Hemorrhage** may occur as infiltration of large numbers of red cells at the edge of infarcts, in hemorrhagic fever, in acute transplantation rejection, and in other conditions. Hemosiderin-laden macrophages may appear after hemorrhage. **Mixed infiltrates** (lymphocytes, neutrophils, plasma cells, and macrophages) appear in most chronic renal diseases. Polymorphonuclear cell infiltration is observed in acute processes (acute pyelonephritis, acute glomerulonephritis, and necrotizing angiitis) and also in chronic pyelonephritis. **Para-amyloid deposits** See under INTERSTITIAL DEPOSITS. **Tuberculoid granulomata**

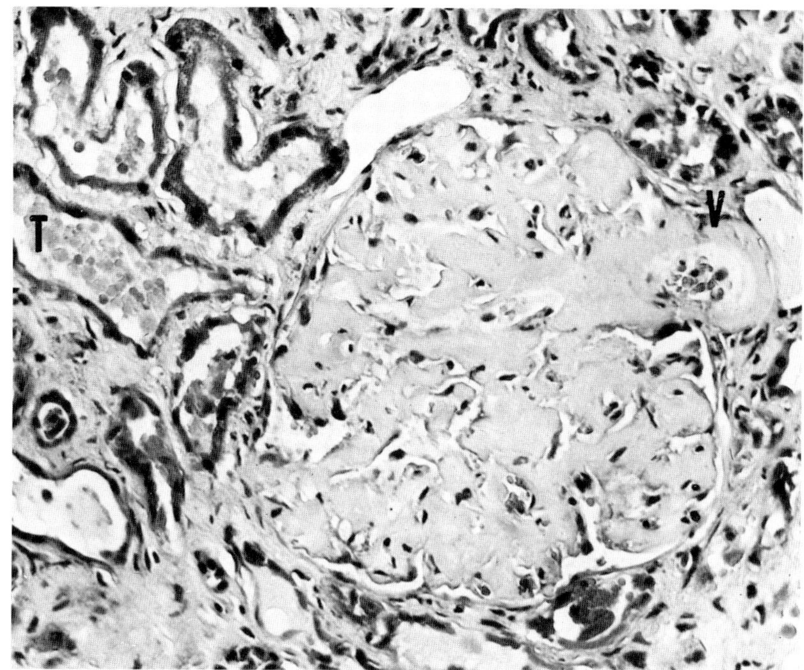

Fig. 46. Amyloid deposits in the glomerular capillary walls from the vascular pole (V) to the periphery of the glomerulus. Protein casts and low, regenerating epithelium can be seen in the proximal tubules (T). (From A. F. Bergstrand and H. Bucht, Renal Amyloidosis, in Becker [1].)

in the form of giant cell and epitheloid granulomata are most often found in tuberculosis and sarcoidosis and occasionally in specific infections such as schistosomiasis.

intracapillary cell   A mesangial or an endothelial cell.

intranuclear cell inclusions   See under INCLUSIONS.

iron in tubular cells   See under INCLUSIONS.

juxtaglomerular cell atrophy   See under ATROPHY.

juxtaglomerular cell hypertrophy   See under HYPERTROPHY.

karyorrhexis   Fragmentation of the cell nucleus, seen in necrotizing glomerular lesions (particularly lupus nephritis).

kidney atrophy   See KIDNEY, CONTRACTED in Clinical Glossary.

lesions   See the following entries:

    Armanni-Ebstein lesion   See under INCLUSIONS. **calyceal lesions**   See PELVIC AND CALYCEAL LESIONS. **diffuse glomerular lesion** or **exudative**

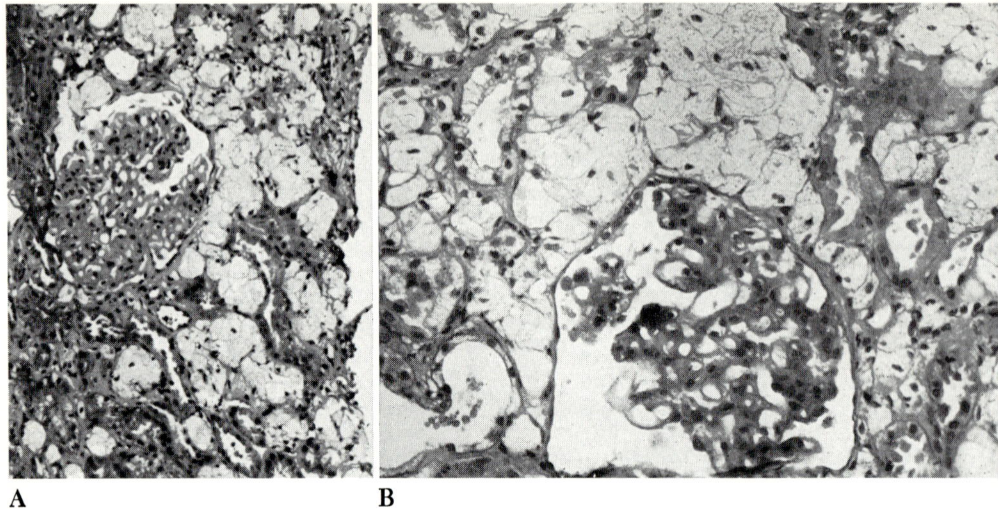

Fig. 47. Severe membranous glomerulonephritis in a 14-year-old girl. Two years prior to initial biopsy she developed edema and proteinuria, accompanied by a mild hypertension, hematuria, and decreased urea clearance. Two full courses of daily steroid therapy, followed by intermittent steroid therapy, achieved very little improvement. At the time of biopsy, she had no edema and only mild hypertension but had proteinuria (up to 10 gm per day), hypercholesterolemia, hypoproteinemia, and moderately reduced urea clearance. A. In addition to severe glomerulonephritis, there was marked diffuse accumulation of foam cells; the material, presumably lipid, appeared to occupy a large percentage of the renal cortex, producing a more extensive deposition of foam cells than has been seen in any case of hereditary glomerulonephritis; no family history of renal disease could be elicited. B. Foam cells in more detail, and marked thickening of the capillary basement membranes. H&E. (From H. G. Worthen, Renal Disease in Children and Hereditary Renal Diseases, in Becker [1].)

lesion See HYALINE LESION. **focal glomerular lesion** or **hyaline lesion** or **insudative lesion** See HYALINE LESION. **local glomerular lesion** See SEGMENTAL GLOMERULAR LESION. **membranoproliferative lesion** or **mesangiocapillary lesion** See MEMBRANOPROLIFERATIVE LESION. **pelvic and calyceal lesions** or **segmental glomerular lesion** or **swan-neck tubular lesion.**

leukocyte accumulation

glomerular leukocyte accumulation Excessive number of neutrophils and of a few eosinophils in the glomerular capillaries and to a lesser extent in the mesangium and in the glomerular capsular space. Lymphocytes and plasma cells are rarely, if ever, seen. Monocytes, if present, are difficult to distinguish from pathologically altered endothelial and mesangial cells. Leukocyte accumulation may be accompanied by exudation of plasma proteins into the urinary space. **tubular leukocyte accumulation** Leukocytes found between the lining cells of degenerated, necrotic, or atrophic tubules. Polymorphonuclear leukocytes may be present in large numbers in the tubular lumina and may form leukocytic casts, as in acute pyelonephritis of either the ascending or the descending variety.

lipid droplet See under DROPLETS.

lipofuscin granule See under DROPLETS.

lipomatosis, medullary See MEDULLARY LIPOMATOSIS.

lobulation, glomerular See GLOMERULAR LOBULATION.

local glomerular lesion See SEGMENTAL GLOMERULAR LESION.

lymphatic capillary dilatation Swelling of the lymphatic capillary, usually associated with interstitial edema. It may be seen in acute glomerulonephritis, acute renal failure, acute pyelonephritis, hydronephrosis, renal vein thrombosis, and transplantation rejection. The dilatation is then compensatory and is secondary to the edema and consequently to the increased lymph flow.

medullary lipomatosis Partial replacement of renal tissue by proliferating hilar fat.

membranoid material See under SCLEROSIS OF GLOMERULI, GLOMERULAR DEPOSITS; BASEMENT MEMBRANE ABNORMALITIES; and also MESANGIAL MATRIX in Anatomy Glossary.

membranoproliferative lesion (also *mesangiocapillary lesion*) Proliferation of mesangium in the glomerular capillary wall between endothelium and basement membrane (also called *ingrowth* or *interposition*) (Fig. 30).

membranous transformation The presence of slender, elongated, irregular projections (**spikes**) of basement membrane-like material on the external surface of the basement membrane. They are usually separated by subepithelial or sometimes intermembranous deposits but may occur without them (Figs. 29 and 68 [p. 183]).

mesangiocapillary lesion See MEMBRANOPROLIFERATIVE LESION.

mesangiolysis Dissolution or attenuation of mesangial matrix and degeneration of mesangial cells, caused by Habu snake poisoning, radiation, and some other conditions.

microangiopathy, thrombotic Alteration of small blood vessels, such as capillaries and arterioles, by deposition of fibrinogen or its derivatives in the vascular wall, aneurysmal dilatation, and thrombosis of the lumen. It often affects the kidneys, occurring in association with thrombotic thrombocytopenic purpura, hemolytic uremic syndrome, and malignant hypertension, and occasionally with systemic lupus erythematosus and preeclampsia or eclampsia.

microvillus See PSEUDOVILLUS.

necrosis Irreversible change leading to death of the affected cell or tissue.
glomerular necrosis Necrosis of the whole or a part of the glomerular tuft, indicated most clearly by nuclear fragmentation (*karyorrhexis*) and presence of debris. Total necrosis or infarction of the glomerulus follows occlusion of the blood vessels supplying the glomerulus and is often accompanied by hemorrhage into the glomerular capsular (Bowman's) space. **Segmental necrosis** is often caused by localized thrombosis and is manifested by structureless, intensely eosinophilic areas. **tubular necrosis** Tubular cells undergoing degeneration or death show severe changes in the mitochondria (swelling, pyknosis, distortion), coalescing areas of opacification and condensation of cytoplasm (**coagulation necrosis**), and nuclear pyknosis, karyolysis, or karyorrhexis. The cells may shed their apical portion, including the brush border (**potocytosis**), or may desquamate in toto, leaving denuled areas of basement membrane. With widespread desquamation the tubules tend to collapse. The denuded basement membrane is often thickened. In focal tubular necrosis complicating acute renal insufficiency, the denuded basement membrane may fragment (**tubulorrhexis**).

nodular glomerulosclerosis See SCLEROSIS OF GLOMERULI.

obsolete glomerulus See SCLEROSIS OF GLOMERULI.

particle, virus-like See VIRUS-LIKE PARTICLE.

PAS Periodic acid–Schiff reagent stain.

PAS-positive droplet, interstitial See under DROPLETS.

PASM periodic acid–silver methenamine stain.

pelvic and calyceal lesions

Lesions involving *changes in configuration:* **Constriction** is usually the result of tumor, inflammation, fibrous scarring, or tuberculosis. **Dilatation** is the principal feature in hydronephrosis. In extrarenal hydronephrosis (in which the pelvis is mainly located extrarenally) the pelvis alone may become dilated and the calyces remain unaffected. In intrarenal hydronephrosis both pelvis and calyces are affected.

Lesions involving *changes in the mucosa:* Congestions, small hemorrhages, and acute inflammation may be present in acute or chronic pyelonephritis. Ulcerations are seen in tuberculosis, fungus infections, and malakoplakia.

phagosome, phagolysosome See under DROPLETS.

podocyte abnormalities See under EDEMA; INCLUSIONS; FOOT PROCESS LOSS.

potocytosis See under NECROSIS.

primitive glomerulus See GLOMERULUS, PRIMITIVE, in Anatomy Glossary.

protein droplet See under DROPLETS.

pseudotubule A segment of the glomerular capsular (Bowman's) space that forms between adhesions and is lined by hypertrophied epithelial cells derived from the glomerular capsule.

pseudovillus   A slender cell projection arising from the surface of the glomerular epithelium that faces the glomerular capsular space. Pseudovilli are seen particularly in heavy proteinuria and the nephrotic syndrome. Some may represent true microvilli whereas others are probably segments of thin cytoplasmic bridges (Fig. 35).

pyuria   Occurrence of excessive numbers of leukocytes in the urine.

regeneration, tubular cell   Renewal following desquamation of damaged tubular lining cells. Regeneration is first manifested by the appearance of very flat cells with basophilic cytoplasm rich in ribosomes and vesicles. The new cells become successively cuboidal and columnar and differentiate with development of mitochondria, endoplasmic reticulum, small microvilli, and basal infoldings of the plasma membrane. Regeneration of cells in a damaged tubule is rapid (days or weeks), but differentiation to mature cells is slow (months).

renal atrophy   See KIDNEY, CONTRACTED in Clinical Glossary.

sclerosis of glomeruli   Replacement of all or part of a glomerulus by fibrillar scleroproteins such as mesangial matrix, basement membrane or basement membrane-like material, and collagen. It may be considered a glomerular equivalent of scarring. Other terms frequently used for this process are less desirable: **Glomerular hyalinization** refers to a process that does occur with sclerosis but is an inconstant and minor constitutent. **Glomerular obsolescence** is a functional rather than a morphologic term. **Glomerular fibrosis** refers to possible further augmentation of sclerosis by fibrous crescents or by fibrous tissue derived from the glomerular capsule and apparently also from mesangial matrix.

Sclerosis may arise from several causes. Sclerosis due to **increase of mesangial matrix** is at first predominantly confined to the mesangium, causing widening of the stalk (**diffuse glomerulosclerosis**) and of the centers of peripheral lobules (**nodular glomerulosclerosis**) (Fig. 48). It may follow inflammation of cellular proliferation as in glomerulonephritis, or it may occur with little cell proliferation as in diabetes, hypertensive sclerosis, and other systemic diseases such as certain forms of idiopathic nephrotic syndrome and hapatic glomerulosclerosis. Progression leads to obliteration of capillaries and eventually conversion of the glomerulus into homogeneous acellular structure. Sclerosed glomeruli sometimes undergo resorption. Sclerosis due to **capillary collapse** leads to replacement of a whole or part of the glomerulus by wrinkled, sometimes thickened, basement membrane (Fig. 49). Sclerosis due to **glomerular fibrosis** is seldom pure. Small amounts of collagen are often found in mesangial sclerosis on electron microscopy,

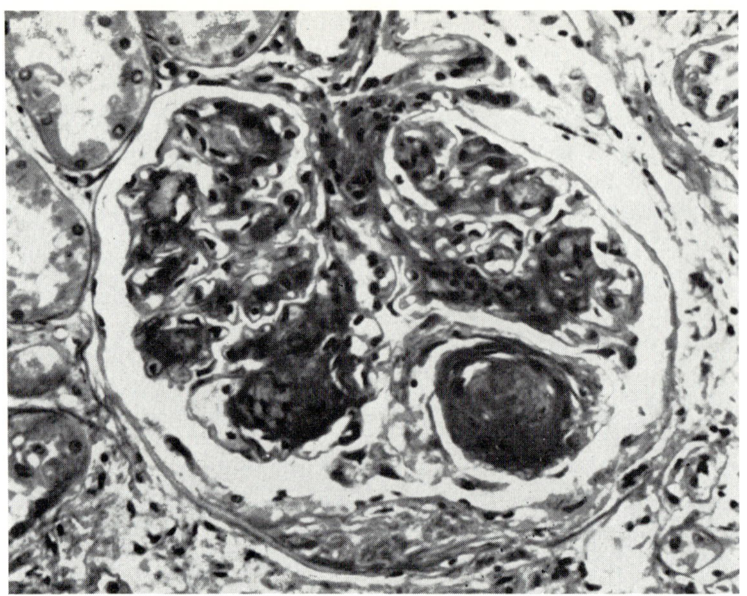

Fig. 48. Nodular and diffuse intercapillary glomerulosclerosis. (From P. Kimmelstiel, Diabetic Nephropathy, in Becker [1].)

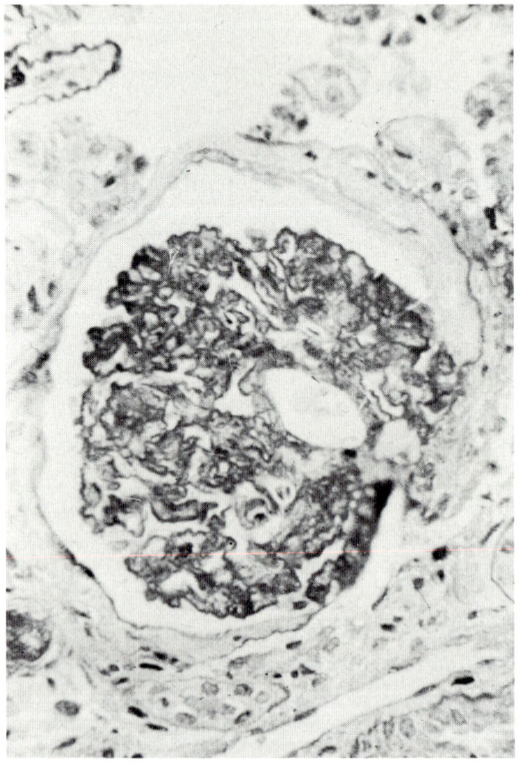

Fig. 49. Capillary collapse. A contracted glomerulus showing collapse and wrinkling of the capillary basement membrane and loss of capillary lumina. (Courtesy of J. Churg.)

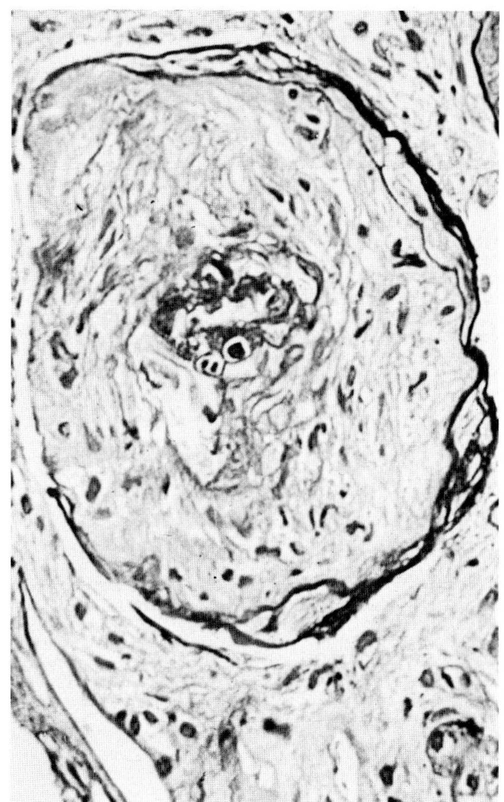

Fig. 50. Glomerular sclerosis due to formation of a fibrous crescent. The crescent fills almost the entire glomerular capsular (Bowman's) space. A few collapsed capillaries (dark staining) are seen in the center. (Courtesy of J. Churg.)

but extensive collagen replacement recognizable by light microscopy is unusual. Collagen is more commonly found in fibrous crescents and in the inner layer of thickened Bowman's capsule and may be seen in scars following segmental necrosis of the tuft (Fig. 50).

segmental glomerular lesion   A lesion involving a portion of a glomerulus; term preferred to *local glomerular lesion* (Figs. 51 and 52).

smudging   See FOOT PROCESS LOSS.

spikes   see BASEMENT MEMBRANE ABNORMALITIES; MEMBRANOUS TRANSFORMATION.

splitting of basement membrane   See BASEMENT MEMBRANE ABNORMALITIES.

storage   See INCLUSIONS.

swan-neck tubular lesion   Deformity of the proximal convoluted segment

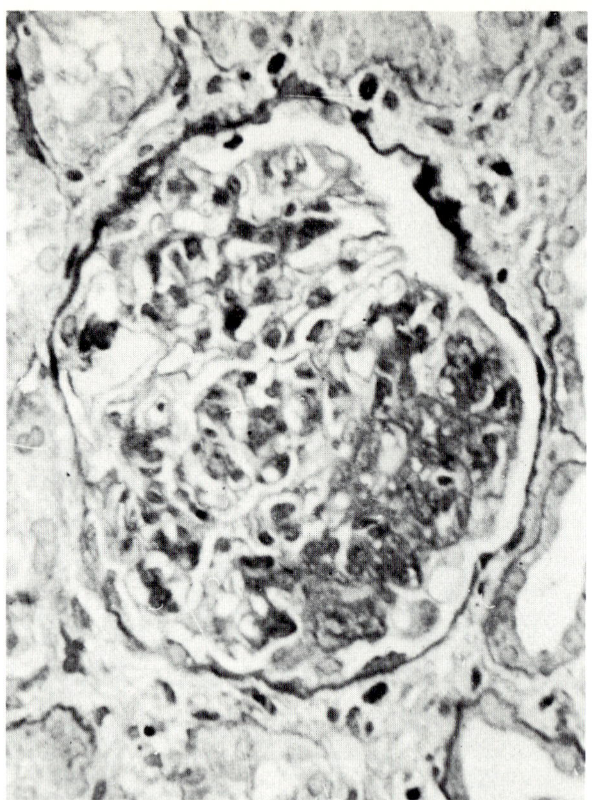

Fig. 51. Segmental glomerular sclerosis. About one-third of the glomerulus appears nearly solid with loss of capillary lumina. (Courtesy of J. Churg.)

of the renal tubule due to marked thinning with shortening of the first part of the segment. It is best demonstrated by microdissection but may also be observed histologically.

swelling, glomerular cell An abnormal increase in cell volume with or without hypercellularity. Generally there is swelling of mesangial and endothelial cells together (e.g., preeclampsia or eclampsia). Swelling of visceral epithelial cells is often seen in proteinuria. See also EDEMA.

swelling, tubular cloudy See under EDEMA.

thickening See GLOMERULAR CAPSULAR THICKENING; CAPILLARY WALL THICKENING, GLOMERULAR; and under BASEMENT MEMBRANE ABNORMALITIES.

thrombosis Clotting of blood in a vascular lumen with precipitation of fibrin, often with agglutinated platelets, erythrocytes, and leukocytes. Fibrin thrombi may be difficult to distinguish from thrombotic emboli; both are intensely eosinophilic and also finely fibrillar. The term

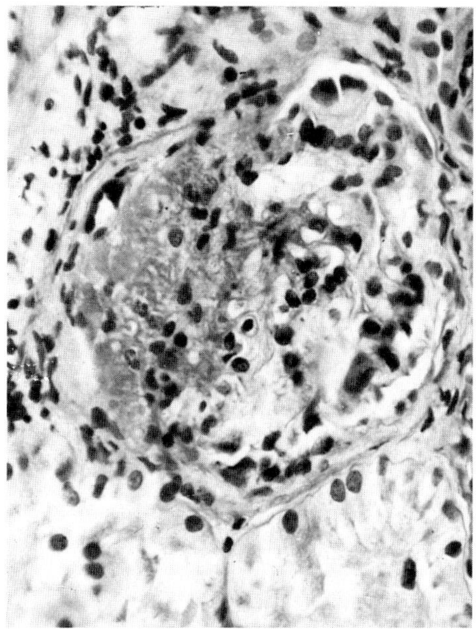

Fig. 52.   Sclerosis of part of a glomerulus in the second biopsy of a patient 35 months after the onset of the nephrotic syndrome. The first biopsy had shown focal proliferative lesions. PAS. (From D. B. Brewer, *Renal Biopsy*. London: Edward Arnold Ltd., 1965.)

hyaline thrombi is often used to denote large subendothelial and intraluminar deposits of hyaline material. Thrombi must be distinguished from conglutinated erythrocytes and cellular debris.

thrombotic microangiopathy   See MICROANGIOPATHY, THROMBOTIC.

thrombus, hyaline   See under THROMBOSIS.

tuberculoid granuloma   See under INTERSTITIAL INFILTRATES.

tubular atrophy   See under ATROPHY.

tubular cell calcification   See CALCIFICATION, RENAL.

tubular cell edema   See under EDEMA.

tubular cell regeneration   See REGENERATION, TUBULAR CELL.

tubular necrosis   See under NECROSIS.

tubulorrhexis   A necrosis of tubular cells accompanied by fragmentation of the supporting basement membrane.

tumors

extrarenal malignant and invasive tumors

Adrenal tumors occasionally invade the upper pole by direct extension. Neuroblastomas in infants and children most commonly exhibit this type of involvement. **Hepatomas** occasionally invade the right kidney. **Sarcomas** from the **retroperitoneal space** may extend through the renal capsule into renal tissue. **Carcinomas of the pancreas**

seldom invade the kidney. **Gastric carcinomas** not infrequently metastasize to the kidney but seldom involve it by direct extension.

metastatic tumors

Carcinomatous tumors commonly metastasize to the kidney but rarely present diagnostic problems or cause clinical insufficiency. The most common primary sites are the lung and breast. Malignant melanoma frequently metastasizes to the kidney. Renal metastases are usually multiple. With the exception of lymphosarcoma, which may form sizable nodules within the kidney, renal involvement by metastatic **sarcoma** is uncommon. Metastasis to the contralateral kidney from **renal cell carcinoma** sometimes occur.

renal and benign tumors

Adenoma is the most common benign renal tumor. It is usually small and seldom gives rise to clinical symptoms. The tumor takes the form of a yellow nodule, usually composed of small uniform basophilic columnar cells, and is often multiple and most often in a subcapsular location. A **capillary hemangioma** is composed of capillary-sized, thin-walled blood vessels lined by endothelium and containing red cells. Capillary hemangiomas tend to remain small and are therefore difficult to diagnose when they cause hematuria. A **cavernous hemangioma** is a collection of dilated vascular spaces containing red cells and lined by endothelium. It may arise in any part of the kidney and may be single or multiple. **Fibromas** are small, circumscribed, spherical, firm, gray nodules, most often seen in the medulla, in which case they are presumed to arise from interstitial connective tissues. The benign fibroblastic tissue may be myxomatous and contain entrapped renal tubules. Superficial cortical fibromas arise from the connective tissue of the renal capsule and less commonly contain renal tubules. **Infantile mesenchymal hamartomas** are bulky, circumscribed, but nonencapsulated renal tumefactions characteristically presenting in infants. Microscopically the lesions consist of whorled masses of spindle-shaped cells with scant intracellular material variously characterized as smooth muscle cells, fibroblasts, or simply mesenchymal cells. The lesions do not metastasize. **Leiomyomas** may arise from muscle fibers in the capsule or media of blood vessels. Usually small and subcapsular, they form tan-white rounded nodules with compression of surrounding tissues. Microscopically they are composed of interlacing bundles of well-differentiated smooth muscle cells containing myofibrils and elongated, plump, blunt-ended nuclei. **Lipomas** are small single tumors of the renal cortex composed of mature adipose tissue which is usually not encapsulated. An **angiomyolipoma** contains a combination of adipose tissue, smooth muscle, and blood vessels, and is often associated with tuberous sclerosis. **renal malignant tumors** See CARCINOMA, RENAL CELL, WILMS' TUMOR in Clinical Glossary.

vacuolar change Formation of large vacuoles in the cytoplasm, similar to those seen after administration of hypertonic solution of carbohydrates but larger, more persistent, and accompanied by disturbances of tubular function. Their origin and the nature of their contents have not been determined. Vacuolar degeneration is typically seen after administration of toxic substances such as ethylene glycol, propylene glycol, and dioxane. It is also seen in potassium deficiency in man, although in this instance at least some of the vacuoles may not be intracytoplasmic but are caused by distention of subbasilar and intercellular compartments (Fig. 53). See also HYPOKALEMIC NEPHROPATHY in Clinical Glossary.

virus-like particle Term applied to two types of structures in renal glomeruli. One is **spherical,** with a diameter of 500 to 600 Å, often showing a central core and a darker outer envelope. Spherical particles occur in clusters located extracellularly under the epithelium, under the endothelium, or in the capillary basement membrane. They may represent either protein deposits, derivatives of cell organelles, or true viral structures, although the evidence for the latter is inconclusive. The second type is an intracytoplasmic branching **microtubule** measur-

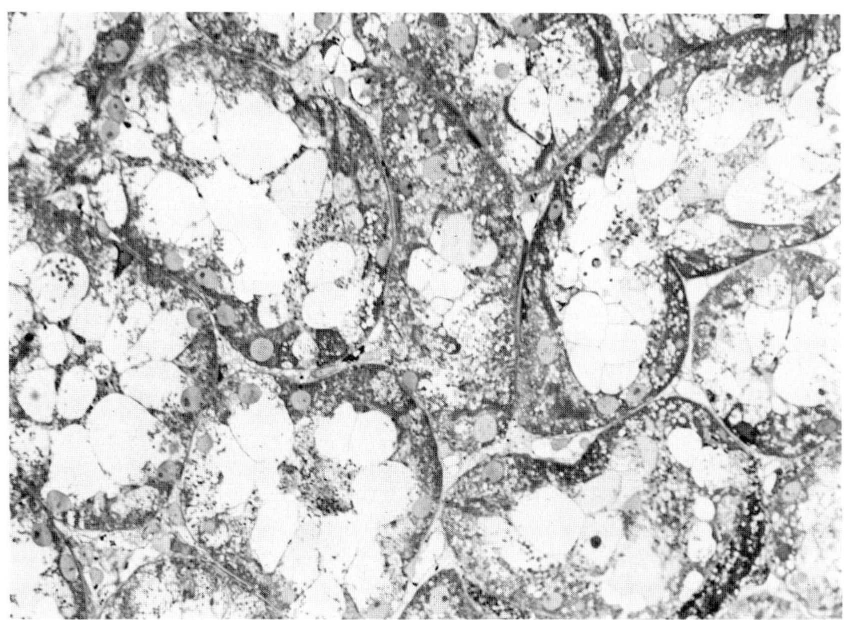

Fig. 53. Biopsy specimen from a patient with severe potassium depletion. The conspicuous proximal tubular vacuolization demonstrated may be characteristic, but not pathognomonic, of the condition. Osmium-fixed, epon-embedded, toluidine blue stain. (From B. H. Spargo, Renal Changes with Potassium Depletion, in Becker [1].)

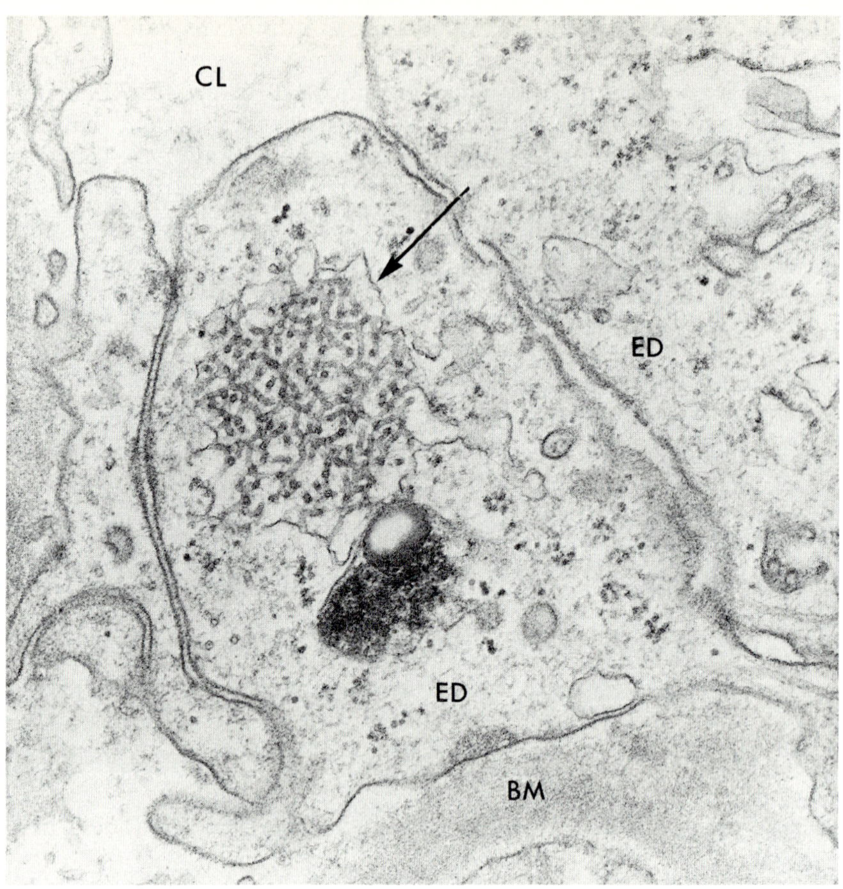

Fig. 54. Electron micrograph showing myxovirus-like structures (*arrow*) in an endothelial cell of a glomerular capillary. Such structures are commonly encountered in lupus nephritis but also occur, though less frequently, in other glomerular diseases. *BM,* basement membrane; *ED,* endothelial cells; *CL,* capillary lumen. (Courtesy of Y. Suzuki in J. Churg and E. Grishman, Ultrastructure of immune deposits in renal glomeruli. *Ann. Intern. Med.* 76:479, 1972.)

ing 200 to 250 Å in diameter and occurring in interlacing bundles. The tubules bear some resemblance to the nucleocapsids of myxoviruses, but so far their viral origin has not been proved. It has been suggested that they arise by budding of the inner lining of the endoplasmic reticulum (Fig. 54).

Physiology

acidemia   Term used by some to indicate an abnormally low pH in whole blood. Mean normal whole blood pH at 38°C is 7.42 in systemic arterial samples with a standard deviation of 0.016. See also ACIDOSIS.

acidifying ability   The capacity of an organism to lower the pH of its urine in response to specific stimuli under standard conditions. Normal man is able to lower urinary pH at least as far as 5.0 in response to systemic acidosis produced by administration of ammonium chloride in a dose of 0.1 gm per kilogram body weight.

acidosis   A state of the body in which physiologic mechanisms at work tend to lower the pH of body fluids. This is in contrast to the term *acidemia,* which describes the actual composition of blood or other body fluids.

   metabolic acidosis   A condition resulting from accumulation of acid (other than carbonic acid) in, or loss of bicarbonate from, extracellular fluid. Compensatory chemical and physiologic changes occur to a variable degree and tend to mask the lowering of pH. In this sense it is possible to have acidosis with a normal blood pH. **respiratory acidosis** A condition resulting from a primary decrease in alveolar ventilation relative to the existing level of carbon dioxide production. As with metabolic acidosis, there is a variable degree of biochemical and physiologic compensation. Metabolic and respiratory acidosis may coexist.

active transport   See ACTIVE TRANSPORT, under TRANSPORT.

Addis count   A method no longer in extensive use, devised for quantifying the number of formed elements contained in urine passed over a 12-hour period. The values reported by Addis in normal subjects are as follows:

Formed Elements	Mean	Range
Casts	1,040	0–4,270
Erythrocytes	65,750	0–425,000
Leukocytes and epithelial cells	322,500	32,400–1,835,000

ADH   See VASOPRESSIN.

aldosterone   A mineralocorticoid produced by the adrenal cortex which accelerates the reabsorption of sodium ions in the kidney, salivary and sweat glands, and gastrointestinal tract. The major site of action in the kidney is in the distal tubule, where sodium reabsorption is linked with secretion of potassium and hydrogen ions. The production of aldosterone is regulated by adrenocorticotrophic hormone (ACTH), serum potassium concentration, and the renin-angiotensin system.

aldosteronism   See Syndrome Glossary.

alkalemia   Term used by some to indicate an abnormally high pH in whole blood. Mean normal whole blood pH at 38°C is 7.42 in systemic arterial samples with a standard deviation of 0.016. See also ALKALOSIS.

alkalosis   A state of the body in which physiologic mechanisms at work tend to raise the pH of blood fluids. This is in contrast to the term *alkalemia,* which describes the actual composition of blood or other body fluids.

metabolic alkalosis   A condition resulting from loss of acid (other than carbonic acid) from, or gain of bicarbonate in, extracellular fluid. Compensatory chemical and physiologic changes occur to a variable degree and tend to mask the rise of pH. In this sense it is possible to have alkalosis with a normal blood pH. **respiratory alkalosis**   A condition resulting from a primary increase in alveolar ventilation relative to the existing level of carbon dioxide production. As with metabolic alkalosis, there is a variable degree of biochemical and physiologic compensation. Metabolic and respiratory alkalosis may coexist.

angiotensin I   A decapeptide formed from angiotensinogen (renin substrate) by the proteolytic action of the enzyme renin. It is devoid of vasoconstrictive activity but stimulates catecholamine release.

angiotensin II   An octapeptide formed from angiotensin I primarily in plasma and in the lung by the splitting off of histidyl-leucine from angiotensin I under the catalytic action of *converting enzyme.* It is the most potent vasoconstrictor currently known and is one of the tropic factors stimulating aldosterone secretion.

angiotensinase   An enzyme present in human blood and tissue that is capable of destroying angiotensin. The chief of these in serum is called **angiotensinase A** and has a pH optimum of 7.5. There are a number of other angiotensinases, referred to as **endopeptidases,** with lower pH optima. It is doubtful that, under normal circumstances in vivo, angiotensinase concentration is of much importance in regulation of angiotensin levels.

angiotensinogen (also *renin substrate*)   A protein synthesized in the liver and contained in the alpha-2-globulin fraction of plasma. It has a molecular weight of around 58,000 and is acted upon by the enzyme renin to form angiotensin I.

antidiuretic hormone   See VASOPRESSIN.

anuresis An obsolete term synonymous with retention. See RETENTION, URINARY.

anuria Absence of formation of urine. This term should not be used to refer to retention.

autoregulation of renal blood flow Ability of the kidney to maintain a constant renal blood flow rate in response to a wide range of renal arterial pressures. This is assumed to be under the control of an intrinsic regulatory system.

baroreceptor A stretch receptor serving to modulate systemic blood pressure. Baroreceptors are found in the carotid sinus, aortic arch, and subclavian and common carotid arteries.

base deficit The negative value of base excess, measured by titration with a strong base of pH 7.4 at a P_{CO_2} of 40 mm Hg at 37°C. This parameter is expressed in milliequivalents per liter.

base excess The base concentration in blood as measured by titration with strong acid to pH 7.4 at a P_{CO_2} of 40 mm Hg at 37°C. This parameter is expressed in milliequivalents per liter.

bicarbonate ion concentration By rigorous chemical definition, simply the concentration of the bicarbonate ion. In many current physiologic studies, however, bicarbonate ion concentration is calculated as the total carbon dioxide concentration minus the product of the partial pressure of carbon dioxide and a coefficient which is temperature dependent and relates the sum of the concentrations of dissolved carbon dioxide and carbonic acid to the partial pressure of carbon dioxide. Therefore, bicarbonate ion concentration as used in physiologic studies includes carbamino compounds and carbonate plus bicarbonate. The error introduced by the use of this physiologic definition is not great for extracellular fluid but may be large for intracellular fluid. See also CARBON DIOXIDE CONCENTRATION, TOTAL.

blood flow, renal See RENAL PLASMA FLOW.

blood flow distribution, renal The partitioning of total renal blood flow throughout the different areas of the renal parenchyma. In studies of dogs and man using radiographic and dye-dilution techniques, two, three, or four compartments of renal blood flow may be distinguished.

buffer base The sum of buffer anions of blood, expressed in milliequivalents per liter. From a practical standpoint, this quantity is usually the sum of bicarbonate and proteinate.

carbon dioxide concentration, total The carbon dioxide extractable from biological fluids, such as plasma and urine, in the presence of a strong acid. The total represents dissolved carbon dioxide, carbonic acid, bicarbonate ion, carbonate ion, and carbamino compounds. It is measured in millimols per liter. See also BICARBONATE ION CONCENTRATION.

carbonic anhydrase A zinc-containing enzyme with a molecular weight of 30,000, which catalyzes the hydration of carbon dioxide to form carbonic acid and also catalyzes the reverse reaction, i.e., the breakdown of carbonic acid to carbon dioxide and water. The dissociation of carbonic acid to a bicarbonate ion and a proton is exremely rapid and requires no catalysis. In tubular cells this process provides the protons which are exchanged for sodium ions across the luminal membrane and the bicarbonate ions which move down an electric gradient into peritubular fluid, thereby indirectly accomplishing net bicarbonate reabsorption (since bicarbonate is coverted in the tubule to carbon dioxide). Dehydration of carbonic acid is catalyzed in the proximal tubule but not in the distal tubule, thereby generating what has been termed a **disequilibrium pH** in the distal convolution. The presence of carbonic anhydrase in the brush border of the proximal tubules facilitates the bulk of reabsorption of bicarbonate by reducing tenfold the gradient against which protons must be secreted, concomitantly reducing the energy expenditure of bicarbonate conservation. See also REABSORPTION.

carbonic anhydrase inhibitor Any of a number of N′-unsubstituted sulfonamides of which the best known is acetazolamide. This compound, by virtue of inhibiting carbonic anhydrase, depresses the reabsorption rate of bicarbonate and thereby increases its excretion rate along with that of sodium. The urine becomes alkaline, and potassium secretion is enhanced.

clearance The volume of plasma which would yield its entire content of a substance for renal excretion in one minute's time and which is thus cleared of the substance during this time. This is a virtual volume rather than a real one, since blood is not completely cleared of a substance during one passage through the kidney. Therefore, the practice is to take the amount of a given substance removed per minute and express it as though it were derived from the complete clearing of a smaller volume of blood. Thus, if 200 ml of plasma yields half its content of a given substance in one minute, this is equivalent to 100 ml of plasma yielding its entire content. Clearance is calculated from the formula

$$C = UV/P$$

where C = clearance
    U = concentration of the substance in the urine (mg/ml)
    V = urine volume per minute (ml/min)
    P = plasma concentration of the substance (mg/ml)

Endogenous **creatinine clearance** is used clinically as a rough approximation of glomerular filtration rate (GFR). Production of creatinine is fairly constant in any one individual but varies from person to person, being roughly proportional to the total muscle mass. In man it is also secreted by the tubules, a factor tending to make creatinine clearance higher than the actual GFR. Noncreatinine chromogen, on the other hand, is not filtered, and therefore its clearance tends to be somewhat lower than the GFR. Therefore standard methods measure noncreatinine chromogen in addition to creatinine, and the two errors tend to cancel out. Creatinine clearance, nevertheless, is not an exact measure of GFR, particularly in the diseased kidney. The most accurate measure of GFR is **inulin clearance.** (See FILTRATION RATE, GLOMERULAR.) **mannitol clearance** was formerly used as a measure of glomerular filtration rate but is now known to be about 10 percent less than the simultaneously determined inulin clearance, indicating a significant degree of reabsorption by the tubules. Because of low plasma concentration (less than 5 mg/100 ml) **sodium *p*-amino-hippuric acid (PAH)** is almost completely cleared from the blood in one passage through the kidney. PAH clearance (C_{PAH}) has therefore been used as a measure of renal plasma flow. (See EFFECTIVE RENAL PLASMA FLOW.) **Urea** is produced in amounts proportional to the rate of protein catabolism, of which it is an end product. When an individual is in nitrogen balance, urea production is therefore proportional to the daily dietary intake of protein. Urea is reabsorbed in the renal tubules, usually to the extent of 40 to 60 percent of the amount filtered. However, under extreme conditions of diuresis or antidiuresis the reabsorption of urea may be greatly increased or decreased. Therefore urea clearance is dependent in part upon urine flow. Under steady state conditions with urine flows of 3 to 6 ml per minute, the urea clearance is about 60 percent of the GFR. A so-called **standard urea clearance** has been employed in the past to correct for variation of urea clearance with urine flow when the latter is 2 ml per minute or less. The empirical formula $U\sqrt{V}/P$ for calculating clearance is not satisfactory since the variation of clearance with urine flow is quite wide and collections at low urine flows tend to be incomplete. See also FREE WATER CLEARANCE; OSMOLAR CLEARANCE.

cold pressor test An obsolete test thought at one time to indicate overactivity of the sympathetic nervous system and consisting of measurement of the rise in blood pressure in response to immersion of the hand in water at 4°C. Although a large literature has been generated by applications of this test, its differential diagnostic significance is uncertain and its prognostic implications negligible.

colligative property A property of a solution that depends on the number of particles of solute per unit mass of solvent and is independent of the chemical nature of the nondissociating solute. Examples are freezing point depression, osmotic pressure, and vapor pressure depression.

competitive transport inhibition See COMPETITIVE TRANSPORT, under TRANSPORT.

concentrating ability (also *concentrating power*) The ability of the kidney to produce urine hypertonic to plasma.

countercurrent exchanger This term relates to the passive diffusion of water across the walls of the vasa recta as this structure traverses the hypertonic medullary interstitium. The process plays no active part in the establishment of an osmotic gradient. The countercurrent arrangement in the exchanger decreases the rate at which the concentration gradient is dissipated by blood flowing through the medulla.

countercurrent multiplier The hairpin configuration of the loop of Henle as a means by which a small concentration difference is enhanced by the countercurrent flow. The descending and ascending limbs of the loop are sufficiently close to be considered contiguous. Fluid flows in opposite directions in the two limbs. The renal epithelium is considered capable of establishing a small concentration difference (or **single effect**) between the two limbs at each level along the course of the loop. As fluid flows down one limb and up the other, the single effect is multiplied, since it operates in fluid of increasing osmolality as the bend of the loop is approached. The net gradient at any given level is small, but the movement of the fluid produces a high osmolality at the tip of the loop. The concentration gradient between the inflow-outflow level (corticomedullary junction) and the flow reversal level (bend of loop near papillary tip) is therefore large.

The osmolal gradient established by the epithelial cells of the loop is considered due to active pumping of sodium by cells of the ascending limb from the luminal fluid into the interstitium. The cells of the ascending limb are considered impermeable to water, whereas those of the descending limb are considered permeable to water and relatively so to sodium.

creatinine See under CLEARANCE.

cryoscopy Determination of osmolality by freezing point depression. Since freezing point depression is a colligative property, it can be used as a measure of the number of osmotically active particles in solution. See also COLLIGATIVE PROPERTY; OSMOLALITY.

dead space error Clearance studies depend upon the measurement of the excretory rate of a given substance over a measured time interval and the relation of this rate to the plasma concentration during that time interval. When tests are made, constant-speed infusions are given in an an attempt to achieve a steady state of plasma concentration during the clearance. In practice slight variations in plasma concentration occur, and therefore blood samples are taken at the midpoint of the clearance period.

Elaboration of the urine occurs during the passage of glomerular filtrate down the nephron from the glomerular (Bowman's) capsule to the collecting duct. However, urine specimens are taken between the bladder emptying of one period and the bladder emptying of the next period. The time required for the urine to traverse the path from collecting duct to urethral orifice is not, strictly speaking, related to the actual process of urine formation during a given clearance. It actually belongs to the previous clearance period, since the urine is formed during the prior clearance interval.

Under steady state conditions and when urine flow is not undergoing marked fluctuations in rate, errors due to this so-called dead space are negligible. However, when plasma concentration is changing markedly or urine flow undergoes rapid increase or decrease, the dead space error may be appreciable. For example, at the initiation of diuresis, the washout of inulin in the dead space of urine that had been formed prior to the diuresis will give a spuriously high urinary excretion rate for inulin, and therefore a falsely high glomerular filtration rate.

dialysance　A concept modelled on renal clearance and introduced to quantitate the functional efficiency of dialysis procedures. It is an expression of the rate of removal of a substance per unit difference in concentration between blood and bath.

dialysis　See Clinical Glossary.

diffusion　The spontaneous movement of atoms or molecules from an area of higher to one of lower electrochemical potential. In biologic systems a semipermeable membrane usually separates such areas. For noncharged molecules chemical activities determine the direction of movement and can be approximated from concentrations and activity coefficients. See DIFFUSION, NONIONIC.

diffusion, nonionic　Since many weak acids and bases exist in solution in both the ionized and the un-ionized state, their ability to traverse biologic membranes tends to be primarily a function of the concentration of the un-ionized molecule. The dissociation of weak acids and bases is strongly influenced by the $[H^+]$ (hydrogen ion concentration) of the solution; consequently, their movement across membranes will be strongly influenced by pH. At diffusion equilibrium, the concentration of un-ionized substance is equal on each side of the membrane, but the total concentration of substance will be determined by the relative pH in the two solutions separated by the membrane. Weak bases will accumulate on the more acid side, while weak acids will accumulate on the more alkaline side of the membrane. The quantitative distribution of a substance between two compartments can be predicted from the pK of the substance and the pH of the two compartments. A physiologic example is the non-ionic diffusion of NH_3 out of the cell where it is produced into tubular lumen, where it is trapped as NH_4^+ in the acidic tubular fluid. Total ammonium (NH_4^+) excretion is increased as urine pH is lowered and is depressed by alkalinizing the urine.

diluting power   The capacity of the kidney to excrete a urine hypoosmolal to plasma.

disappearance curve   See WASHOUT CURVE.

diuresis   Increase, either spontaneous or provoked, in urine flow over that which would ordinarily be expected under given metabolic conditions. When used clinically, the term usually connotes a negative water balance.

induced diuresis   Diuresis occurring for a variety of reasons, chief of which is the use of drugs which diminish sodium reabsorption in the renal tubules.   **osmotic diuresis**   Diuresis resulting when a nonreabsorbable or poorly reabsorbable solute is introduced into the nephron. An example is the diuresis following intravenous infusion of mannitol.   **spontaneous diuresis**   Diuresis occurring in any patient with overt or occult edema, for reasons that are poorly understood. The diuresis that is sometimes observed when patients with mild congestive heart failure are put at bed rest has been referred to as spontaneous, but in fact it is induced by reduction of tissue requirements for oxygen.   **water diuresis**   Increase in urine flow following ingestion of water. It is attributable to decreased output of ADH secondary to the reduction in osmotic pressure detected by osmoreceptors located within the area of distribution of the internal carotid artery.

Many other factors may induce diuresis. The most important of these is extracellular fluid volume expansion. (See FACTOR III.)

diuretic   A drug which produces diuresis.

divided renal function studies   See SPLIT RENAL FUNCTION TESTS.

dysuria   Painful micturition.

effective renal plasma flow   The amount of plasma perfusing the secretory renal tubular cells. Assuming that renal tubular cells are capable of removing all the PAH at low plasma concentrations offered to them from the blood during one passage through the kidney, then the PAH clearance must equal effective renal plasma flow. This is about 10 percent less than true renal plasma flow, the extraction of PAH in the kidneys being about 90 percent complete in man. See also SODIUM P-AMINOHIPPURATE (PAH), under CLEARANCE.

enuresis   Involuntary discharge of urine, usually at night (bed-wetting). See also NOCTURIA.

erythropoietin   Protein, primarily produced by the kidney, which stimulates erythropoiesis.

exchangeable potassium   That amount of potassium in equilibrium with a known quantity of injected radioactive potassium. It is calculated by subtracting the radioactive potassium excreted from the amount of radioactive potassium injected and then dividing this by the ratio of the serum radiopotassium to the total serum potassium. It is necessary that a period of equilibration, usually 18 to 24 hours, elapse to allow the radiopotassium to become distributed throughout the body tissues. This method makes no distinction between extracellular and intracellular potassium. Erythrocytes, brain, and bone exchange potassium less rapidly than other areas of the body. However, 98 percent of the total body potassium (42 mEq/kg body weight) is intracellular and readily exchangeable.

exchangeable sodium That amount of sodium in equilibrium with a known quantity of injected radioactive sodium. It is calculated by subtracting the radioactive sodium excreted from the amount of radioactive sodium injected and then dividing this by the ratio of the serum radiosodium to the total serum sodium. It is necesary that a period of equilibration, usually 18 to 24 hours, elapse to allow the radiosodium to become distributed throughout the body tissues. This method makes no distinction between extracellular and intracellular sodium. Exchangeable sodium is about 42 mEq per kilogram body weight, or about 70 percent of the total body sodium. It includes all the sodium of the extracellular and intracellular fluids and somewhat less than half of bone sodium. Brain and some parts of bone are areas of slow exchange. The 18 mEq of nonexchangeable sodium is thought to exist on the surfaces of the hydroxyapatite crystals of the denser long bones.

excretion, fractional That fraction of a filtered substance that finds its way into the urine, i.e., the excretory rate of the substance in question divided by its rate of filtration at the glomerulus. This is mathematically the same as the ratio between the clearance of the given substance and the clearance of inulin.

extracellular water See under WATER.

extraction ratio The renal arteriovenous difference of any substance. It is commonly expressed as

$$E = \frac{RA - RV}{RA} \times 100$$

where   E = percentage of extraction
       RA = arterial concentration
       RV = renal venous concentration

Such a ratio may be positive, negative, or zero.

factor III An unidentified mechanism or group of mechanisms presumed to regulate sodium excretion independently of GFR (factor I) and aldosterone (factor II).

filtered load The quantity of a substance that gains access to tubular fluid via glomerular filtration per unit time. It is derived by multiplying the glomerular filtration rate (expressed in milliliters per minute) by the concentration of a given substance in the plasma (expressed in weight per milliliter), with appropriate corrections if necessary for binding to plasma protein and plasma water and for Donnan effects in the case of electrolytes. The product is expressed as a mass per minute.

filtration fraction That fraction of effective renal plasma flow that is filtered.

filtration pressure The pressure available to overcome frictional resistance to filtration through the glomerular membrane. The **net filtration pressure** is derived from the glomerular capillary hydrostatic pressure, which is estimated to be 80 mm Hg in man, minus the intracapsular pressure and the colloid oncotic pressure, which total 40 mm Hg.

filtration rate, glomerular (GFR) The volume of plasma ultrafiltrate filtered by the glomeruli in unit time. In man, while the glomerular filtration rate can be accurately measured by the clearance of inulin, the endogenous creatinine clearance approximates the inulin clearance for most practical clinical purposes. In the presence of an increased serum creatinine concentration, the GFR is spuriously elevated due to excessive creatinine secretion. See also CLEARANCE.

fractional excretion See EXCRETION, FRACTIONAL.

free water clearance The volume of water excreted in excess of that required to render urine isosmotic with plasma. Free water clearance is calculated as the difference between urine flow and osmolal clearance:

$$C_{H_2O} = V - \frac{U_{osm}V}{P_{osm}}$$

where C_{H_2O} = free water clearance
V = urine flow
U_{osm} = osmolality of urine
P_{osm} = osmolality of plasma
and osmolal clearance (C_{osm}) is equal to $U_{osm}V/P_{osm}$.

Free water clearance is therefore measured in milliliters per minute. When the urine is concentrated, the osmolal clearance is greater than the urine volume, and the free water clearance has a negative value. Under these circumstances it is referred to as $T^c_{H_2O}$:

$$T^c_{H_2O} = - C_{H_2O}$$

$T^c_{H_2O}$ can be regarded as the tubular reabsorption rate of water in excess of that which would result in a urine isosmotic with plasma.

frequency Frequent emptying of the bladder.

GFR See FILTRATION RATE, GLOMERULAR.

glomerular filtration rate See FILTRATION RATE, GLOMERULAR.

glomerular intermittence See INTERMITTENCE, GLOMERULAR.

glomerulotubular balance The physiologic observation that changes in glomerular filtration rate are associated with similar changes in the tubular reabsorption of salt and water. The term has been applied to alterations in reabsorption which are attributable to changes in GFR. Such alterations result in a relative constancy of fractional reabsorption in the proximal tubule and the delivery of a relatively constant fraction of filtrate to the more distal tubular segments.

glomerulotubular imbalance A physiologic concept introduced to explain evidence of functional heterogeneity in the nephron population. Should a nephron have relatively greater glomerular filtration potential than tubular reabsorptive capacity, a reabsorbed solute such as glucose might appear in the urine at a relatively low plasma level. In contrast, a nephron with a low glomerular filtration rate but with average tubular reabsorptive capacity will saturate and spill only at relatively high plasma levels. This serves as a partial explanation for the splay found in experimentally determined curves for reabsorptive maximum (Tm). See also REABSORPTIVE MAXIMUM; SPLAY.

glucose titration See under SPLAY.

hematocrit, renal (also *intrarenal hematocrit*) The ratio of the volume of erythrocytes to that of plasma in the blood perfusing the kidney. It is determined by measuring the intrarenal red cell mass by radioisotope-labeled erythrocytes and measuring the renal plasma by radioiodine or dye-labeled albumin. The renal hematocrit is lower than large vessel hematocrits elsewhere in the body. Although whole kidney hematocrits probably do not differ from those of other organs, the hematocrit for the renal medullary areas is lower than for cortical regions. See also PLASMA SKIMMING.

hemoconcentration Diminution in the water content of blood leading to an abnormally high concentration of formed elements and solutes.

hemodialysis See under DIALYSIS, KIDNEY in Clinical Glossary.

hydrogen secretion The quantity of H^+ excreted in the urine in unit time in excess of that filtered at the glomerulus. It is calculated as the sum of the NH_4^+ excretion and the titratable acidity minus HCO_3^- excretion and is expressed in microequivalents per minute.

hyposthenuria Impairment of the ability to concentrate the urine appropriately in response to a given stimulus of fluid deprivation for a definite period. It may be measured by the urine-to-plasma osmolality ratio (U/P_{osm}). See also FREE WATER CLEARANCE; CONCENTRATING ABILITY.

inhibition, competitive See COMPETITIVE TRANSPORT, under TRANSPORT.

intact nephron hypothesis The concept that the functional disturbances encountered in renal disease result from a progressive reduction in the number of functioning nephrons rather than from the separate impairment of glomerular and tubular functions. As the number of nephrons diminishes, the remaining units undergo structural and functional hypertrophy.

intermittence, glomerular The assumption that only part of the total nephron population functions at any one time. This has been demonstrated directly only in lower species.

interstitial pressure See PRESSURE, INTERSTITIAL.

intracellular water See under WATER.

intrarenal blood flow See BLOOD FLOW DISTRIBUTION, RENAL.

intrarenal hematocrit See HEMATOCRIT, RENAL; PLASMA SKIMMING.

intrarenal pressure See PRESSURE, INTERSTITIAL.

inulin A polysaccharide of fructose with a molecular weight of about 5000. Derived from plant sources, it is metabolically inert in animals. In mammals it is distributed throughout the extracellular fluid volume. It does not bind to plasma protein, is freely filtered at the glomeruli, and is neither reabsorbed nor secreted by the renal tubules. Therefore its excretory rate is linearly related to its plasma concentration no matter how high the latter is raised, and its clearance is numerically equal to the glomerular filtration rate. See also FILTRATION RATE, GLOMERULAR.

ion exchange mechanism A process in which the net flux of an ion through a biological membrane is quantitatively coupled with the flux of another ion of the same charge but taking place in the reverse direction. Ion exchange may result from either passive or active transport mechanisms.

isosthenuria A condition, occurring in severe renal disease, in which there is impairment of both concentrating ability and diluting ability. In most forms of renal disease maximum concentrating ability is decreased at an earlier stage than maximum diluting ability. When both functions are severely impaired, the urinary specific gravity becomes relatively fixed at 1.010 (approximately 285 mOsm/kg, the osmolality of glomerular filtrate). In contrast, the normal kidney can produce dilute urine with specific gravity as low as 1.001 (50 mOsm/kg) and concentrated urine with specific gravity as high as 1.040 (1300 mOsm/kg). When tests of concentrating and diluting ability are performed under conditions of water diuresis, water deprivation, or vasopressin administration, the existing conditions should be specified, and tests results should preferably be given in terms of U/P osmolality rather than specific gravity.

lymphatic circulation, kidney There are two sets of renal lymphatics in the mammal. One plexus is an abundant anastomotic system which parallels the blood vessels as far as the intralobular segments. The second plexus drains the outer subcapsular cortex and communicates with the hilar system. In the dog lymph flow is quite variable and probably has an upper limit of less than 1 ml per minute. Total flow is difficult to measure because of the variation in number of channels and flow in each. Lymphatic function is poorly understood but may be of considerable importance in kidney function. It has recently been shown that renin and angiotensin II occur in high concentration in renal lymph.

mannitol clearance   See under CLEARANCE.

microperfusion   A micropuncture technique in which small fluid samples are introduced into the renal tubule through a micropipet and continuous infusion by pump and are subsequently reaspirated after a given period of time, from the same or a more distal site, and analyzed.

micropuncture   An experimental technique permitting the study of an individual nephron in situ by penetration of the wall of the tubule with a micropipet. It is generally used in order to collect tubular fluid from selected portions of the nephron.

micturition   The act of urination.

net reabsorption   See REABSORPTION.

nocturia (also *nycturia*)   Increase in elaboration of urine during sleep with resultant increase in frequency of micturition. Nocturia may be part of a generalized polyuria such as occurs in chronic renal insufficiency or may be due to increased mobilization of excess body fluid during rest in bed (such as occurs in myocardial insufficiency). Although nocturia may be an occasional cause of enuresis, the terms should not be used interchangeably.

nonprotein nitrogen (NPN)   Serum nitrogen from nonprotein sources such as nitrogen of urea, free amino acids, and creatinine. Serum urea nitrogen constitutes the main component, amounting to approximately 50 percent of the total NPN at normal levels of serum urea.

NPN   See NONPROTEIN NITROGEN.

nycturia   See NOCTURIA.

oliguria   Decrease in the rate of urine formation with resultant development of abnormalities of body fluid composition.

oncotic pressure   The effect of colloids on the chemical potential of water molecules. Because of their high molecular weight, colloids contribute much less to total osmotic pressure than does an equal weight of smaller molecules. In vivo, however, they do contribute to the effective osmolality of biologic solutions and, since they do not pass through cell membranes readily, they may be responsible for the major difference in total osmotic pressure of two fluids separated by a biologic membrane. The largest class of colloids in biologic fluids is protein. See also OSMOLALITY; OSMOTIC PRESSURE.

opsiuria   Delayed excretion of water after a water load.

osmol The gram-molecular weight of any nondissociating solute. One osmol contains 6.06×10^{23} particles. See also OSMOLALITY.

osmolality The number of osmols in 1 kilogram of water; also the osmotic pressure in osmols or milliosmols per kilogram of water.

When 1 osmol of solute is present in 1 kilogram of water, the resulting aqueous solution is said to be a **one osmolal solution.** The osmolality of a solution containing a given gram-molecular weight of a dissociating solute will vary depending on the degree of dissociation and the number of osmotically active particles resulting from such dissociation. (The greater the degree of dissociation and the larger the number of particles, the greater is the osmolality.) The osmolality of biologic fluids is quite low and is therefore usually expressed in units of milliosmols (mOsm) (0.001 osmol). Osmolality can be measured in terms of osmotic pressure, freezing point depression, or boiling point elevation. The method in common use for biologic fluids is freezing point depression. See also COLLIGATIVE PROPERTY; CRYOSCOPY; OSMOTIC PRESSURE.

osmolar clearance The virtual volume of plasma which is cleared of osmotically active substances in unit time. It is calculated from the equation:

$$C_{osm} = \frac{U_{osm}V}{P_{osm}}$$

where C_{osm} = osmolar clearance (in ml/min)
U_{osm} = urinary osmolarity (in mOsm/liter)
V = urine volume per minute
P_{osm} = plasma osmolarity (in mOsm/liter)

osmolarity The number of osmols in 1 liter of solution. When 1 osmol of solute is dissolved in water to form 1 liter of solution, the resulting aqueous solution is termed a **one osmolar solution.**

osmometry Measurement of the osmolality of a solution. See CRYOSCOPY; OSMOL; OSMOLALITY.

osmotic diuresis See under DIURESIS.

osmotic pressure The pressure that would be required to prevent entry of a solvent into a solution that is separated from the solvent by a membrane permeable to the solvent but impermeable to the solute. If external pressure is applied to a solution to oppose the volume increase consequent upon the net addition of solvent to it, this pressure is numerically equal to the osmotic pressure of the solution.

The vapor pressure of pure water is depressed when a solute is dissolved in it (see COLLIGATIVE PROPERTY). In more rigorous thermodynamic terms, the osmotic pressure is the force per unit area deriving from the lowering of the chemical potential of a solvent by the presence of a solute. This pressure is equal to the hydrostatic pressure that would have to be applied to the solution to restore the normal chemical potential of the solvent.

para-aminohippuric acid clearance   See SODIUM P-AMINOHIPPURIC ACID CLEARANCE under CLEARANCE.

peritoneal dialysis   See under DIALYSIS, KIDNEY in Clinical Glossary.

phenolsulphonphthalein test (PSP test)   See TEST, PHENOLSULPHONPHTHALEIN.

plasma flow, renal   See RENAL PLASMA FLOW; also SODIUM P-AMINOHIPPURIC ACID CLEARANCE under CLEARANCE.

plasma skimming   A phenomenon that may occur in the kidney if the deep glomeruli receive blood richer in plasma than the superficial glomeruli. Blood flow through most arteries of the body is laminar, consisting of a central stream rich in red cells and a peripheral stream rich in plasma. If this is so in the interlobular arteries of the kidneys, the deep glomeruli are supplied by the peripheral stream and the superficial glomeruli are mostly supplied by the central stream. This would account for the difference in the renal hematocrit from the hematocrit of the peripheral blood.

pollakiuria (also *pollakisuria*)   Frequency of micturition.

polyuria   Increase in the rate of urine formation above what would be expected in normal individuals.

potential difference, transtubular   The resting potential difference in millivolts (mv) between luminal fluid and interstitial fluid across the epithelial layer of the renal tubule. Under appropriate conditions this difference can be measured with reversible microelectrodes.

pressure, interstitial   The hydrostatic pressure of the interstitial fluid of the kidney. Its actual value results both from hydrodynamic conditions along blood vessels and urinary tubules and from the tension of the kidney capsule. Interstitial pressure is often referred to as **intrarenal pressure,** which is less exact since pressure distribution is not uniform throughout the different extracellular compartments of the kidney.

pressure, osmotic   See OSMOTIC PRESSURE.

pressure, partial, of carbon dioxide   The equivalent of carbon dioxide tension for biologic fluids such as plasma and urine. It is the partial pressure of carbon dioxide in a gas phase in equilibrium with the biologic fluid in question. The symbol used is P_{CO_2}, and the usual units are millimeters of mercury.

prostaglandins   A group of substances formed in many organs, primarily at the site of cell membranes. Basically they are variants of a 20-carbon carboxylic fatty acid incorporating a cyclopentane ring. Prostaglandins of the 1, 2, and 3 series, respectively, incorporate 1, 2, and 3 double bonds. The PGE structures have an oxygen atom attached to the cyclopentane ring at site 9, whereas the PGF structures have a hydroxyl group at that position. Dehydration of a PGE molecule will lead to either a PGA or a PGB compound. The different prostaglandins can be looked upon as variations on the structure of prostanoic acid, which in turn is mostly formed from arachidonic acid.

Although occurring in small amounts, the prostaglandins constitute a ubiquitous group of substances, being found in many animals and even in a type of coral. They have a wide range of biologic actions, and their effects may be quite different depending on small changes in chemical structure. For instance PGE_2 lowers blood pressure, whereas PGF_2-alpha raises it. PGE_1 and PGA_1 are natriuretic. Because prostaglandins are found in the extractable fat of the renal medullary area, and because of their vascular effects and their effects on sodium, they are suspected of having a role in the normal regulation of blood pressure.

PSP See TEST, PHENOLSULPHONPHTHALEIN.

puncture, tubular See MICROPUNCTURE.

reabsorption Transport of material from the tubular fluid to the peritubular fluid and blood. It may be **passive**, effected only by physical force, or **active**, effected by energy produced by the tubular cells. The term **net reabsorption** applies to substances that undergo bi-directional tubular transport, and it indicates the difference between the two opposing processes. Reabsorption is calculated as the difference between the quantity filtered per minute and the quantity excreted per minute in the bladder urine. "Net" indicates that this is not necessarily the absolute quantity reabsorbed by the tubule. For example, urate is concomitantly secreted and reabsorbed. The apparent rate of reabsorption (net reabsorption) would, therefore, be less than the actual rate. **fractional reabsorption** The proportion of a filtered substance that has been reabsorbed.

reabsorptive maximum (also *transport maximum*) The maximum reabsorptive rate of the renal tubules for a substance, expressed in milligrams per minute. For example, as the filtered load of glucose is increased by elevation of the plasma concentration, the rate of **tubular reabsorption** (T_G) regains equal to the increment in filtered load, and, therefore, no glucose appears in the urine. At a certain point, however, further increases in filtered load of glucose bring no further increment in T_G. This maximal limit in the rate of reabsorptive activity for glucose is designated as Tm_G, or the transport maximum for glucose. Other substances displaying a reabsorptive maximum include sulphate, inorganic phosphate, and some amino acids.

renal blood flow distribution See BLOOD FLOW DISTRIBUTION, RENAL.

renal fraction of cardiac output That portion of the cardiac output perfusing the kidney (renal blood flow/cardiac output). In man, under resting conditions and with a normal mean blood pressure, this is approximately one-fifth of the cardiac output.

renal plasma flow The amount of plasma perfusing the kidneys. It may be approximated by the clearance of PAH. See also EFFECTIVE RENAL PLASMA FLOW.

renin A proteolytic enzyme found primarily in the juxtaglomerular apparatus of the kidney and having a molecular weight of between 40,000 and 50,000. Renin cleaves angiotensinogen at a leucyl-leucyl bond and will also act upon degradation products of angiotensinogen to produce angiotensin I. Renin substrate (See ANGIOTENSINOGEN) may be degraded with trypsin to produce a 14-amino-acid polypeptide which will yield angiotensin I when incubated with renin.

resistance Total renal vascular resistance, calculated as effective perfusion pressure divided by renal blood flow.

$$R = \frac{P_A - P_V}{RBF} \times 1328$$

where R = total renal resistance (dynes sec cm^{-5})
P_A = mean renal arterial pressure (mm Hg)
P_V = mean renal venous pressure (mm Hg)
RFB = renal blood flow

The conversion factor 1328 is used to convert pressure in torrs (mm Hg) to CGS units (baryes, or dynes cm^{-2}). When divided by the RBF (ml sec^{-1}), this yields the resistance in dynes (sec cm^{-5}). Resistance can also be expressed in arbitrary units by dividing mean perfusion pressure by renal blood flow.

For clinical purposes R may be approximated by using mean peripheral blood pressure in place of $P_A - P_V$. Formulas also exist for calculating the partial resistances across the various parts of the renal vascular bed. The greatest pressure gradients (and therefore the largest components of the total renal resistance) occur in the afferent and efferent arterioles.

retention, urinary Absence of micturition despite the presence of urine in the distended bladder.

secretion, tubular The net transport of a given solute from peritubular capillaries to tubular lumen. Excluding the inorganic monovalent cations the renal tubules possess two distinct transport mechanisms for secretion; one for certain organic anions and the other for organic cations.
active secretion Secretion of a substance against chemical and/or electrical gradients. **competitive secretion** Secretion of several substances under conditions of mutual interference. See also TRANSPORT, ACTIVE; TRANSPORT, COMPETITIVE.

secretory maximum The maximum rate of secretory transport of a substance, given an excess of substrate. For example, as the amount of *p*-aminohippurate presented for tubular transport is increased by increasing its concentration in the plasma perfusing peritubular capillaries, the amount secreted increases only to a given point. The transport mechanism then becomes saturated, and the rate of transfer which has been achieved does not increase with further increments in the concentration of PAH.

shrinking drop technique A micropuncture technique for the measurement of transtubular flux. Oil is injected into the lumen of the tubule through a double-barreled micropipet, and the oil column is then split by injection of a droplet of the aqueous solution under study. As the droplet is reabsorbed, the ends of the oil columns approximate; with time-lapse photography, the volume of fluid present and the area of tubular epithelial lumen utilized for reabsorption can be estimated and the transtubular net flux of water and solutes calculated. The half-time for disappearance of the aqueous solution is generally measured.

shunts, intrarenal Postulated intrarenal arterial or arteriovenous connections making it possible for blood to bypass the capillaries. The term has also been used to describe bypass of the glomerular capillaries of deep nephrons through the diversion of blood from the cortex to the medulla, as reported in some species during shock (**Trueta shunts**).

skimming See PLASMA SKIMMING.

solvent drag Transfer of solute through a membrane by action of the net flux of solvent.

specific gravity The ratio of the density of a liquid to the density of water under standard conditions of temperature and pressure. The density of a liquid is defined as the mass of a unit volume of the liquid at standard temperature and pressure expressed in ml^{-3}.

splay In a graph of filtered load against reabsorption, the alteration that occurs in the expected curve when a lower than threshold concentration of a substance begins to appear in the urine (See THRESHOLD).

When the filtered load of glucose, for example, is plotted on the abscissa against glucose reabsorption (derived from excretion minus filtered load) on the ordinate (T_G), a theoretical reabsorptive curve is obtained. The experimental determination of such a curve for glucose transport is termed a **glucose titration** of the renal tubules. Theoretically, a sharp break in this curve should occur at a plasma glucose concentration of approximately 300 mg per 100 ml (given a normal glomerular filtration rate), since at that point glucose reabsorption (T_G) should become maximal (Tm_G) and should show no further increase at higher plasma glucose concentrations. (See REABSORPTIVE MAXIMUM). In actuality, however, this does not occur. Glucose begins to appear in the urine when the load presented to the tubules is only approximately 70 percent of their capacity to reabsorb glucose. Furthermore, the full capacity to reabsorb glucose is not used until the amount filtered is approximately 50 percent greater than the theoretical reabsorptive capacity.

The moderate degree of splay found in normal man may reflect the fact that not all nephrons have the same balance of glomerular filtration rate against reabsorptive capacity. It would appear that some heterogeneity in the ratio of filtration rate to reabsorptive capacity exists among nephrons. Whether this glomerulotubular imbalance has a kinetic or a morphologic basis is unknown.

split renal function tests Methods of demonstrating the lower rate of excretion of water and sodium displayed by the diseased kidney in hypertension secondary to unilateral renal artery stenosis. The tests measure urine flow rates and sodium concentrations and employ various modifications and criteria to accentuate these abnormalities for diagnostic purposes. All methods require catheterization with its attendant discomfort and risk of infection. Among the modifications are intravenous infusions of hypertonic saline, mannitol, PAH, ADH, and urea.

The physologic mechanism for the increased sodium and water reabsorption is not definitely known, but since a stenotic arterial lesion will diminish blood flow through an initially normal nephron population, the GFR per nephron may be presumed to be low, and this is evidenced by a delayed transit time. This could increase the reabsorption rates of sodium and water, while nonreabsorbable solutes, such as creatinine, would thereby become more concentrated in the urine from the affected side. (It is not clear whether additional hormonal or hemodynamic factors are operative.)

stop-flow analysis A method of studying the tubular transport of a given substance and its localization in the nephron. It is used exclusively in experiments with animals. The method is based on two steps:
1. The creation of a stationary column of tubular fluid to provide prolonged contact between the fluid and the tubular cells (*stop*).
2. The free outflow of the tubular fluid (*flow*) after the period of prolonged contact. The composition of the fluid, withdrawn rapidly and sequentially in a series of small samples, may be regarded as an approximation of the pattern of tubular activity with regard to the given substance.
Assuming there is no tubular water reabsorption during the free outflow and no movement of the stationary column during the stop time, it is possible to determine the existence and localization of tubular transport of a given substance and partially to quantify the data. The evaluation is commonly made by means of graphs. The method is open to much criticism.

test, phenolsulfonphthalein An obsolete test of renal function based on the rate of excretion of injected dye by the kidneys.

tetany   A disorder of neuromuscular transmission or excitability characterized by intermittent tonic muscular contractions and characteristically exemplified by carpopedal spasm. In the hands this is characterized by flexion at the carpometacarpal joints, flexion of the phalanges at the phalangometacarpal joints, and extension of the interphalangeal joints. Usually it is associated with a diminution in concentration of ionized calcium such as accompanies the hypocalcemia of renal insufficiency or alkalosis. It may also be associated with magnesium deficiency.

third factor   See FACTOR III.

threshold   That plasma level of a substance (such as glucose) at which tubular reabsorption can no longer completely extract the substance from tubular fluid and at which, therefore, it begins to appear in the urine. The threshold for glucose is approximately 180 mg per 100 ml in health. However, this threshold is highly variable in the presence of renal disease, since it is dependent upon glomerulotubular balance (see SPLAY). For example, the patient with diabetic glomerulosclerosis may appear to have a high threshold as glucose will not appear in the urine until the plasma glucose concentration becomes greatly elevated. This actually may be a reflection of a relative decrease in glomerular filtration rate per nephron without a proportional change in Tm_G.

titratable acid   The amount of acid in urine in excess of that in blood, measured by the number of milliequivalents of alkali necessary to titrate the urine from its initial acid reaction to the pH of the blood. Customarily it is obtained from 24-hour urine collections and is expressed in units of milliequivalents of acid excreted per day. If the initial urinary pH exceeds that of the plasma, strong acid is used in the titration and the titratable acid is said to be negative.

titratable acidity of urine   See TITRATABLE ACID.

transit time   The time it takes a short pulse of a tracer substance to flow between two selected points of a channel system. The context in which this term is used must be specified (transit time from renal artery to renal vein or from renal artery to ureteral urine, proximal tubular transit time, loop of Henle transit time, and so forth).

transport

active transport   Movement of a substance across a biologic membrane, such as the epithelial layer of the tubules, which is not the result of external driving forces such as osmotic, hydrostatic, electric, or chemical gradients. This process therefore requires energy input from cell metabolism. **competitive transport** (also *competitive inhibition*)   Transport of a substance across a biologic membrane under conditions of interference from simultaneous transport of another substance. This may occur by competition for a common carrier or common energy source, particularly if the other substance has a greater affinity for the carrier. A depression in rate of transport results. An example of this phenomenon is the inhibition of glucose reabsorption by the glycoside phlorizin. Adequate doses of this compound may completely abolish glucose transport, so that glucose clearance becomes equal to that of inulin.

transport maximum   See REABSORPTIVE MAXIMUM.

Trueta shunts   See under SHUNTS, INTRARENAL.

tubular reabsorption   See REABSORPTION.

urate   See URIC ACID.

urea clearance   See under CLEARANCE.

uric acid   An end product in the purine metabolic pathway. Clinical interest in uric acid and **urate** arises from their etiologic role in gout and their potential nephrotoxicity. Physiologic interest in renal tubular transport of urate is concerned with its bi-directional flux and the large number of factors influencing reabsorption or secretion.

urine   A solution of variable composition elaborated by the kidney and involving the separate processes of glomerular filtration and subsequent modification of filtrate by selective tubular reabsorption and secretion. The excretory function of the kidney may be regarded as the homeo-static preservation of the composition of body fluid. Thus, the composition of urine is best explained as varying according to the content of the remnant of extracellular fluid discarded after the kidney has selectively retained the solvent and solutes necessary to preserve a solution appropriate for the environment of body cells. In this sense the function of the kidney is to regulate the composition of what the body retains rather than what it excretes.

vasopressin (also *antidiuretic hormone; ADH*)   An octapeptide consisting of a five-membered ring made up of tyrosine, phenylalanine, glutamine, asparagine, and cystine plus a three-membered side chain made up of proline, glycinamide, and (in man and in some other mammals) arginine. Its secretion is regulated by the supraopticohypophyseal system in response to change in osmotic pressure of body fluid but also to a variety of other stimuli. It increases the permeability of the membranes of the distal convoluted tubule and collecting ducts to allow the increased passage of a variety of small molecules, chief of which is water.

washout curve (also *disappearance curve*)   The graphic depiction of the disappearance of a tracer substance from the kidney. Curves obtained with krypton or xenon give information about renal blood flow.

water

    extracellular water   That fraction of total body water which is external to cell membranes. It consists of the sum of plasma water and interstitial water but excludes cerebrospinal fluid, fluid within the collecting system of the urinary tract, the gastrointestinal tract, and the exocrine glands, and the aqueous humor of the eye. It is determined by measuring the distribution of a substance which diffuses freely through the cell membranes. Chemicals commonly used for this are inulin and radioactive sulphate. It is not certain, however, whether these substances, or others used for this measurement, are in fact limited to the extracellular compartment or whether they penetrate connective tissue fluid within the time allowed for equilibration. Depending upon what test substance is used, estimates of extracellular fluid volume vary from 16 to 20 percent of total body weight. **intracellular water** The total water content of body cells, taken as the difference between total body water and extracellular water. **total body water** The total amount of water contained in the body. It is usually estimated in vivo by determining the amount of a substance which is distributed throughout the total body water, e.g., tritiated water.

Clinical Terms

abscess, kidney   Small, raised, yellowish-white focus on the kidney surface, usually surrounded by a thin hemorrhagic zone, ordinarily representative of an abscess or marked chronic inflammation. Such lesions may also be seen in the cortex and may become confluent, forming large, yellowish-red areas.   **streak abscesses**   Yellow streaks which may be seen in the medulla in such cases. The parenchyma between the affected areas often appears to be normal.

acidosis, diabetic   See under DIABETES MELLITUS, MAJOR RENAL COMPLICATIONS OF.

acidosis, renal distal tubular (also *acidosis, renal tubular: distal adult type; gradient; permanent; type 1*)   A functional disturbance of the distal tubule, possibly hereditary in origin, characterized by the inability of the tubular cell to secrete enough hydrogen ion to ensure an appropriate gradient between urine and blood. Urinary pH is inappropriately high under conditions of an acid stimulus. Metabolic acidosis develops. (See ACIDOSIS in Physiology Glossary). Patients begin to show symptoms in infancy, chiefly lethargy, anorexia, apathy, and stunted growth. In some cases the disease may not be overt until maturity. Adult symptoms and signs are those of bone disease, hypokolemia, nephrocalcinosis, and nephrolithiasis. Interstitial nephritis is a common complication which may lead to a secondary reduction in glomerular filtration rate. About two-thirds of patients are female, sometimes with definite familial incidence, suggesting autosomal dominant inheritance with greater preponderance in females.

acidosis, renal proximal tubular (also *acidosis, renal tubular, type 2*)   A functional disturbance of the proximal tubule in which there is a defect in bicarbonate reabsorption. The clinical picture in children is mainly one of retarded growth. Bone lesions and nephrocalcinosis are absent, and there is only slight hypercalciuria.

acidosis, renal tubular   A condition in which there is a defect in renal excretion of hydrogen ion, or reabsorption of bicarbonate, or both (**mixed renal tubular acidosis**), which occurs in the absence of, or out of proportion to, an impairment in the glomerular filtration rate. See

also ACIDOSIS, RENAL DISTAL TUBULAR, and ACIDOSIS, RENAL PROXIMAL
TUBULAR.

acute nephritis See ACUTE POSTSTREPTOCOCCAL GLOMERULONEPHRITIS
under GLOMERULONEPHRITIS.

adenocarcinoma See CARCINOMA, RENAL CELL.

adenoma See RENAL AND BENIGN TUMORS under TUMORS in Pathology
Glossary.

adenomyosarcoma See WILMS' TUMOR.

ADH Antidiuretic hormone. See VASOPRESSIN in Physiology Glossary. See
also VASOPRESSIN, INAPPROPRIATE SECRETION OF in Syndrome Glossary.

adrenal tumor with renal involvement See EXTRARENAL MALIGNANT AND
INVASIVE TUMORS under TUMORS in Pathology Glossary.

adrenal-renal fusion Fusion of otherwise histologically and functionally
normal adrenal and renal masses without interposition of a connective
tissue capsule.

agenesis, renal Absence of the kidney or a grossly identifiable metanephric
structure. Agenesis may be unilateral or bilateral.

Unilateral renal agenesis is, per se, asymptomatic and associated with
normal renal function. **Bilateral renal agenesis** (the Potter syndrome)
is associated with a characteristic, if not completely specified, spec-
trum of abnormalities and with prenatal, intrapartum, or neonatal
death.

albuminuria Often used incorrectly for proteinuria. See PROTEINURIA.

aldosteronism See Syndrome Glossary.

alkaptonuria The excretion of alkaptones in the urine as a result of the
imperfect metabolism of tyrosine and phenylalanine. The incomplete
oxidation of these acids may recur and subside at irregular intervals
or may persist as a result of a congenital hereditary defect. If the urine
of alkaptonuric patients is left to stand or is alkalinized, it darkens.

Alport's disease (also *Alport's syndrome*) See NEPHRITIS, HEREDITARY
CHRONIC.

alveolar carcinoma See CARCINOMA, RENAL CELL.

amino acid storage disease Classified according to the specific amino
acid, e.g., glycogen storage disease.

aminoaciduria An abnormal elevation in the urinary amino acid excretion
rate. This may consist of an increase in a single amino acid, a specific
group of amino acids, or a generalized increase in many amino acids.

amyloidosis A condition in which there is extracellular deposition of abnormal proteinaceous material, which may or may not be associated
with antecedent or coexisting disease. Amyloid consists of fine fibrils
about 75 to 100 Å wide. It is characterized by metachromatic staining
with certain basic aniline dyes (e.g., crystal violet); by dichroic polarization following Congo red and similar stains; and by focal deposition
of IgG and C3. The deposition of amyloid may occur in any organ of
the body, and the kidney is very commonly involved. The glomerulus

is usually affected; in early lesions there is diffuse or nodular thickening of the mesangium and, to a lesser degree, of the capillary basement membrane. Massive deposits may compress and occlude capillary lumens. Clinically, renal amyloidosis may be completely asymptomatic; proteinuria is usually present, and occasionally a nephrotic syndrome develops. Uremia is often a terminal event.

amyloidosis, familial (also *hereditary amyloidosis*) Amyloidosis occurring in members of a family.

analgesic nephropathy (See Fig. 55 in Part II, Criteria for Diagnosis.) The fully developed stage of analgesic abuse, characterized in the kidney by papillary necrosis with secondary obstructive damage to the cortex. The columns of Bertin are frequently spared from this secondary change and stand out as ridges on the subcapsular surface. The condition is brought about by ingestion of large amounts of mixtures of analgesics, but the noxious agent cannot be pinpointed at the present time. Impairment of urinary concentrating ability is an early finding and hematuria and pyuria are common. Renal colic may follow sloughing of the papilla. Many of the patients have psychiatric problems. See also PHENACETIN TOXICITY.

anaphylactoid purpura nephritis See SCHÖNLEIN-HENOCH PURPURA NEPHRITIS.

anasarca Massive retention of fluid, including peripheral edema and serous effusions in the peritoneal and pleural spaces. The protein content of the fluids is low.

anesthetic agent toxicity Decreased perfusion pressure correlated with hypotension induced by general anesthetic agents, resulting in a decrease in glomerular filtration rate and renal blood flow. The use of halogenated compounds such as Fluothane may be toxic under certain circumstances, leading to high urinary output and renal failure.

aneurysm, renal arterial See under ARTERIES, RENAL, ABNORMALITIES OF.

angiitis, necrotizing See POLYARTERITIS.

angiokeratoma corporis diffusum universale See FABRY'S DISEASE.

antibiotic toxicity Damage to renal tissue as a result of antibiotic therapy. Diagnosis may be difficult because of the effects of the underlying disease on the kidney. Penicillins rarely cause a hypersensitivity nephritis. Systemic use of bacitracin or neomycin or excessive dosage of kanamycin, amphotericin, or polymyxins may be directly toxic and result in tubular necrosis. Renal damage due to vancomycin and cephaloridine has also been described. Tetracyclines may increase blood urea concentrations (liver effect), and when outdated and degraded, may cause a reversible aminoaciduria. Dimethylchlortetracycline has induced transient renal diabetes insipidus.

antidiuretic substance (ADH), inappropriate secretion of See VASOPRESSIN, INAPPROPRIATE SECRETION OF in Syndrome Glossary.

aplasia, renal Severe corticomedullary dysplasia in which the kidney is extremely small and structurally disorganized. The usual gross architectural arrangement is lacking, and dysplastic and primitive elements are apparent histologically. Sometimes, a few well-differentiated nephrons may be identified. Small cysts are frequently present. The ureter is commonly atretic, but patency may be encountered, and even megaureter may accompany rudimentary kidneys. The condition is usually unilateral. If bilateral, it is often associated with multiple congenital malformations. **lobular aplasia** (also *hypoplasia*) Aplasia in which the kidney has a markedly reduced number of reniculi and calyces, five or fewer. See also DYSPLASIA, RENAL.

arteries, renal, abnormalities of

Compression Very rarely, the main renal vessels are compressed by extrinsic tumors, muscle, or fibrous bands. The renal effects will depend on the degree of narrowing and the location—whether in the main renal artery or in primary branches.

Dilatation Dilatations of the main renal arteries, primary branches, and accessory arteries often occur in association with occlusive diseases. There are two main types: **aneurysmal** and **poststenotic.**

aneurysmal dilatation There are two types of aneurysmal dilatation. A **true aneurysm** results from a deficiency of the internal elastic membrane and media. It occasionally complicates atherosclerosis and polyarteritis nodosa, while it occurs regularly in medial fibroplasia. The aneurysm looks like a bead, and when two or more are found together, the arteriographic picture suggests a string of beads. The main renal physiologic derangements result from the hypertrophied ridges of media between aneurysms. The dilatations probably add to the distortions of these segments but otherwise have little hemodynamic significance. A **dissecting aneurysm** is due to localized disintegration of the internal elastic membrane which permits a hematoma to form. Dissecting aneurysms can complicate atherosclerosis but more commonly are found in intimal fibroplasia and fibromuscular hyperplasia. On the arteriogram the aneurysm is seen as an irregular dilatation that often follows abruptly after the area of stenosis. A dissecting aneurysm is, potentially, a severely occlusive lesion, particularly if arterial branches are affected.

poststenotic dilatation This characteristically accompanies atherosclerosis, intimal fibroplasia, and fibromuscular hyperplasia. On arteriography the dilatation appears as a smooth, usually symmetrical widening that tapers toward the proximally located stenosis.

Embolism This is a rare disorder of the renal circulation, usually found in patients with rheumatic heart disease with atrial fibrillation and subacute bacterial endocarditis. Cholesterol emboli can also occur, but these usually affect smaller arteries (see CHOLESTEROL EMBOLI). Embolism causes the signs, symptoms, and physiologic changes that are associated with sudden, complete obstruction.

Inflammation   Inflammatory lesions of the main renal artery are rare. The main renal artery can be narrowed just at its origin by arteritis extending from the aorta. This arteritis usually has histologic characteristics of "pulseless disease," or Takayashu's syndrome, and patients may or may not have symptoms suggesting occlusive disease of the aortic arch. The lesion produces stenosis because of intimal proliferation, but aneurysms can develop, since destruction of the media and internal elastic lamina can occur. Polyarteritis may affect the primary branches of the renal artery, although it usually involves smaller arteries. Thrombosis occurs frequently during the acute phase, producing segmental infarction. In addition, areas of the wall may be so weakened by fibrinoid necrosis that aneurysms result.

Ligation   Occasionally, an accessory lower polar renal artery is ligated in the course of a surgical repair of hydronephrosis, resulting in infarction.

Stenosis   This is almost entirely due to atherosclerosis or fibromuscular disease. When mild, it may be an incidental finding of no consequence. When severe, it may cause renovascular hypertension.

Thrombosis   Thrombosis of the main renal artery or primary branches occurs as a complication of other renal artery lesions. It may occur suddenly, causing acute infarction, with flank pain and hematuria. With less rapid development, the renal effects may be minimal.

arteriolar nephrosclerosis (also *arteriolonephrosclerosis* See RENAL ARTERIOSCLEROSIS under NEPHROSCLEROSIS.

arterionephrosclerosis   See RENAL ARTERIOSCLEROSIS under NEPHROSCLEROSIS.

arteriovenous fistula   See under DIALYSIS, KIDNEY.

arteritis, giant cell   See POLYARTERITIS.

arteritis, necrotizing (also *necrosing arteritis*)   See POLYARTERITIS.

arthritis, rheumatoid, renal disorders associated with   Proteinuria may occur in patients with advanced disease. The renal complications of rheumatoid arthritis are papillary necrosis secondary to treatment, and amyloidosis. There is frequently a low filtration fraction. In all cases, analgesic abuse must be excluded. See also GOLD NEPHROPATHY; ANALGESIC NEPHROPATHY.

artificial kidney   A device which removes or reduces the levels of waste products and other substances from the blood of patients with renal failure. Most equipment operates on the principle of dialysis across a semipermeable membrane. See also DIALYSIS, KIDNEY.

Ask-Upmark kidney   See SEGMENTAL HYPOPLASIA under HYPOPLASIA, RENAL.

atheroma (renal) with hypertension   See under HYPERTENSION, RENOVASCULAR.

auditory lesion   See under NEPHRITIS, HEREDITARY CHRONIC.

azotemia   Increased concentration of nonprotein nitrogen (NPN) in blood. In some countries it denotes only the concentration of NPN. **asymptomatic azotemia** Retention of nitrogenous products in renal insufficiency or severe dehydration.

bacteremic shock   See ENDOTOXIN SHOCK in Syndrome Glossary.

bacteriuria   The presence of bacteria in the urine.   **significant bacteriuria** The presence of more than 10^5 bacterial organisms per milliliter in freshly voided noncontaminated urine.

Baron Münchausen syndrome   See HEMATURIA, SELF-INDUCED.

Bartter's disease   See BARTTER'S SYNDROME in Syndrome Glossary.

Bence-Jones proteinuria   See PROTEINURIA. See also MYELOMA, RENAL INVOLVEMENT IN.

benign hematuria   See HEMATURIA, RECURRENT, WITH NEPHRITIS, ASSOCIATED WITH INFECTIOUS AGENTS.

benign Wilms' tumor   See NEPHROMA, MULTILOCULAR, CYSTIC.

Besnier-Boeck-Schaumann disease   See SARCOIDOSIS, RENAL INVOLVEMENT IN.

bichloride of mercury intoxication   See MERCURY TOXICITY.

bilharziasis   See SCHISTOSOMIASIS.

bilirubinuria   The presence of bilirubin in the urine. In excessive amounts it may stain the whole kidney and its casts. Its effect on the tubular cells is controversial.

bismuth toxicity   Soluble bismuth salts produce hyposthenuria, glycosuria, proteinuria, desquamation of tubular epithelial cells, and granular cylindruria, possibly followed by anuria or the nephrotic syndrome.

black-water fever   High fever, associated with dark (black) urine due to hemoglobinuria, occurs in patients living in or recently sojourning in malarious (falciparum) areas. See also RENAL FAILURE, ACUTE ANURIC OR OLIGURIC in Syndrome Glossary; HEMOGLOBINURIA; MALARIA, RENAL INVOLVEMENT IN.

blastomal tumor   See WILMS' TUMOR.

Boeck's sarcoid   See SARCOIDOSIS, RENAL INVOLVEMENT IN.

Bright's disease   Formerly used to describe any renal disorder characterized by proteinuria. The English physician Richard Bright (1789–1858) pioneered the modern clinical-pathologic approach to renal disease through his careful observations of symptoms and postmortem examinations. He linked coagulable urine, dropsy, and anasarca with pathologic changes in kidney structure, and described the course of nephritis with great accuracy. Bright thought that the varied appearance of the kidney noted in such disorders might represent successive stages of the same disease.

brucellosis   Any of a variety of pathologic changes produced by *Brucella* organisms: (1) a chronic granulomatous disease of the urinary tract and kidney, with necrosis, abscesses, and caseation resembling tuberculosis; if less intense, it mimics interstitial nephritis with infection (chronic pyelonephritis); (2) a transient renal infection resembling acute nephritis or acute pyelonephritis, sometimes with residual diffuse interstitial nephritis; (3) a diffuse interstitial nephritis with focal and segmental glomerular involvement, usually, but not always, associated with *Brucella* endocarditis.

Burnett's syndrome (also *milk-alkali syndrome*) See MILK-ALKALI in Syndrome Glossary.

cake kidney malformation See KIDNEY, CAKE.

calculi, renal See NEPHROLITHIASIS.

calculi, xanthine See XANTHINURIA AND XANTHINE CALCULI.

carbon tetrachloride toxicity Acute renal failure caused by dermal absorption, inhalation, or ingestion of carbon tetrachloride, with necrosis most apparent in proximal tubules and limbs of Henle. Alcohol increases the hazard by increasing absorption and possibly affecting metabolism. Hepatic necrosis may occur. Other halogenated hydrocarbons and organic solvents may also cause nephrotoxicity.

carcinoid tumor See METASTATIC TUMORS, under TUMORS in Pathology Glossary.

carcinoma, renal cell (also *hypernephroma; Grawitz's tumor; hypernephroid tumor* [obsolete]; *adenocarcinoma; clear cell tumor; alveolar carcinoma*) A malignant tumor of renal tubular origin and the most common of primary renal malignancies. It is more common in males than in females, with the highest incidence in the sixth and seventh decades.

casts See Pathology Glossary; see also CYLINDRURIA.

cephalopathia splanchnocystica See MICHEL'S SYNDROME in Syndrome Glossary.

cerebrohepatorenal syndrome See STILLWEDGER'S SYNDROME in Syndrome Glossary.

cerebro-oculorenal syndrome See OCULOCEREBRORENAL SYNDROME in Syndrome Glossary.

childhood nephrosis An obsolete term. See LIPOID NEPHROSIS.

cholesterol emboli Needle-shaped cholesterol crystals causing partial or complete obstruction of small parenchymal renal arteries and thought to originate from soft atheromatous aortic lesions, frequently following surgical procedures on the aorta. They may result in infarcts.

chyluria The presence of chyle in the urine. Chyle is a creamy suspension of fat globules and protein originating from intestinal absorption into the central lacteals and draining into the thoracic duct.

clear cell tumor See CARCINOMA, RENAL CELL.

colic, renal An intermittent, severe pain, lasting one or more hours. It is caused by obstruction of the upper urinary collecting system, which distends with urine and contracts with intermittent peristalsis. If the obstructing agent is a calculus which causes local ureteral muscle spasm, the pain is intensified. Pain distribution is over the kidney from back to front and along the ureter, with referral to the labioscrotal area.

congenital hepatic fibrosis   See HEPATIC FIBROSIS, CONGENITAL.

congenital medullary cystic disease   An obsolete term. See CYSTIC DISEASE, MEDULLARY.

copper storage disease (also *Wilson's disease; hepatolenticular degeneration*)   An autosomal recessive inborn error of metabolism in which excessive and toxic deposits of copper are found in almost all organs and tissues. Pathologic effects occur primarily in the liver and central nervous system, but renal plasma flow, glomerular filtration, tubular secretion, and tubular reabsorption may all be impaired by accumulations of copper in the kidney. Aminoaciduria, glycosuria, uricosuria, phosphaturia, hypercalciuria, defects in acidification, and the Fanconi syndrome are encountered. Nephrocalcinosis occurs rarely.

Coxiella burnetti (Q fever)   See under RICKSETTSIA DIAPORICA.

crush injuries   See under RENAL FAILURE, ACUTE ANURIC OR OLIGURIC in Syndrome Glossary.

crystalluria   The appearance of crystals in the urine. Characteristic crystals may appear in the course of certain metabolic diseases or during administration of certain drugs. These include sulfonamides, cystine in the various cystinurias, and other amino acids (such as leucine and tyrosine), which sometimes appear during the massive aminoaciduria occurring in hepatic necrosis. Other crystals may be found in urine, depending on the pH of the urine. In alkaline urines the following crystals may be found: ammonium urates, ammonium magnesium phosphates, calcium carbonate, and calcium phosphate. In acid urines, uric acid crystals or calcium oxalate crystals may occur. When urine has been refrigerated or is standing at room temperature, most crystalluria has little clinical significance.

cylindruria   The presence in the urine of an abnormal number of casts. See also CASTS in Pathology Glossary.

cystic disease, medullary (also *familial juvenile nephronophthisis; familial nephronophthisis; juvenile familial nephropathy with tapetoretinal degeneration; familial nephropathy with retinitis pigmentosa*) (See Figs. 56 to 58.) A diffuse nephropathy, either genetic or congenital in origin, usually seen in children or young adults and characterized by the insidious onset of anemia or uremia. There is little or no proteinuria and few or no formed elements in the urinary sediment. Polyuria or nocturia may precede onset by several months or years. Renal salt-wasting is frequently encountered, and serum sodium may be low. Acidosis with or without relative hyperchloremia is often seen. Retarded growth and evidence of bone disease are common in children. The course of the disease is variable, but is usually fatal within months or years following the appearance of anemia and uremia. Tapetoretinal degeneration may occur in some cases, and retinitis pigmentosa may occur in others. Medullary cystic disease is inherited as an autosomal dominant trait. If inheritance is autosomal recessive, the disease is called *familial juvenile nephronophthisis.*

cystic nephroblastoma See NEPHROMA, MULTILOCULAR, CYSTIC.

cystinosis A condition in which cystine is deposited in most tissues. It produces a generalized aminoaciduria, but not a selective cystinuria. It is often associated with the Fanconi syndrome. It is a serious and often fatal disease but is much rarer than cystinuria.

cystinuria A congenital and familial chronic tubular disease with reduced reabsorption of cystine, arginine, lysine, and ornithine. Two genetic varieties exist. Heterozygotes with the classic recessive type do not have excess cystine in the urine. Heterozygotes of less common incomplete recessive type do have increased cystine, and homozygotes have marked cystinuria. Cystinuria is asymptomatic, except when cystine calculi are formed.

cystitis A bladder infection with lower urinary tract symptoms such as frequency, urgency, dysuria, nocturia, or difficulty in completely emptying the bladder. The disorder is most common in women, and the incidence increases with age. The infection may also involve the ureters and kidneys.

cystocele A hernia of the bladder. The term is usually applied to the downward protrusion of the bladder into the vagina or introitus and subjacent anterior vaginal wall.

cysts

> **endometrial cysts** Cysts of müllerian origin arising in the midline below the bladder. They may enlarge retroperitoneally to the renal area and are differentiated from other cysts by the presence of endometrium and myometrium in the walls. They are discovered usually in the second and third decade of life. **multilocular renal cysts** Cysts which are split into multiple minor compartments. Those of congenital origin are very rare, unilateral, and do not communicate with the pelvis. They are usually discovered in children because of flank mass or hematuria, but may be present until old age without causing harm. They may be mistaken for tumor. **multiple bilateral cysts** Bilateral macroscopic simple cysts are commonly found in 50 percent of adult kidneys at autopsy and may be difficult to distinguish from early cystic disease. Urographic defects from larger cysts, when multiple and bilateral, may suggest polycystic disease. **pyelocalyceal cysts** See PELVIS, RENAL, ANOMALIES OF. **retroperitoneal cysts** Cysts that may arise from aberrant wolffian or müllerian anlage and may be single, multiple, or multilocular. They are usually unilateral, may attain a large size and may contain urine, lymph, blood, or seromucinous material. **simple renal cysts** Multiple bilateral cysts; single cysts; unilateral multicystic disease. **single cysts** Solitary congenital cysts of varying size and unknown origin which occur in the cortex, contain a fluid

resembling a transudate of plasma, and do not communicate with
the pelvis. They are significant clinically chiefly due to confusion with
parenchymal tumors. **teratodermoid cysts** Cysts containing ecto-
dermal material such as hair, teeth, and sebaceous material. They may
be attached to the kidney and adherent to the aorta. **unilateral multicystic disease** A congenital lesion in which the kidney is replaced by
varying-sized cysts. Remnants of atrophic nephrons or dilated tubules
may be the only renal tissue recognizable. Such kidneys are usually
discovered as a palpable flank mass in infants (see DYSPLASIA, RENAL).
cytomegalic inclusion disease A systemic disease of viral origin which is
characterized by granular acidophilic inclusion bodies due to an intrinsic defect of the distal tubule, which may be congenital or acquired.
congenital cytomegalic inclusion disease Renal diabetes insipidus
may be the sole manifestation of a familial disorder, probably sex-
linked, which occurs mostly in males and develops early in infancy. It
may also be associated with other inborn defects of tubular function as
in the Fanconi syndrome. **acquired cytomegalic inclusion disease**
Renal diabetes insipidus may develop in the course of chronic renal
disease of varying etiology, including infiltrative lesions of the kidney
and urinary tract obstruction. Diabetes insipidus-like symptoms unresponsive to vasopressin have also been noted in potassium deficiency,
in hypercalciuria from a variety of causes, and perhaps also following
excessive doses of salt-retaining steroids.

diabetes mellitus, major renal complications of
arterionephrosclerosis and arteriolonephrosclerosis These are more
commonly seen in the diabetic than in the nondiabetic population.
diabetic acidosis with acute renal functional impairment Severe diabetic acidosis is accompanied by acute impairment of renal function, including glomerular filtration rate and renal blood flow. Although blood
urea nitrogen may increase significantly, urine flow is maintained by
the osmotic effect of the glycosuria. The renal functional impairment
appears to be secondary to dehydration, increased blood viscosity,
hypovolemia, and cardiovascular collapse. It is readily reversed by
correction of the acidosis and dehydration. **diabetic glomerulosclerosis**
(See Figs. 59 and 60) This is one of the most common serious complications of diabetes. The lesion may antedate the development of proteinuria and clinical evidence of renal disease, which generally do not
appear until diabetes has been present for some years. Proteinuria
usually is the first sign. This may gradually increase to a sufficient degree to result in the nephrotic syndrome. Microscopic hematuria is
not uncommon. Although progression may take years, gradual decline
in renal function eventually leads to renal insufficiency and uremia.
Hypertension often develops as renal function declines. Histologically,
the earliest and commonest lesions are diffuse but irregular and variable

thickening of the mesangium and of the capillary basement membrane. Nodular lesions are less common but coexist with the diffuse lesions. They represent striking accumulations of mesangial matrix in the centers of peripheral lobules. The nodules vary in size and number and often are strongly acidophilic and positive to periodic-acid Schiff. Diffuse and nodular lesions may be accompanied by hyaline deposits (so-called exudative or insudative lesions). Arteriosclerosis and arteriolosclerois are almost the rule in diabetic patients with renal insufficiency. Diabetic glomerulosclerosis is part of a more generalized disease, diabetic microangiopathy, which involves small blood vessels in various parts of the body, including those of the retina. **papillary necrosis** Diabetes predisposes to papillary necrosis. **pyelonephritis** Some investigators believe that pyelonephritis is seen more commonly in the diabetic than in the non-diabetic population.

diabetic microangiopathy A disease of small blood vessels characterized by thickening of basement membranes and frequently by aneurysmal dilatations. It is most commonly seen in the kidney (see DIABETES MELLITUS, MAJOR RENAL COMPLICATIONS OF) and the retina, but also occurs in other locations.

dialysis disequilibrium syndrome See Syndrome Glossary.

dialysis, kidney The process by which molecules are removed from the blood of uremic patients by diffusion through a semipermeable membrane into a surrounding dialysis fluid.
hemodialysis Dialysis in which the blood of the uremic patient is brought into contact with an inert membrane. The diffusible molecules pass through the membrane into the dialysis fluid, loosely termed **dialysate.** Access to the circulation is gained through an external arteriovenous fistula (Quinton-Scribner shunt) or an internal, surgically induced arteriovenous fistula (Bresco-Cimino shunt). **peritoneal dialysis** Dialysis in which the dialysis fluid is introduced into the peritoneum of the uremic patient, and the living membrane serves passively to separate the smaller from the larger molecules. See also ARTIFICIAL KIDNEY.

dialysis, peritoneal See DIALYSIS, KIDNEY.

distal adult type renal tubular acidosis See ACIDOSIS, RENAL DISTAL TUBULAR.

doll kidney See SIMPLE HYPOPLASIA under HYPOPLASIA, RENAL.

doughnut kidney See under KIDNEY, FUSED.

dwarf kidney See SIMPLE HYPOPLASIA under HYPOPLASIA, RENAL.

dwarfism, renal See RENAL RICKETS.

dysplasia, renal A malformation of the kidney marked by microscopic abnormalities variously attributed to developmental arrest or failure to differentiate, with persistence of fetal structures or mesonephric tissue, or both. Dysplasia can be unilateral or bilateral, cortical or medullary, focal, segmental, or total (aplasia). It is often associated with urinary tract malformation, especially obstructive anomalies of the ureter. Dysplastic kidneys may be large or small, normally shaped or misshapen, cystic or not cystic. The dysplastic elements present may include: (1) primitive ducts, lined by relatively tall columnar epithelium, often ciliated, and surrounded by fibromuscular collars; (2) nests of metaplastic cartilage, principally in the cortex; (3) primitive glomeruli, in which the tuft is covered by cuboidal epithelium. These glomeruli undergo hyalinization and sclerosis; (4) primitive tubules, lined by crowded columnar epithelium resembling that of undifferentiated fetal tubules; (5) primitive ductules, surrounded by narrow collars of lamellated connective tissue; and (6) cysts of glomerular, tubular or ductular origin. See also APLASIA, RENAL; HYPOPLASIA, WITH DYSPLASIA; KIDNEY, MULTICYSTIC.

dysproteinemia A nonspecific generic term for a group of diseases involving metabolic abnormalities in plasma proteins. These abnormalities are usually qualitative, as in the case of multiple myeloma, but may also be simply quantitative, as in the case of Waldenström's macroglobulinemia, in which there is excess production of IgM immunoglobulin. Qualitative or quantitative alterations in plasma proteins may affect any protein fraction and have been reported to involve not only the globulins and albumins but also the lipoproteins.

dystrophy, cerebro-oculorenal See OCULOCEREBRORENAL SYNDROME in Syndrome Glossary.

eclampsia and preeclampsia See Syndrome Glossary.

ectopia, renal The congenital malposition of one or both kidneys. Ectopic kidneys may be asymptomatic throughout life.

simple ectopia A lumbar, iliac, or pelvic malposition involving one or both kidneys. Pelvic kidneys may be fused, forming a flat mass from which two ureters arise. **crossed ectopia** Ectopia in which the ureter crosses the midline before draining distally.

Displacement of one or both kidneys to the thorax or posterior mediastinum through defects in the diaphragm is an acquired rather than a congenital defect. Renal ptosis, the hypermobility of the kidney in the retroperitoneal space, is not considered renal ectopia.

embryoma See WILMS' TUMOR.

encephalopathy, hypertensive Acute cerebral manifestations, especially convulsions, associated with severe hypertension and accompanied by papilledema and renal failure.

endocarditis, subacute bacterial, nephritis associated with Two classes of glomerular lesions occur frequently in patients with subacute bacterial endocarditis, those of focal embolic glomerulonephritis and those of diffuse glomerulonephritis (indistinguishable from poststreptococcal glomerulonephritis).

endometriosis See METASTATIC TUMORS under TUMORS in Pathology Glossary.

endotoxin shock See Syndrome Glossary.

enuresis Micturition during sleep (bed-wetting).

epidemic hemorrhagic fever (also *Far East hemorrhagic fever; Songo fever; Korean fever; epidemic hemorrhagic nephrosonephritis; Kokka disease; Nidoko disease*) An acute febrile, probably viral, infection associated with loss of plasma, hemorrhagic phenomena, and acute renal insufficiency due to extreme congestion of the renal medulla.

epidemic hemorrhagic nephrosonephritis See EPIDEMIC HEMORRHAGIC FEVER.

essential hypertension See PRIMARY HYPERTENSION under HYPERTENSION.

ethylene glycol nephrotoxicity Rapidly fatal poisoning associated with sheaves of needle-shaped calcium oxalate crystals in the tubular lumen may follow ingestion of ethylene glycol. Patients not succumbing at once may suffer acute renal failure, with death in uremia. In addition at the oxalate deposition, severe swelling of the proximal convoluted tubules and focal hemorrhagic necroses in the cortex are found in these patients.

exercise proteinuria See PROTEINURIA.

Fabry's disease (also *angiokeratoma corporis diffusum universale*) An inborn sex-linked error of metabolism with accumulation of glycolipid (ceramide plus two or three molecules of monohexose) intracellularly in all organs, especially in the muscle cells of the smaller arteries. The characteristic dermal vascular lesions, which appear around puberty, are papillary telangiectatic lesions, most conspicuous on lower abdomen, upper thighs, buttocks, and scrotum; they may regress during early adulthood. Diffuse limb pains are a common complaint. The kidneys are severely affected, with inevitable kidney failure and death in uremia in affected males. Renal disease may occur in the absence of skin lesions. Carrier females may have vascular lesions and, rarely, renal involvement.

failure, acute renal See RENAL FAILURE, ACUTE OLIGURIC; RENAL FAILURE, ACUTE POLYURIC in Syndrome Glossary.

familial congenital hemorrhagic nephritis See NEPHRITIS, HEREDITARY CHRONIC.

familial juvenile nephronophthisis See CYSTIC DISEASE, MEDULLARY.

familial Mediterranean fever (FMF) A hereditary disease mainly affecting Middle Eastern or North African ethnic groups. It is characterized by fever, repeated acute episodes of pain in the joints, abdomen, and thorax, and, more rarely, an enlarged spleen, pericarditis, and purpura. Onset may be during childhood, with the disease persisting over several decades. Renal involvement is most often due to renal amyloidosis. The clinical signs include proteinuria, the nephrotic syndrome, and renal failure. The renal failure is usually progressive, leading to death several years after onset. The amyloid disease may be a familial amyloidosis genetically associated with FMF rather than a complication of the latter.

familial nephronophthisis See CYSTIC DISEASE, MEDULLARY.

familial nephropathy with retinitis pigmentosa See CYSTIC DISEASE, MEDULLARY.

familial renal diabetes (also *familial renal glycosuria*) Glycosuria due to familial renal tubular anomaly.

Fanconi syndrome, idiopathic, infantile, and adult See Syndrome Glossary.

Far East hemorrhagic fever See EPIDEMIC HEMORRHAGIC FEVER.

febrile proteinuria See PROTEINURIA.

fetal lobulation Separation of the kidney into lobes by residual clefts (shallow linear indentations). Fetal lobulation may persist in adults.

fibroma, kidney See RENAL AND BENIGN TUMORS under TUMORS in Pathology Glossary.

fibromuscular disease A general term for a variety of nonatherosclerotic renal artery lesions, primarily affecting the intima or media.

Intimal fibroplasia usually occurs in children or young adults. It produces stenosis by a segmental circumferential accumulation of fibrous tissue applied to the internal elastic membrane. In younger patients, the elastica is usually intact, while in older ones it is often broken, with dissecting aneurysms resulting. **Fibromuscular hyperplasia** or **dysplasia** represents various gross and microscopic alterations in the development and relations of the intima, media, elastic tissue, and adventitia of the renal arterial wall. Usually, there is a localized or generalized overgrowth of the media, comprising smooth muscle, fibrous tissue, or both. The artery may be tortuous, internally corrugated, and frequently stenotic. The internal corrugation can give rise to a "string-of-beads" appearance in the angiogram. The lesion is found primarily in women between the ages of 30 and 50 and is commonly bilateral (see also HYPERTENSION, RENOVASCULAR). **Medial fibroplasia** with microaneurysms produces the string-of-beads arteriogram (see DILATATION under ARTERIES, RENAL, ABNORMALITIES OF). The lesion is found primarily in women between the ages of 30 and 50 and is commonly bilateral. **Subadventitial fibroplasia** is also a disease of women but expresses itself at an earlier age, usually between 20 and 40 years. It produces severe stenosis through deposition of dense collagen in the outer portion of the media. It occurs more frequently on the right than on the left; when it is bilateral, the right side is always more severely affected.

fibromuscular hyperplasia See FIBROMUSCULAR DISEASE.

fibromuscular hypoplasia Dysplasia of the renal artery, intimal, medial, or adventitial. See also HYPERTENSION, RENOVASCULAR.

fibroplasia, intimal; medial; subadventitial See under FIBROMUSCULAR DISEASE.

fibrosis, retroperitoneal A disease manifested by the formation of dense fibrous tissue in the retroperitoneum. The fibrous tissue may displace and obstruct the ureter(s) and inferior vena cava, thus leading to renal impairment and inferior vena cava obstruction. It may spread to involve the mediastinum. In some instances the disorder follows administration of methysergide for the treatment of migraine.

fistula, arteriovenous See under DIALYSIS, KIDNEY.

flea-bitten kidney See KIDNEY, FLEA-BITTEN.

Fluothane toxicity See under ANESTHETIC AGENT TOXICITY.

FMF See FAMILIAL MEDITERRANEAN FEVER.

focal glomerulitis with recurrent hematuria See HEMATURIA, RECURRENT, WITH NEPHRITIS, ASSOCIATED WITH INFECTIOUS AGENTS.

focal glomerulonephritis See HEMATURIA, RECURRENT, WITH NEPHRITIS, ASSOCIATED WITH INFECTIOUS AGENTS.

foot process disease See LIPOID NEPHROSIS.

frequency Abnormally frequent urination.

fusion, renal See KIDNEY, FUSED.

galactosemia A metabolic disorder in which there is a deficiency in galactose 1-phosphate-uridyl transferase. The disorder is transmitted as a hereditary recessive trait. Clinical signs include physical and mental retardation, liver disorders, and cataract development. Tubular dysfunction in this disorder results in proteinuria, hyperaminoaciduria, and hypokalemia. Clinical signs may be prevented by eliminating lactose and galactose from the diet.

giant cell arteritis See POLYARTERITIS.

glomerular capillary endotheliosis See PREECLAMPSIA AND ECLAMPSIA in Syndrome Glossary.

glomerulonephritis

  acute benign hemorrhagic glomerulonephritis An infectious disorder, presumably viral in origin, in which focal glomerulitis and transient hematuria occur in association with nonstreptococcal pharyngitis. **acute poststreptococcal glomerulonephitis** (See Fig. 61.) A disorder characterized by the abrupt onset of proteinuria, hematuria, and often cylindruria, which may or may not be associated with edema, circulatory congestion, hypertension, or evidence of renal functional impairment, either alone or in combination, five days to six weeks after onset infection due to certain strains of group A streptococci. Rarely, similar disease may occur following or concurrently with onset of infection. The histologic features include diffuse proliferative or exudative glomerulitis, or both, with or without crescent formation. Characteristic electron-dense subepithelial deposits ("humps") are apparent on electron microscopy. **focal glomerulonephritis** See HEMA-

TURIA, RECURRENT, WITH NEPHRITIS, ASSOCIATED WITH INFECTIOUS
AGENTS; also ACUTE BENIGN HEMORRHAGIC GLOMERULONEPHRITIS under
GLOMERULONEPHRITIS. **hereditary glomerulonephritis** See CHRONIC
HEREDITARY NEPHRITIS under NEPHRITIS. **hypocomplementemic glomerulonephritis** See MEMBRANOPROLIFERATIVE GLOMERULONEPHRITIS
under GLOMERULONEPHRITIS. **lobular glomerulonephritis** See GLO-
MERULAR LOBULATION in Pathology Glossary; also MEMBRANOPROLIFER-
ATIVE GLOMERULONEPHRITIS under GLOMERULONEPHRITIS. **membranoproliferative glomerulonephritis** (also *hypocomplementemic glomerulonephritis; mesangial proliferative glomerulonephritis; mesangiocapillary glomerulonephritis*) A chronic glomerulonephritis of unknown
origin, most commonly appearing in late childhood or early adolescence. The complement level is usually depressed but fluctuates. The
histologic findings consist of proliferation and sclerosis of the mesangium and thickening of the capillary wall, the latter apparently due
to circumferential mesangial extension between the endothelium and
basement membrane and to deposits of complement (C3), gamma
globulin, and sometimes fibrin. When there is a striking mesangial
proliferation, the lesion assumes a lobular pattern. **mesangial proliferative glomerulonephritis** See MEMBRANOPROLIFERATIVE GLOMERU-
LONEPHRITIS under GLOMERULONEPHRITIS. **mesangiocapillary glomerulonephritis** See MEMBRANOPROLIFERATIVE GLOMERULONEPHRITIS under
GLOMERULONEPHRITIS **rapidly progressive glomerulonephritis** See
Syndrome Glossary.

glomerulosclerosis

congenital glomerulosclerosis A condition observed in autopsies of
some infants in which small, involuting, and scarred glomeruli are
seen scattered in the cortex. Usually, there are no alterations in the
corresponding tubules unless the lesion is widespread. If a large part
of the cortex is affected, tubular atrophy and fibrosis of the interstitium
may be found as well, and the condition is known as **congenital nephrosclerosis** or **congenital chronic glomerulonephritis.** It is a cause of
renal insufficiency in the first year of life. **intercapillary glomerulosclerosis** See DIABETIC GLOMERULOSCLEROSIS under DIABETES MELLI-
TUS, RENAL COMPLICATIONS OF.

glycinuria The excretion of abnormal quantities of glycine in the urine;
a type of aminoaciduria. **hereditary glycinuria** A rare hereditary condition, transmitted as a dominant, which is characterized by hyper-
glycinuria without hyperglycemia, apparently due to diminished reabsorption of glycine in the renal tubules. Some patients with this defect
suffer from recurrent calcium oxalate stones containing small amounts
of glycine.

glycogen in proximal tubules Glycogen inclusions may occur in poorly
controlled diabetes, primarily in the pars recta of the proximal convo-

luted tubules. The morphologic finding is termed the *Armanni-Ebstein lesion*. See also INCLUSIONS in Pathology Glossary.

glycogen storage disease (also *Von Gierke's disease*) A disorder characterized by deficiency of the enzyme glucose 6-phosphatase and accumulation of glycogen in the liver and kidney. Clinical signs usually appear in the first year of life and include hepatomegaly, hyperlipemia, glycosuria, aminoaciduria, and episodes of acidosis. Morphologic findings in the kidneys include enlargement and pallor seen grossly, and tubular vacuolization due to glycogen deposition microscopically. Occasionally, patients with glucose 6-phosphatase deficiency may manifest some or all of the features of the Fanconi syndrome.

glycosuria The excretion of abnormal quantities of glucose in the urine. Normally, 100 to 200 mg per 24 hours of reducing substances may be found in the urine. This includes glucose, other sugars, and non-sugar-reducing substances such as ascorbic acid. Glycosuria is usually secondary to plasma glucose elevations that exceed the reabsorptive capacity of the tubule. It may also occur in association with lowered renal tubular reabsorptive capacity for glucose (normoglycemic or renal glycosuria). **self-induced glycosuria** Glycosuria in patients who add or cause to be added surreptitiously to their urine glucose or other sugars, or who ingest or absorb other substances which induce glycosuria. The abnormality may be ascribed to spontaneous disease, and the patient may thereby gain sympathy, admission to a hospital, or other ends.

gold nephropathy Disease occurring in a small percentage of patients treated with organic gold salts. Proteinuria and eventually a nephrotic syndrome appears. Subendothelial immune deposits or gold deposits, or both, may be present in the lysosomes of the proximal segment of the tubules. Cessation of therapy usually clears up the lesions. In some cases systemic lupus erythematosus rather than gold therapy may be the cause of arthritis and proteinuria. See also ARTHRITIS, RHEUMATOID, RENAL DISORDERS ASSOCIATED WITH.

Goodpasture's syndrome See LUNG PURPURA WITH NEPHRITIS.

gouty kidneys See HYPERURICEMIC NEPHROPATHY; also INFARCTS, URIC ACID.

gradient acidosis See ACIDOSIS, RENAL DISTAL TUBULAR.

gram-negative shock See ENDOTOXIN SHOCK in Syndrome Glossary.

granulomata, urate Accumulations of needle-shaped urate crystals in collecting tubules, associated with destruction of tubular cells and surrounded by mononuclear and giant cells. The granulomata may result in tubular obstruction and secondary pyelonephritis. They are commonly found in gout and less frequently in other conditions associated with hyperuricemia.

granulomatosis, Wegener's A chronic disease of unknown etiology affecting the nasopharynx, lungs, and kidneys. The renal lesion is characterized by vasculitis and focal proliferative glomerular lesions with occasional necrotic lobules. Granulomas also are common in the kidney. The rate of development of renal insufficiency is variable. Hypertension is common. Pulmonary lesions may represent granulomas, vasculitis, or cavities. Nasopharyngeal lesions vary widely.

Grawitz's tumor   See CARCINOMA, RENAL CELL.

halogenated hydrocarbon toxicity   See CARBON TETRACHLORIDE NEPHROTOXICITY.

hamartoma, infantile mesenchymal   See RENAL AND BENIGN TUMORS under TUMORS in Pathology Glossary.

Hartnup disease   A rare inborn error of renal tubular amino acid transport involving decreased reabsorption of the monoamine monocarboxylic acids except glycine, proline, and hydroxproline. No other tubular functions are impaired. It is inherited as a mendelian autosomal recessive gene. The disorder appears to lead to an increased requirement of nicotinamide, so that only moderately deficient diets produce a pellagra-like rash. This is often accompanied by cerebellar ataxia, diarrhea, and psychotic symptoms, all abating with large doses of nicotinamide.

heart disease, hypertensive   A disorder of the heart in which left ventricular hypertrophy occurs in response to the increased work load imposed by arterial hypertension. It is characterized by electrocardiographic changes involving left axis deviation, increase of left ventricular voltage in the precordial leads, S-T wave alterations, and, often, signs of left atrial enlargement. With further progression, cardiac enlargement becomes apparent on chest x-ray, and left ventricular failure may occur. Coronary insufficiency may accompany hypertensive heart disease, secondary to hypertrophy to the left ventricle and atherosclerosis of the coronary arteries.

hemangioma, capillary   See RENAL AND BENIGN TUMORS under TUMORS in Pathology Glossary.

hemangioma, cavernous   See RENAL AND BENIGN TUMORS under TUMORS in Pathology Glossary.

hematuria   The occurrence of excessive numbers of red blood cells in the urine. It may be gross (evident on mere inspection of the urine) or microscopic (evident only when examining the urinary deposit by microscope.)

Initial hematuria refers to the excretion of blood only at the onset of micturition, which is characteristic of a urethral lesion; **terminal hematuria** is most notable at the end of micturition and indicates a lesion of the posterior urethra or base of the bladder. **Total hematuria** indicates an excretion of blood throughout the micturition, and its origin is usually above the bladder.

hematuria, hereditary See CHRONIC HEREDITARY NEPHRITIS under NE-
PHRITIS.

hematuria, recurrent, with nephritis, associated with infectious agents
(also *focal glomerulonephritis with recurrent hematuria; benign hematuria*) A form of glomerulonephritis with recurrent attacks of gross
or microscopic hematuria, often associated with a variety of infections,
usually of the upper respiratory tract. Edema and hypertension are
uncommon prior to the terminal stages. Histologically, the appearance
of the kidneys is most often like that seen in focal glomerulonephritis,
but sometimes a diffuse lesion is found. One form, which is benign, is
associated with the presence of IgA in the mesangium.

   self-induced hematuria (also *Baron Münchausen syndrome*) Macroscopic or microscopic hematuria stimulated by patients who, by themselves or with the help of others, cause their urine to be contaminated
with human or animal blood. Many of these patients have underlying
psychiatric disturbances.

hemodialysis See DIALYSIS, KIDNEY; also ARTIFICIAL KIDNEY.

hemoglobinemia The presence of free hemoglobin in the blood plasma,
as when intravascular hemolysis occurs.

hemoglobinuria The appearance of free hemoglobin or its derivatives in
the urine in excess of the saturation of plasma haptoglobin. Hemoglobinuria must be differentiated from the lysis of erythrocytes due to
a very dilute or alkaline urine during hematuria. The chief varieties of
hemoglobinuria are as follows:

1. Hemoglobinuria from acute intoxications. Examples are arsine inhalation, naphthalene injections, ingestion of certain mushrooms
   such as *Amanita phalloides*, and sensitivity to fava bean.
2. Hemoglobinuria due to entry of fresh water into the blood.
3. Hemoglobinuria from septicemia with hemolytic bacteria such as
   Clostridium perfringens.
4. Hemoglobinuria in black-water fever, a complication of malaria.
5. Hemoglobinuria from incompatible transfusion.
6. Hemoglobinuria from extensive burns.
7. Paroxysmal cold hemoglobinuria. In this syndrome the attacks are
   provoked by cold followed by rewarming.
8. Paroxysmal nocturnal hemoglobinuria (also *Marchiafava-Micheli
   syndrome*). This form of hemoglobinuria is associated with hemosiderinuria, which continues between attacks.
9. Effort hemoglobinuria (also *march hemoglobinuria*). This occurs
   in long-distance runners, although it may also appear after short
   sudden marches in those unaccustomed to such exercise.

hemolytic uremic disease See Syndrome Glossary.

hemosiderosis Deposits of hemosiderin in many organs, including renal
tubules. It is associated with hemosiderinuria.

hepatic fibrosis, congenital, renal lesions in A familial (usually recessive) syndrome characterized by manifestations of portal hypertension in childhood or adolescence or subsequently associated with immature mesenchymatous expansion of hepatic portal spaces and irregularly branching portal biliary ductules (virtually never by cystic expansion of portal bile ducts). In about half of reported cases, the patients have cystic or polycystic kidneys. Some few of these appear to be examples of infantile polycystic disease in which the patients survive the newborn period. In about half of reported cases the kidneys are normal.

hepatolenticular degeneration   See COPPER STORAGE DISEASE.

hereditary chronic nephritis   See CHRONIC HEREDITARY NEPHRITIS under NEPHRITIS.

hereditary glomerulonephritis   See CHRONIC HEREDITARY NEPHRITIS under NEPHRITIS.

hereditary hematuria   See CHRONIC HEREDITARY NEPHRITIS under NEPHRITIS.

hereditary nephritis   See CHRONIC HEREDITARY NEPHRITIS under NEPHRITIS.

high altitude sickness, chronic   See HYPOXIA, HIGH ALTITUDE.

Hodgkin's disease, renal involvement in   Compression of the pedicle and ureteral constriction by tumor are the more common renal complications of Hodgkin's disease. The infiltrate rarely involves the kidney directly but more often involves the periureteral tissue, retroperitoneal lymph nodes, and nodes in the vicinity of the renal vascular pedicle. There may also be hypercalcemia with nephrocalcinosis, secondary amyloidosis, urate nephropathy, or nephrotic syndrome.

horseshoe kidney   See under KIDNEY, FUSED.

hydronephrosis   Dilatation of the renal pelvis and calyceal system, with varying degrees of reduction of the renal parenchyma. The dilatation is the result of obstruction to urine flow, which may come about from a tumor or a number of congenital causes, including Calarbon's disease, congenital narrowing at the pelviureteric junction, neuromuscular disorders such as spina bifida, congenital valves in the posterior urethra, and congenital narrowing of urethra or ureter.

hypercalcemia   An increased level of calcium in the serum. Among the causes of hypercalcemia are hyperparathyroidism, hyperthyroidism, vitamin D intoxication, malignancies with or without bone metastases, and immobilization, usually associated with bone fractures. A hormone originating in the thyroid gland, thyrocalcitonin, appears to help prevent hypercalcemia by inhibiting osteoclastic bone resorption.

hypercalciuria   An excess of calcium in the urine. Hypercalciuria may be found in any condition associated with hypercalcemia. It occurs without hypercalcemia in renal tubular acidosis, in an idiopathic form and in normocalcemic hyperparathyroidism.

hyperkalemia   An increased level of potassium in the serum. It may result from the inadequate renal excretion that occurs in a variety of renal diseases, or following too rapid infusion of potassium salts. It may also be induced by using outdated blood. No specific effects on the kidney are known.

hyperlipidemia Excess amounts of fats and related lipids in the blood, often seen in the nephrotic syndrome.

hypernatremia An increased level of sodium in the blood.

hypernephroid tumor An obsolete term. See CARCINOMA, RENAL CELL.

hypernephroma See CARCINOMA, RENAL CELL.

hyperparathyroidism, secondary to impaired renal function Overactivity of the parathyroid glands secondary to diminution in ionized serum calcium. This may lead to autonomous overactivity of the parathyroid glands (**tertiary hyperparathyroidism**).

hyperparathyroidism, tertiary See under HYPERPARATHYROIDISM, SECONDARY TO IMPAIRED RENAL FUNCTION.

hyperphosphatemia An increased level of phosphorus in the serum. This occurs most often in chronic renal insufficiency due to reduced glomerular filtration rate. In hypoparathyroidism, excessive tubular reabsorption of phosphorus occurs because of insufficient parathyroid hormone, leading to hyperphosphatemia.

hypersensitivity Nephropathies resulting from hypersensitivity to therapeutic agents are described under ANESTHETIC AGENT TOXICITY; ANTIBIOTIC TOXICITY; BISMUTH TOXICITY; GOLD NEPHROPATHY; IRON DEXTRAN TOXICITY; OSMOTIC DIURETIC TOXICITY; SALICYLATE TOXICITY; and SULFONAMIDE TOXICITY. See also ANALGESIC NEPHROPATHY; NEPHRITIS, CHRONIC INTERSTITIAL; PAPILLARY NECROSIS.

hypertension

arterial hypertension An elevation of the arterial blood pressure above the normal range. Although no sharp distinction exists between normal and abnormal values, a systolic blood pressure of about 140 mm Hg may be considered **systolic hypertension,** while a diastolic pressure above 90 may be regarded as **diastolic hypertension.** Most population studies show increases with age. Transient elevation of diastolic pressure may represent a physiologic fluctuation or an early manifestation of disease. Persistent diastolic hypertension may be related to a variety of underlying conditions and is frequently associated with the development of cardiomegaly and arterial and arteriolar vascular disease.

diastolic hypertension with renal involvement Disease of the renal blood vessels regularly accompanies diastolic hypertension that is either of long duration or of the **malignant** type. It seems to be related to elevated arterial pressure because it occurs in association with most **secondary** forms of hypertension, as well as in the **primary** type. It is lacking in young people with mild hypertension and in patients with thoracic aortic coarctation. Further, in unilateral arterial stenosis, the unaffected kidney can show the characteristic lesions, but these are lacking in the affected one, which is perfused at a lower arterial pressure.

Intrarenal vascular disease is primarily arteriolar and is termed either **benign** or **malignant arteriolonephrosclerosis,** depending on the type of lesion found. Arteriosclerosis also occurs, but it is usually not so prominent as is arteriolosclerosis. In the **benign** form, arterioles show a patchy hyaline thickening of the entire wall, with afferent arterioles being more affected than efferent. Probably as a consequence, some glomeruli undergo changes that finally result in complete sclerosis. In addition to these lesions, there may be fibroelastic intimal thickening of interlobular arteries, associated with reduplication of the internal elastic lamina. In arteries of larger size, the lumen is sometimes narrowed by intimal thickening and increased width of the media. In hypertension of long duration, these arterial lesions can be so severe that patchy cortical atrophy results. The hyaline arteriolar change that characterizes this vascular disease can occur in older people in the absence of hypertension; however, in the presence of hypertension it occurs at a younger age and is more severe.

In the **malignant** form of arteriolonephrosclerosis, two types of arterial lesions occur. One of these (which mainly involves small and medium-sized arteries) is an "onion-peel" lamellar hyperplasia produced by endothelial proliferation and reduplication of the elastica. The other (which mainly affects arterioles) is fibrinoid necrosis of the wall, which often contains lipid-laden histocytes and red blood cells. This necrosis can extend into the glomerulus. Although this is a diffuse disease, the extent of involvement is extremely variable. The lesions of malignant hypertension can occur alone in the case of severe hypertension of brief duration, but are usually found in conjunction with benign arteriolosclerosis because the malignant phase often develops in the course of hypertension rather than de novo.

Renal function is variably affected by benign and malignant nephrosclerosis, depending on the degree of arteriolar and glomerular involvement. In some patients with the benign form, there may be no evidence of renal disease throughout a long course. In others, excretory function decreases very slowly over many years, with proteinuria eventually developing. Renal failure rarely occurs; when it does, it is often accompanied by cortical scarring, resulting from obliterative sclerosis of small and medium-sized arteries.

The effect of malignant nephrosclerosis on renal function is vastly different from the benign form. This is potentially a rapidly advancing vascular disease; as afferent arterioles and glomeruli become progressively affected, excretory function decreases progressively, and renal failure usually ensues. Proteinuria is present, except in the early stages of the disease. Cylindruria is common, and microscopic hematuria is frequent. See also RENAL ARTERIOLOSCLEROSIS under NEPHROSCLEROSIS.

essential hypertension   See PRIMARY HYPERTENSION.

malignant hypertension (also *accelerated hypertension*)   A disorder characterized by severe hypertension with rapidly progressive vascular damage. Malignant hypertension may arise de novo, be superimposed on primary hypertension of long duration, or be secondary to other, renal and extrarenal, causes of hypertension. The diastolic pressure is usually greater than 140 mm Hg, and there is marked neuroretinopathy, resulting in flame hemorrhages, soft cotton-wool exudates, and papilledema. Congestive heart failure, hypertensive encephalopathy, intracerebral hemorrhage, and malignant nephrosclerosis are frequent sequelae.

postpartum hypertension   Transient hypertension occurring several days to a week after delivery.

primary hypertension (also *essential hypertension*)   An increase of diastolic blood pressure for which no recognizable cause may be found. Primary hypertension is the most common type of elevated blood pressure, showing a strong familial tendency. The age of onset is generally between 20 and 50 years. There is an increased incidence of primary hypertension in women, in blacks, and in patients with diabetes mellitus. Although affected patients may be asymptomatic and free of complications for a number of years, cardiomegaly and arterial and arteriolar vascular disease frequently develop. Hypertension with a prolonged course is often referred to as benign; with a rapidly progressive course as malignant.

renal hypertension   An elevation of diastolic blood pressure secondary to renal parenchymal disease, occlusive disease of the renal arteries, or obstruction of the urinary tract. Renal hypertension may be associated with an increased concentration of renin in the renal venous blood and sometimes in the peripheral blood.

renoprival hypertension   An elevation of diastolic pressure found in the anephric patient. Renoprival hypertension in man is very sensitive to alterations of intravascular or extravascular fluid volume.

renovascular hypertension   An increase of diastolic blood pressure secondary to occlusive disease of the main renal artery, its primary branches, or aberrant renal vessels. Renovascular hypertension is most commonly caused by atherosclerotic lesions and by fibrous and fibromuscular dysplasias. Aneurysm, thrombosis, embolism, arteritis, and extrinsic compression of the renal artery are uncommon causes.

secondary hypertension   An elevation of diastolic blood pressure for which a specific cause may be found. Conditions associated with secondary hypertension include renal arterial and parenchymal diseases, endocrine disorders, diseases of the central nervous system, preeclampsia, and coarctation of the aorta.

hyperthermia, renal trauma due to   Exposure to high environmental temperatures and severe exercise may result in impaired renal function varying from mild proteinuria and increased urinary cellular excretion to acute oliguric renal failure. Recovery is usually complete, but sequelae of interstitial fibrosis with proteinuria and diminished function can occur.

hyperuricemic nephropathy Renal damage associated with elevation of serum uric acid, whether primary or secondary. Several types of damage occur: (1) Deposition of sodium bi-urate crystals, mainly in the renal medulla; (2) formation of uric acid calculi (patients with uric acid stones show a persistently low urinary pH, which may contribute to the stone formation); (3) a greater degree of arterionephrosclerosis and arteriolonephrosclerosis than expected for age and blood pressure.

hypervitaminosis D An excess of vitamin D. This may cause hypercalcemia, which may result in nephrocalcinosis.

hypocomplementemic glomerulonephritis See MEMBRANOPROLIFERATIVE GLOMERULONEPHRITIS under GLOMERULONEPHRITIS.

hypokalemia A decrease in serum concentration of potassium in the blood.

hypokalemic nephropathy (also *kaliopenic nephropathy*) Potassium deficiency resulting from a variety of causes. Among these are vomiting, diarrhea, small bowel suction, repeated enemas, and loss of fluid through intestinal fistulas. It may be induced by endocrine disorders (e.g., aldosterone-secreting tumors), diuretic drugs, and following the use of steroid hormones. It may be one result of chronic renal disease (potassium-losing nephritis). Both acute and chronic potassium deficiency affect the kidney.

acute hypokalemic nephropathy Initially, the potassium deficiency state produces reversible functional and anatomical defects in the kidney. These are nocturia, hyposthenuria, conspicuous vacuolization of proximal convoluted tubule cells, and dilatation of subbasilar extracellular compartments. **chronic hypokalemic nephropathy** With prolonged potassium deficiency, a progressive chronic interstitial nephritis develops, with nocturia, hyposthenuria, and loss of concentrating ability. **self-induced hypokalemic nephropathy** (also *purgative hypokalemic nephropathy*) Patients ingest purgatives, usually surreptitiously, to produce watery diarrhea day after day. Sometimes this is done in the mistaken belief that daily purgation cleanses the bowel and body. Enemas may also be taken each day, or less frequently, to "wash the bowel clean." The result is a chronic hypokalemia with alkalosis, and chronic hypokalemic nephropathy develops. Many of these patients have neuroses or psychiatric disturbances and may complicate their water and electrolyte problems by self-induced vomiting or anorexia or by taking diuretics.

hyponatremia A decrease in the level of sodium in the blood. See SALT-WASTING NEPHRITIS in Syndrome Glossary.

hypophosphatemia A decrease in the level of phosphorus in serum. As in the case of calcium, serum phosphorus concentration is maintained by numerous interacting variables, including phosphorus absorption from the gut, renal tubular reabsorption of phosphorus as determined by parathyroid hormone, glomerular filtration rate, and acid-base balance. Hypophosphatemia occurs in sprue, rickets, hyperparathyroidism, and in certain types of renal disease in which tubular reabsorption of phosphrous is impaired.

hypoplasia, renal A congenital anomaly in which one or both kidneys appear externally normal but are very small. Hypoplasia may occur with or without dysplasia.

lobular hypoplasia See APLASIA, LOBULAR. **oligonephronic hypoplasia** A bilateral condition characterized by extremely small kidneys without evidence of dysplasia or malformation of the urinary tract. There is a reduced number of pyramids and nephrons, with hypertrophy of the nephrons present. (Glomeruli may be two to three times larger than in normal infants.) The condition leads to interstitial fibrosis and nephronal atrophy. Glomerular sclerosis, initially focal, is progressive. **pluricystic hypoplasia** Very small kidneys with no evidence of dysplasia and with regular, intense, and diffuse dilatations of all tubules. **segmental hypoplasia** (also *Ask-Upmark kidney*) Hypoplasia of varying degree without dysplasia, often associated with hypertension and usually occurring in one kidney only. The affected lobe is distinguished by a transverse groove on the capsular surface, which marks the site of a thin hypoplastic segment overlying an elongated calyx-like recess of the renal pelvis. The hypoplastic lobe contains both malformed cortex and medulla and histologically appears to consist entirely of thyroid-like, cystically dilated tubules, numerous tortuous and thickened arterioles, and sclerosed or resorbed glomeruli. Glomeruli may also be completely absent. The vascular pattern indicates primary malformation rather than acquired disease, since the cortex of affected areas consist entirely of juxtamedullary nephrons. **simple hypoplasia** (also *miniature kidney, doll kidney, dwarf kidney*) The renal mass is significantly reduced without parenchymal maldevelopment; the tissue is histologically normal. **hypoplasia with dysplasia** A significant reduction in renal mass accompanied by all gradations of malformation and dysplasia, which may be generalized or segmental in distribution. A semblance of normal architecture is retained: renal lobes, calyces, and pelvis are recognizable. The diagnosis of dysplasia is based on the findings of primitive ducts and metaplastic cartilage. Other primitive elements are also present in the cortex, which often contains small cysts. The cysts are frequently peripheral, subcapsular, and along the interlobular tissues.

hypothermia, renal trauma due to Cold-induced injury is usually functional, with reversible lowering of PAH clearance, Tm_{PAH}, and

Tm$_G$. Tubular abnormalities predominate, so that polyuria may result, with urine approaching the composition of glomerular ultrafiltrate. The main effects are presumed due to decreased metabolic activity and increased blood viscosity.

hypoxia   A condition in which insufficient oxygen is delivered to a tissue or organ, permanently or temporarily causing dysfunction and secondary adjustments designed to increase oxygenation.

anemic hypoxia   In chronic anemia (and absence of heart failure) the increase in hematocrit is associated with a rise in renal plasma flow and glomerular filtration but a fall in the filtration fraction. **hemorrhagic hypoxia**   Moderate sudden hemorrhages produce a drop in systemic arterial pressure with a rise in renal vascular resistance and fall in renal blood flow. A temporary oliguria with urine of high specific gravity is followed by diuresis associated with vasodilation and a lowered blood viscosity as hemodilution occurs. If hemorrhage is severe, with prolonged hypotension (and, presumably, prolonged hypoxia), acute oliguric renal failure may follow. In both cases, glomerular filtration is greatly reduced. **high altitude hypoxia**   Moderate hypoxia in unacclimatized subjects causes an increase in glomerular filtration rate, renal blood flow, and urine flow, but severe acute hypoxia depresses all these functions. In acclimatized subjects born at high altitudes, inulin and para-amino hippurate clearances are depressed. This is most marked in subjects with chronic high altitude sickness (Monge's disease), some of whom show proteinuria. **hypoxia associated with chronic hypoxic lung disease**   Glomerular and tubular sizes increase; glomerular filtration rate and renal blood flow decrease. Oliguria and proteinuria may occur acutely, with diminished clearances. **hypoxia associated with cyanotic heart disease**   Subjects with this condition develop glomerular enlargement and mesangial hyperplasia, together with proteinuria and depression of glomerular filtration rate and para-amino hippurate. The severity of the histologic and functional alterations is proportional to the degree of arterial hypoxia and the length and extent of compensatory polycythemia. In a few subjects the nephrotic syndrome may develop.

idiopathic nephrotic syndrome in children   See LIPOID NEPHROSIS.

iminoglycinuria   Increased excretion of imino acids (especially iminoglycine) in patients with chronic renal insufficiency and osteodystrophy.

inclusion disease, cytomegalic   See CYTOMEGALIC INCLUSION DISEASE.

incontinence   Inability to prevent the discharge of urine.

Stress incontinence results from an increase in intraabdominal pressure through coughing, lifting, sneezing, or bending over. **Overflow incontinence** occurs when the bladder is overdistended as a result of urethral or prostatic obstruction or faulty vesical innervation. **Urgency**

incontinence usually is associated with inflammatory disease of bladder or urethra. **Sphincteric incontinence** results from mechanical damage to the urethral sphincters.

infarct, kidney surface   See Pathology Glossary.

infarct, renal   Necrosis caused by interruption of the circulation, either arterial or venous. Arterial obstruction is usually dependent on pre-existing vascular disease (cardiac disorders producing embolism or local arteriosclerotic narrowing). Trauma, congenital aneurysms, vasculitis, and compression by adjacent tumors are rare causes. Venous thrombosis may be associated with amyloidosis, sepsis, and dehydration (especially in infants) or with neoplasma (especially those invading or compressing the renal veins or cava). Hypercoagulable states seem to be a major factor in some; others seem idiopathic. Venous infarcts are hemorrhagic, usually massive, and often bilateral. See also RENAL VEIN THROMBOSIS.

infarcts, uric acid   Amorphous urate deposits in the collecting tubules commonly found in the kidneys of infants during the first few days of life. They are easily recognized grossly by the pale yellow, streaked appearance of the renal pyramids.

insufficiency, acute renal   See RENAL FAILURE, ACUTE in Syndrome Glossary.

insufficiency, chronic renal   See RENAL INSUFFICIENCY, CHRONIC in Syndrome Glossary.

internal radiation   See RADITION NEPHRITIS under NEPHRITIS.

interstitial nephritis   See under NEPHRITIS.

iron dextran toxicity   Interstitial nephritis caused, on rare occasions, by iron dextran in sensitized individuals.

iron storage disease   Renal iron pigment deposition and interstitial fibrosis caused, occasionally, by hemosiderosis or hemochromatosis.

juvenile familial nephropathy with tapetoretinal degeneration   See CYSTIC DISEASE, MEDULLARY.

kaliopenic nephropathy   See HYPOKALEMIC NEPHROPATHY.

kidney, artificial   See ARTIFICIAL KIDNEY.

kidney, Ask-Upmark   See SEGMENTAL HYPOPLASIA under HYPOPLASIA, RENAL.

kidney, cake   A form of crossed renal ectopia in which the posterior surface of the organ is smooth and concave, while the anterior surface, from which the ureters emerge, is lobulated.

kidney, coarsely granular   Irregular, uneven, usually large depressed scars separated by irregular elevations on the surface of diseased kidneys. See also KIDNEY, FINELY GRANULAR.

kidney, contracted   A small, markedly shrunken kidney with a thick adherent capsule and diffuse scarring of the surface, which is usually both finely and coarsely granular. In addition, the surface may show haphazardly scattered large elevations of varying sizes measuring from 0.5 to 2 cm and separated by deep V-shaped or wedge-shaped scars. Small cysts are usually present.

kidney, doll   See SIMPLE HYPOPLASIA under HYPOPLASIA, RENAL.

kidney, dwarf   See SIMPLE HYPOPLASIA, under HYPOPLASIA, RENAL.

kidney, ectopic   See ECTOPIA, RENAL.

kidney, failure, acute oliguric   See RENAL FAILURE, ACUTE ANURIC OR OLIGURIC in Syndrome Glossary.

kidney, failure, acute polyuric   See RENAL FAILURE, ACUTE POLYURIC in Syndrome Glossary.

kidney, finely granular   Appearance sometimes noted when a diseased kidney is stripped of its capsule. Small, pale, fairly uniform elevations measuring up to 0.2 cm are seen, separated by dark, shallow, thin depressions. The elevations are due to small foci of dilated tubules, and the depressions are areas of atrophy and scarring.

kidney, flea-bitten   Fine petechial venous hemorrhages distributed haphazardly in the kidney. They are usually associated with subacute bacterial endocarditis or bacteremia.

kidney, fused   The connection of normally lateralized renal organs or renal masses on the same side of the body (crossed ectopia with fusion) (see ECTOPIA, RENAL). The most common form of renal fusion, the **horseshoe kidney,** may be characterized as inferior polar fusion with mild caudal ectopia and hyporotation. The isthmus between normally lateralized renal masses may be other than caudal (e.g., cephalic, giving rise to horseshoe kidney; concave downward-medium; or multiple, producing the **ring** or **doughnut kidney**). Fusion often occurs between pelvic or sacral ectopic kidneys and also somewhat inhibits normal medial rotation of the renal masses.

kidney insufficiency, chronic   See RENAL INSUFFICIENCY, CHRONIC in Syndrome Glossary.

kidney, large white (also *large pale kidney*)   A condition associated with the nephrotic syndrome. The kidney is enlarged and swollen, the capsule tense, the surface smooth and pale, a cut section bulging, and corticomedullary markings indistinct. The medulla is often darker than the cortex. In some instances, yellow lipid deposits may be present in the cortex (**myelin kidney**).

kidney, medullary sponge   See SPONGE KIDNEY, MEDULLARY.

kidney, microcystic   See MICROCYSTIC DISEASE; also NEPHROTIC SYNDROME, CONGENITAL in Syndrome Glossary.

kidney, miniature   See SIMPLE HYPOPLASIA under HYPOPLASIA, RENAL.

kidney, multicystic   A kidney distorted and enlarged by cysts varying in size, in severe corticomedullary dysplasia. Remnants of atrophic nephrons or dilated tubules may be the only renal tissue recognizable.

Multicystic kidney is usually unilateral, and ureteral atresia is almost always an accompanying finding. Such a kidney is usually discovered as a palpable flank mass in infants. See also DYSPLASIA, RENAL.

kidney, myelin See under KIDNEY, LARGE WHITE.

kidney, papillary necrosis of See PAPILLARY NECROSIS.

kidney, supernumerary A third kidney smaller than normal which is entirely free or only loosely attached to a normal kidney. It usually lies inferior to the normal one, but occasionally lies in the pelvis or above the normal kidney. The blood supply to the extra kidney is variable, usually derived from the closest arterial source. The ureters of the supernumerary and adjacent kidneys usually fuse somewhat along their course, commonly just proximal to their entrance into the bladder. In some cases the ureters may be reduplicated, so that three ureteral orifices may be present. Occasionally, the third ureter ends in the vulva, vagina, or prostatic urethra.

Kimmelstiel-Wilson (nodular) lesion Rounded nodules of hyaline material in the glomerular mesangial areas almost characteristic of diabetic glomerulosclerosis.

Kokka disease See EPIDEMIC HEMORRHAGIC FEVER.

Korean fever See EPIDEMIC HEMORRHAGIC FEVER.

lead toxicity A tubular syndrome with proteinuria, glycosuria, aminoaciduria, and increased excretions of lead, delta aminolevulinic acid, coproporphyrin, urobilinogen, and bile pigments. Chronic interstitial nephritis leading to small fibrotic kidneys has been associated with chronic exposure to lead. Pathologic changes may include nephrosclerosis, tubular degeneration, and scarring and concretions within the tubules believed to be lead salts incrusted with calcium. Acid-fast intranuclear inclusion bodies have also been described. Encephalopathy, anemia, hypertension, mild proteinuria, tophaceous gout, and renal insufficiency are usual clinical findings.

leiomyoma See RENAL AND BENIGN TUMORS under TUMORS in Pathology Glossary.

Leptospira icterohaemorrhagiae, canicola, autumnalis, bataviae A large group of antigenically distinct microorganisms comprising the genus *Leptospira*, some of which cause disease in man. A variety of mammals, including cattle, swine, dogs, and various rodents, are natural hosts for *Leptospira* and excrete them in the urine. Man usually acquires the infection through direct contact with contaminated water. Most infections are benign and self-limiting, characterized by fever, headaches, vomiting, myalgia, and conjunctival infection. Infections with *L. icterohaemorrhagiae* are more often associated with severe disease, with symptoms which may include jaundice, renal failure, hemorrhages, severe prostration, and vascular collapse. The kidneys are involved early in the course of the disease with variable oliguria, proteinuria, hematuria, and renal insufficiency.

leukemia, lymphatic, renal involvement in Lymphatic leukemia may be associated with local or diffuse kidney infiltration. The diffuse type can produce striking renal enlargement but only rarely leads to chronic renal failure. Renal amyloidosis may complicate lymphatic leukemia.

leukemia, myelogenous, renal involvement in Leukemic cells often infiltrate the renal parenchyma. Hemorrhages from renal infiltrates frequently give rise to hematuria. Hyperuricemia is common and may lead to renal insufficiency.

lipoid nephrosis (also *foot process disease, idiopathic nephrotic syndrome of children, minimal change disease, minimal lesion disease, nil disease, pure nephrosis*) A form of the nephrotic syndrome with recurrent edema and highly selective proteinuria. The condition is more common in infants and children, but occurs at all ages. Spontaneous recovery may occur, particularly in children. This disease is associated with a minimal histologic lesion on light and electron microscopy in the glomerulus. The etiology is unknown, but it may be associated in some cases with allergy.

lipoma See RENAL AND BENIGN TUMORS under TUMORS in Pathology Glossary.

lithiasis See NEPHROCALCINOSIS; NEPHROLITHIASIS.

lobular aplasia See under APLASIA.

lobular glomerulonephritis See MEMBRANOPROLIFERATIVE GLOMERULONEPHRITIS under GLOMERULONEPHRITIS. See also GLOMERULAR LOBULATION in Pathology Glossary.

lordotic proteinuria See ORTHOSTATIC PROTEINURIA under PROTEINURIA.

Lowe's syndrome (also *cerebro-oculorenal dystrophy*) See OCULOCEREBRORENAL SYNDROME in Syndrome Glossary.

lung purpura with nephritis (also *Goodpasture's syndrome; hemorrhagic and interstitial pneumonitis with nephritis; hemorrhagic pulmonary renal syndrome*) (See Figs. 62 and 63.) An idiopathic disorder more common in males than females and usually occurring in young adults. Patients usually present with hemoptysis and dyspnea. Anemia and urinary abnormalities are usually discovered incidentally. The course and recurrent pulmonary opacities may be indistinguishable from those of idiopathic pulmonary hemosiderosis until urinary abnormalities appear, but thereafter very rapid progression to uremia ensues.

lupus erythematosus See SYSTEMIC LUPUS ERYTHEMATOSUS.

lupus nephritis See SYSTEMIC LUPUS ERYTHEMATOSUS.

lymphangiectasis, pericalyceal See PELVIS, RENAL ANOMALIES OF.

lymphosarcoma Lymphocytic cells in lymphosarcoma commonly invade the kidney, perirenal, and periureteral tissue. Renal insufficiency is rare, but function may be compromised by extrinsic pressure from lymphatomous nodes and by periureteral fibrosis.

macroglobulinemia with renal involvement See DYSPROTEINEMIA.

malacoplakia A form of chronic inflammation, characteristically of the lower urinary tract, with production of sessile soft polypoid foci of chronic inflammation, including histiocytes with characteristic ferruginous inclusions (Michaelis-Guttman bodies). Exceptionally, the same lesions occur in the renal parenchyma (and in the rectum, gallbladder, or retroperitoneal tissues).

malaria, renal involvement in Various renal disorders, clinical and pathologic, that may be associated with infection with malarial parasites. Among them are the nephrotic syndrome, interstitial nephritis (*Plasmodium malariae*) and black-water fever (*P. falciparum*).

malignant nephroma See WILMS' TUMOR.

maple sugar urine disease A hereditary recessive defect in metabolism of the keto acids that corespond to the branched chain amino acids leucine, isoleucine, and valine. Of the several abnormal organic acids found in serum and urine, the alpha-hydroxyacids probably contribute the odor from which the disorder derives its name. The defect is associated with mental retardation, and the affected children usually die in infancy.

Marchiafava-Micheli syndrome See PAROXYSMAL NOCTURNAL HEMOGLOBINURIA under HEMOGLOBINURIA.

mechanical causes of nephrotic syndrome See NEPHROTIC SYNDROME in Syndrome Glossary.

medullary cystic disease See CYSTIC DISEASE, MEDULLARY.

medullary sponge kidney See SPONGE KIDNEY, MEDULLARY.

membranoproliferative glomerulonephritis See MEMBRANOPROLIFERATIVE GLOMERULONEPHRITIS under GLOMERULONEPHRITIS.

membranous nephropathy A disease of long duration, which mostly affects adults. It is characterized by massive proteinuria and a slowly progressive nephrotic syndrome. There is no known treatment. In some cases, spontaneous cessation of proteinuria occurs. Ultimately, chronic renal insufficiency may supervene. The histologic lesions consist of diffuse membranous changes, with protein deposits mainly on the epithelial side of the capillary basement membrane, separated by projections (spikes) of the basement membrane. The deposits contain gamma globulin and complement (C3) in a characteristic diffuse granular distribution.

mercury toxicity (also *sublimate poisoning; bichloride of mercury intoxication*) Acute renal insufficiency caused by consumption of or exposure to a mercuric salt. Oliguria may occur after ingestion of as little as 0.4 gm (usually more than 2 gm) and lasts an average of two weeks. The urine usually contains protein, epithelial cell casts, and red cells.

Glycosuria and aminoaciduria may occur. Gastrointestinal symptoms, with hemorrhage, tissue necrosis, and increased tissue catabolism, account for a mortality rate approaching 50 percent, despite dialysis therapy. Smaller quantities of inorganic mercury or organic compounds such as mercurial diuretics may cause milder acute renal failure or, on prolonged exposure, the nephrotic syndrome. Inhalation of mercury vapors may also cause renal damage.

microangiopathy, thrombotic   See HEMOLYTIC UREMIC SYNDROME in Syndrome Glossary.

microcystic disease   This manifests in infancy or early childhood as the congenital nephrotic syndrome (see Syndrome Glossary), but in older children it has been reported as a form of slowly progressive renal insufficiency with little change in the urinary sediment or urine except for a concentrating defect. Eventually, anemia, azotemia, and renal osteodystrophy develop. The biopsy lesion may be misinterpreted and called chronic pyelonephritis. Closer scrutiny will demonstrate the dilated tubules to be truly cystic. The glomeruli may also be seen to be cystic.

milk-alkali syndrome   See Syndrome Glossary.

minimal change disease, minimal lesion disease   See LIPOID NEPHROSIS.

Monge's disease   See HIGH ALTITUDE HYPOXIA under HYPOXIA.

Moschcowitz's syndrome   See THROMBOTIC THROMBOCYTOPENIC PURPURA.

multicystic kidney   See KIDNEY, MULTICYSTIC.

multilocular cystic nephroma   See NEPHROMA, MULTILOCULAR, CYSTIC.

multilocular renal cyst   See under CYSTS.

Münchausen, Baron, syndrome   See HEMATURIA, SELF-INDUCED.

myeloma, renal involvement in   Proteinuria in myeloma can be of three kinds: (1) plasma proteins, (2) myeloma proteins (Bence Jones protein), and (3) mixtures of (1) and (2). If the proteinuria is severe enough, a nephrotic syndrome may develop. In patients with myeloma, acute renal insufficiency can supervene if intravenous pyelography is done. This is thought to be due to dehydration and may be the result of interaction between the myeloma proteins in the cells and the contrast medium. Numerous hard, glassy casts are present in the tubule, mainly in the distal, but also in the proximal portion; these are associated with various degrees of giant cell reaction. Protein droplets appear in the tubular cells. Syncytial changes of the epithelial cells is often seen, and plasma cell infiltrates may be present.

myoglobinemia   See MYOGLOBINURIA.

myoglobinuria   The appearance of myoglobin in the urine. This may follow severe physical exertion, especially in the untrained. Myoglobinuria may also occur in various disorders such as the crush syndrome, exposure to toxins and poisons (Haff disease), and in myopathies. See also RENAL FAILURE, ACUTE, ANURIC OR OLIGURIC in Syndrome Glossary; HEMOGLOBINURIA.

necrotizing papillitis See PAPILLARY NECROSIS.

nephritis

> **acute nephritis** See ACUTE POSTSTREPTOCOCCAL GLOMERULONEPHRITIS under GLOMERULONEPHRITIS. **acute interstitial nephritis** This manifests clinically as a form of acute nephritic syndrome or acute renal insufficiency which results from hypersensitivity to drugs. In addition, it may develop as a result of infections (poststreptococcal, and so on) and acute deposition of uric acid. See ACUTE NEPHRITIC SYNDROME and RENAL FAILURE, ACUTE ANURIC OR OLIGURIC in Syndrome Glossary. **Balkan nephritis** A chronic progressive endemic familial nephropathy of unknown origin occurring in the Balkan area of the Danube basin. **chronic hereditary nephritis** (also *hereditary glomerulonephritis, hereditary hematuria, hereditary nephritis, familial congenital hemorrhagic nephritis, Alport's syndrome*) A hereditary diffuse nephropathy more severe in males than in females and characterized by intermittent hematuria or pyuria, or both, and beginning in childhood. The disease usually is progressive, especially in young adult males. Nerve deafness is common, but hypertension and ocular defects are uncommon manifestations. Survival past middle age is rare. The mechanism of inheritance appears to be a dominant gene, though not necessarily an autosomal one, since affected males frequently give rise to disproportionately large numbers of involved females. **chronic interstitial nephritis** A term used to describe renal interstitial cellular infiltration (lymphocytes, plasma cells, and sometimes eosinophils), and fibrosis, with variable degrees of tubular damage, particularly to the lower nephron. Glomerular involvement is late. The disorder is manifested by impaired urinary concentration; there is minimal or no proteinuria. The sediment may be normal or contain only a few white cells and white cell casts unless it is infected. The condition usually progresses very slowly, with hypertension and, eventually, chronic renal insufficiency. It is a picture common to many conditions, such as infections, ischemia, hypersensitivities, analgesic abuse, sickle cell anemia, residue of severe acute renal insufficiency, hypokalemic and hyperkalemic states, and obstruction of the urinary tract. **lupus nephritis** See SYSTEMIC LUPUS ERYTHEMATOSUS. **poststreptococcal nephritis** See GLOMERULONEPHRITIS, ACUTE. **radiation nephritis** Interstitial nephritis resulting from irradiation exceeding 2300 rads. In addition to the interstitial nephritis, arterioles may be affected, hypertension is common, and renal insufficiency is often rapidly progressive. **systemic lupus erythematosus nephritis** See SYSTEMIC LUPUS ERYTHEMATOSUS.

nephroblastoma See WILMS' TUMOR.

nephrocalcinosis The deposition of calcium salts in the renal tissue. This is commonly medullary but also occurs, rarely, on the surface of the kidney (tramline calcinosis following cortical necrosis) or in the cortex (glomerulonephritis). Nephrocalcinosis is usually the result of proximal tubular acidosis. It may also occur in association with hypercalcemic states and vitamin D toxicity. Local calcium deposits occur in tuberculosis or infarcts.

nephrolithiasis (*renal calculi*) A common disorder, especially in hot dry areas, and endemic in certain regions. Calculi are bilateral in about 10 percent of cases and recurrent in the same proportion. The chief organic substances involved are uric acid cystine and xanthine. In many patients, systemic predisposing factors exist, such as hyperparathyroidism, other hypercalcemic and hypercalciuric states (e.g., sarcoidism and prolonged immobilization), hyperuremic states, cystinuria, and xanthinuria. Local factors favoring stone formation include obstruction and infection.

nephroma, multilocular, cystic (also *multilocular renal cyst; cystic nephroblastoma; benign Wilms' tumor*) Circumscribed, unilateral multilocular lesion enclosed in a capsule that often contains dysontogenic mesenchymatous tissue (smooth muscle, cartilage, striated muscle).

nephronophthisis, familial juvenile See CYSTIC DISEASE, MEDULLARY.

nephropathica epidemica A fibrile disease, presumed to be viral in origin, associated with oliguria, heavy proteinuria, moderate renal insufficiency and rapid recovery. It occurs in north central Sweden during the winter, mostly among lumbermen.

nephropathy, hypokalemic See HYPOKALEMIC NEPHROPATHY.

nephropathy, uric acid See HYPERURICEMIC NEPHROPATHY.

nephrosclerosis

renal arteriosclerosis Renal manifestation of general arteriosclerosis. The arteries show atheroma, thickening of the media with duplication of the elastic lamina, and fibroelastic intimal thickening. Narrowing of the lumen may ensue, with ischemic changes in the corresponding segments of the parenchyma, leading to segmental atrophy and scarring. If the main renal artery is severely affected, the whole kidney undergoes atrophy. **renal arteriolosclerosis** Occlusive changes in the renal arterioles associated with hypertension or diabetes mellitus. In the benign form there is hyaline thickening of the walls of the afferent arterioles. When the changes are associated with diabetes, the efferent arterioles are also involved. Slowly progressive renal insufficiency may follow, with glomerulosclerosis, tubular atrophy, and interstitial fibrosis. In the malignant form there is "onion-peel" thickening of the intima of interlobular and arcuate arteries, fibrinoid necrosis of the afferent arterioles, wrinkling of the glomerular capillary walls, and glomerular necrosis. Rapidly progressive renal insufficiency ensues. Histologically identical lesions may occur in a variety of chronic renal diseases. See also HYPERTENSION, DIASTOLIC, WITH RENAL INVOLVEMENT.

nephrosis See LIPOID NEPHROSIS.

neurogenic bladder Dysfunction of the urinary bladder resulting from injury or disease of the central or peripheral nervous system.

Nidoko disease   See EPIDEMIC HEMORRHAGIC FEVER.

nil disease   See LIPOID NEPHROSIS.

obstructive uropathy   See UROPATHY, OBSTRUCTIVE.

oligonephronic hypoplasia   See under HYPOPLASIA, RENAL.

oliguric renal failure   See RENAL FAILURE, ACUTE ANURIC OR OLIGURIC in Syndrome Glossary.

organic solvents toxicity   See CARBON TETRACHLORIDE TOXICITY.

orthostatic proteinuria   See under PROTEINURIA.

osmotic diuretic toxicity   Marked dilatation of tubules with vacuole formation in renal tubular cells, sometimes resulting from the use of osmotic diuretics. These changes are attributed to the effect of increased urinary flow and intraluminal osmotic pressure on renal cellular fluid. They may be seen with hyperglycemia, following infusion of hypertonic sucrose or urea, and in patients given mannitol, dextran, and a variety of other salts and sugars. Functional impairment is rare.

osteitis   See under RENAL OSTEODYSTROPHY.

osteodystrophy, renal   See RENAL OSTEODYSTROPHY.

osteoporosis   See under RENAL OSTEODYSTROPHY.

oxalate deposition   Oxalate deposition occurs in oxalosis, after ingestion of prophyleneglycol, or in association with pentane anesthesia.

oxalosis   Widespread deposition of calcium oxalate crystals. Hyperoxaluria is useful in establishing the diagnosis, but the methods of analysis are difficult and often unreliable. More important is demonstration of the crystalline composition of calculi, which should be mainly calcium oxalate monohydrate on crystallographic analysis. Perhaps most definitive is the demonstration of oxalate crystals on renal biopsy (numerous birefractile crystals in polarized light that do not take up von Kossa's stain). The crystals may be positively identified by polarography or x-ray diffraction. Organs other than the kidneys may demonstrate oxalate infiltration.

papillary necrosis (also *papillary necrosis of the kidney, renal medullary necrosis, papillitis necroticans, necrotizing papillitis*)   Necrosis of one or more renal pyramids or of their distal parts: (1) as a complication of pyelonephritis; (2) in patients with diabetes mellitus; (3) as a complication of an obstructive uropathy; (4) in association with frequent and/or prolonged intake of analgesic drugs, especially phenacetin; (5) in patients with sickle cell disorders; (6) in cyclophosphamide toxicity; or (7) occurring idiopathically.

papillitis necroticans   See PAPILLARY NECROSIS.

pelvis, renal, anomalies of

calyceal diverticulum (pyelocalyceal cysts)   The cysts are usually asymptomatic, but stones or infection may cause complications.

extrarenal anomalies Virtually all the pelvis may be visible outside the kidney parenchyma. This is of no clinical importance. **pericalyceal lymphangiectasis** Dilated lymph channels along the major renal lymph ducts produce single or multiple peripelvic cysts. They may reach a large size and simulate a tumor radiographically.

pentosuria An inborn error of metabolism involving a block in the glucuronic acid oxidative pathway. This is a benign condition, although it may be confused with diabetes. It is transmitted as an autosomal recessive, almost exclusively in Jews. The condition is diagnosed by demonstrating excretion of more than one gram of xylose per 24 hours.

periarteritis nodosa See POLYARTERITIS.

pericalyceal lymphangiectasis See under PELVIS, RENAL, ANOMALIES OF.

perinephric abscess An abscess in the perirenal fat tissue closely associated with the kidney and originating from an inflammatory process in the kidney or renal pelvis. The clinical signs are swelling of the loin on the affected side, sometimes associated with a diaphragmatic elevation, severe pain, fever, chills, rigors, and bacteremia. Radiologic examination is helpful. White cells appear in the urine.

perinephric or retroperitoneal hematoma Massive bleeding in the perirenal tissue, usually due to trauma but sometimes spontaneous, especially in pregnancy. It may be a complication of percutaneous renal biopsy which usually does not necessitate surgical treatment but in exceptional cases makes nephrectomy necessary. There is severe intractable loin and back pain, which may be unaffected by analgesics. Hematuria may be present. There may be associated loin swelling, sometimes mild ileus fever, and increasing white blood cell count. The hematocrit is decreased. The patient should not be moved after biopsy, as is sometimes done for x-ray examination for possible retroperitoneal hemorrhage, as this tends to increase the bleeding.

periodic disease See FAMILIAL MEDITERRANEAN FEVER.

permanent renal tubular acidosis See ACIDOSIS, RENAL DISTAL TUBULAR.

phenacetin toxicity A condition of chronic interstitial nephritis with a high frequency of papillary necrosis, which may result from excessive ingestion of phenacetin or of mixed analgesic compounds. Phenacetin or its metabolites or a manufacturing contaminant, acetic-4 are the suspected toxins. Ingestion causing toxicity usually exceeds 2 kg over 5 years. Clinical manifestations include microscopic hematuria, pyuria, cylindruria, impaired urinary concentration, a high prevalence of bacilluria, and, less often, hypertension and decreased glomerular filtration rate. Sulfohemoglobinuria and methemoglobinuria reflect recent phenacetin ingestion. There often is a background of psychiatric disorders, headaches, peptic ulcer, hemolytic anemia, and arthritis. See also ANALGESIC NEPHROPATHY; NEPHRITIS, CHRONIC INTERSTITIAL.

phenylketonuria A congenital metabolic defect inherited as an autosomal recessive trait in which there is a failure to produce sufficient amounts of phenylalanine hydroxylase. As a result, there is an increase in serum phenylalanine, urinary excretion of phenylpyruvic acid, and accumulation of phenlalanine metabolites, all easily detectable after birth. The metabolites produce brain damage, leading to severe mental retardation, often with seizures, other neurological abnormalities, and eczema.

pluricystic hypoplasia See under HYPOPLASIA, RENAL.

pneumaturia The passage of gas from the urethra during or after micturition. This usually results from an intestinal fistula or, less frequently, from decomposition of bladder urine. It is occasionally seen after catheterization in which air had been injected for bladder washout.

poisons and toxins Nephropathies resulting from contact with or ingestion of poisons or biologic toxins are described under CARBON TETRACHLORIDE TOXICITY; ETHYLENE GLYCOL NEPHROTOXICITY; LEAD TOXICITY; and MERCURY TOXICITY; also under ENDOTOXIN SHOCK (in Syndrome Glossary). See also HEMOGLOBINURIA; HYPERSENSITIVITY; MYOGLOBINURIA.

polyarteritis (also *necrosing arteritis, necrotizing angiitis, periarteritis nodosa*) A systemic disease with variable clinical manifestations. The pathology is characterized by lesions along the course of arteries, segmental in distribution, in various stages of development and involving vessels throughout most of the body. The pathologic features comprise necrosis, fibrinoid degeneration and hyalinization with marked inflammatory infiltration. The arteries may develop aneurysmatic formations which may rupture. The disease occurs more commonly in males with peak incidence from the third to the sixth decade. Etiology and pathogenesis are undefined although infections, allergic reactions and immune mechanisms have been implicated. The renal lesions are of two different types, one involves arteries, the other is of proliferative and necrotizing glomerulonephritis, focal or diffuse. Fever, leukocytosis, hypertension, neuritis, proteinuria and hematuria are common signs. About one-fourth of the patients have eosinophilia and about 15 percent may have evidence of severe renal insufficiency. In addition to polyarteritis, various forms of arteritis involve the renal vessels. Among these are Takayashu's syndrome (pulseless disease), giant cell arteritis, acute arteritis of Zeek. See also GRANULOMATOSIS, WEGENER'S.

polycystic renal disease A hereditary development disturbance in which the renal parenchyma is grossly displaced by cysts. Once manifest, the cysts enlarge, eventually leading to renal insufficiency and death in uremia. The **infantile form** is inherited as an autosomal recessive trait and is characterized by ectasia of collecting ducts. The disorder usually results in death in the perinatal period. Occasional patients survive into childhood or, rarely, adolescence, and may manifest hypertensive cardiovascular disease or portal hypertension. In the **adult form** inherited as an autosomal dominant trait of high penetrance, no symptoms may appear for many years, and the disease is rarely manifest before the age of 20. Cystic nephrons in adults partially retain their functional activity and may contribute to the formation of urine. Increase in kidney size antedates functional deterioration. Symptoms and signs may include pain in the lumbar region, hematuria, hypertension, palpable renal masses, recurrent renal and urinary tract infections, and uremia in the terminal stages. The disease may be associated with cysts in the liver, pancreas, and spleen and aneurysms of the cerebral arteries.

polycythemia, renal involvement in   Polycythemia refers to a variety of conditions associated with an elevated hemoglobin, hematocrit, and red cell count in the peripheral blood. When there is an absolute increase in the measured red cell volume, either primary or secondary polycythemia is responsible; when the red cell mass is normal, the polycythemia is usually spurious, i.e., the high peripheral values reflect a constitutional tendency and not a pathologic process. Renal involvement may be a complication of primary polycythemia or may underly the development of secondary polycythemia. It is not characteristic of spurious polcythemia.

primary polycythemia (also *polycythemia; rubra vera*)   A chronic progressive disorder in which the abnormal proliferation of reticulum-derived cell lines produces a panmyelosis and pancytosis. Although an increased erythroid mass is the most characteristic feature, the presence of leukocytosis, thrombocytosis, and myelofibrosis contributes to the clinical picture and the complications of the disease. An increased tendency for thrombosis reflects both the peripheral vascular congestion and elevated platelet levels. Renal vein thrombosis may complicate the course of primary polycythemia, with the typical presentation of nephrotic syndrome. More commonly, hematuria or proteinuria, or both, occur in the absence of either venous thrombosis or uric acid nephropathy. Uric acid nephropathy may be seen secondary to the increased cell turnover (hypermetabolism) and hyperuricemia. The increased serum uric acid is accompanied by an increase in urinary urate excretion, producing renal lithiasis and uric acid nephropathy in a significant number of patients. Ths predisposes them to repeated attacks of pyelonephritis. **secondary polycythemia**   An erythrocytosis induced by a physiologic erythropoietin-stimulated increase in the red blood cell mass, as in cyanotic cardiopulmonary disease, or by the inappropriate elaboration of erythropoietin in connection with a variety of neoplasma and renal lesions. Increased erythropoietin levels are usually found in the blood and urine. Secondary polycythemia has been seen in association with renal cysts, hydronephrosis, renal ischemia, polycystic renal disease, and hypernephroma and occasionally is seen following renal transplantation. Other neoplasms which have been found with secondary polycythemia include adrenal adenomas, hepatomas, and uterine leiomyomas.

polydipsia, primary See WATER DRINKING, COMPULSIVE.

porphyrinuria A condition characterized by urinary excretion of excess amounts of porphyrins or their precursors. These are colorless in freshly voided urine but turn dark as the urine stands. Porphyrinuria occurs in several clinically different forms, many of which are inherited. Transient hypertension may occur during the acute episodes of acute intermittent porphyria which is associated with an inherited abnormality of pyrrole metabolism. The acute attack is characterized by colicky abdominal pain, fever, leukocytosis, and sometimes diarrhea or constipation, nausea and vomiting, and neurologic disturbances.

postpartum renal failure Similar to thrombotic microangiopathy, but occurring within a few weeks of delivery.

postural proteinuria See ORTHOSTATIC PROTEINURIA under PROTEINURIA.

potassium deficiency, self-induced See HYPOKALEMIC NEPHROPATHY, SELF-INDUCED.

potomania See WATER DRINKING, COMPULSIVE.

preeclampsia and eclampsia (See Fig. 69.) See Syndrome Glossary.

prostatism The symptoms include hesitancy, slow voiding, and incomplete vesical emptying and are the result of prostatic hypertrophy.

prostatitis Bacterial infection of the prostate, which is usually associated with the presence of leukocytes and bacteria in the urine. It is frequently asymptomatic and often resistant to therapy.

proteinuria The finding of abnormal amounts of protein in the urine; up to 150 mg per 24 hours may normally be present. The term *proteinuria* is preferable to albuminuria, since 20 or more proteins may be found in normal urine and are also usually present in diseases in which albumin loss is most prominent. The urinary proteins normally present are in part antigenically similar to serum protein but have additional components believed to be of lower urinary tract origin. Sustained proteinuria, unrelated to posture or exercise, is one of the principle signs of renal disease and may accompany primary renal disease or systemic diseases involving the kidney.

Bence Jones proteinuria The appearance in the urine of proteins chemically identical with the light polypeptide chains of immunoglobulin molecules (kappa and lambda chains with molecular weights 20,000 to 22,000). Their presence in the urine supports the diagnosis of multiple myeloma or a related lymphoproliferative disorder. The Bence Jones proteins arise in the plasma cells in the marrow and seem to be synthesized independently rather than being degradative products of the abnormal myeloma protein. There is extensive catabolism of the light chain prior to excretion, and the chief site of such metabolic activity appears to be renal tissue. **exercise proteinuria** The production of urine with a higher than normal protein content which occurs during and after heavy muscular exercise. It is qualitatively and quantitatively different from orthostatic proteinuria. The physiologic mechanism for exercise proteinuria is speculative, and the clinical significance is uncertain. **febrile proteinuria** Proteinuria which appears only during fever. Referred to in the older literature as "larval nephrosis." It is of doubtful significance. **orthostatic proteinuria** (also *lordotic proteinuria; postural proteinuria*) Proteinuria which is demonstrable during quiet, upright ambulation or standing but not when the patient is recumbent. The excretory pattern of the proteinuria is usually "nonselective." The mechanism and clinical significance of orthostatic proteinuria are still uncertain. **selective proteinuria** Proteinuria characterized according to the molecular size of the urinary proteins as determined by immunoassay or Sephadex column chromatography. The milder renal structural lesions, such as lipoid nephrosis, have been characterized by a "selective" proteinuria, with a loss of albumin and smaller globulins such as transferrin (molecular weight 88,000). With more severe histologic damage, and particularly basement membrane thickening, loss of higher-weight globulins such as IgG (molecular weight 155,000) becomes more prominent. The degree of selectivity has also been suggested to correlate directly with the therapeutic response of the nephrotic syndrome to cortico-steroid therapy. **self-induced proteinuria** Proteinuria resulting when a patient adds or causes to be added surreptitiously to his urine egg white or other proteins, or ingests or absorbs other substances which induce proteinuria. The abnormality may be ascribed to spontaneous disease and the person may thereby gain sympathy, admission to a hospital, deferment from military service, or other ends.

pseudocysts, perinephric   See PERINEPHRIC ABSCESS.

pseudohydronephrosis   See HYDRONEPHROSIS.

psychogenic polydipsia   See WATER DRINKING, COMPULSIVE.

pulseless disease (also *Takayashu's syndrome*)   See POLYARTERITIS; INFLAMMATION under ARTERIES, RENAL, ABNORMALITIES OF.

pure nephrosis   See LIPOID NEPHROSIS.

purpura, Schönelin-Henoch   See SCHÖNLEIN-HENOCH PURPURA NEPHRITIS.

pyelonephritis (See Fig. 70.)

acute pyelonephritis   Renal parenchymal disease caused by bacterial infection. The infecting organisms are usually aerobic gram-negative bacilli (*Escherichia coli, Proteus* species, group D streptococci, staphylococci, and *Pseudomonas* species). The disease may be asymptomatic or manifest only as fever of undetermined origin. But there may also be pain, unilateral or bilateral, gradual or abrupt in onset, often radiating along the course of the ureters to the groin. This may be accompanied by nausea, vomiting, headaches, and lower urinary tract symptoms such as frequency, urgency, dysuria, nocturia, and difficulty in completely emptying the bladder. The disease may occur as a result of a new infection or a recurrent infection, or as a complication in a setting of urinary obstruction due to calculi, prostatic obstruction, congenital anomalies, neurologic disorders, or recent instrumentation of the urinary tract. **chronic pyelonephritis** The presence of renal parenchymal disease in which bacterial infection has played an important role in pathogenesis. In this sense chronic and acute pyelonephritis have the same meaning. See also NEPHRITIS, ACUTE INTERSTITIAL. **xanthogranulomatous pyelonephritis** A distinctive form of pyelonephritis associated with obstruction and usually *Proteus* species infection characterized by the presence of large accumulations of lipid-laden macrophages or foam cells, often arranged as nodules in the renal medulla, especially near the calyces. Renal function is usually severely impaired.

pyonephrosis Distention of the pelvis and calyces of the kidney with pus, in association with obstructive uropathy.

pyuria The presence of pus in the urine.

Q fever See RICKETTSIA DIAPORICA.

radiation, external, injury due to (See Fig. 71.) Following irradiation of one or both kidneys with more than approximately 2300 rads in five weeks following a latent period of up to 6 to 12 months (shorter in children), a patient may manifest one of five clinical syndromes: (1) acute radiation nephritis, which is characterized by proteinuria, edema, renal failure, hypertension, or severe malignant hypertension; (2) chronic radiation nephritis; (3) benign hypertension; (4) late malignant hypertension; or (5) asymptomatic proteinuria. The last four conditions may follow an attack of acute radiation nephritis or may arise months or years later without an acute illness. In some cases, late malignant hypertension may arise from excessive radiation damage to one kidney. The radiation damage primarily affects the renal blood vessels, and an extreme degree of renal interstitial fibrosis may ultimately occur.

reflux, vesicoureteral A condition characterized by decompensation of the valvelike action of the normal ureterovesical orifice, which may be unilateral or bilateral. There is reflux of urine from the bladder into the ureter, particularly during voiding. It is most commonly observed in children.

renal artery embolism See INFARCT, RENAL.

renal calculi See NEPHROLITHIASIS.

renal colic See COLIC, RENAL.

renal cysts See under CYSTS.

renal diabetes insipidus See DIABETES INSIPIDUS, RENAL.

renal dwarfism See RENAL RICKETS.

renal ectopia   See ECTOPIA, RENAL.

renal failure, acute oliguric   See RENAL FAILURE, ACUTE ANURIC OR OLIGURIC in Syndrome Glossary.

renal failure, acute polyuric   See Syndrome Glossary

renal insufficiency, acute oliguric   See RENAL FAILURE, ACUTE ANURIC OR OLIGURIC in Syndrome Glossary.

renal insufficiency, acute polyuric   See RENAL FAILURE, ACUTE POLYURIC in Syndrome Glossary.

renal insufficiency, chronic   See Syndrome Glossary.

renal medullary necrosis   See PAPILLARY NECROSIS.

renal osteodystrophy   A skeletal disorder seen in renal failure. The skeletal pathology may be osteomalacia, osteitis fibrosa, osteosclerosis, osteoporosis, or any combination of these defects. Frequently, there may be associated soft tissue calcification. The etiology appears to be related to multiple metabolic defects. These are secondary or tertiary hyperparathyroidism, effects of acidosis in bone, and multiple defects of vitamin D metabolism. These are due to renal enzymic failure in forming active compounds from vitamin D_3. These defects adversely affect calcium and phosphate metabolism. The severity of skeletal involvement is related to the duration and degree of renal impairment and the degree of secondary hyperparathyroidism. Patients with renal osteodystrophy may be free of symptoms related to the skeletal disease. Long-term dialysis may aggravate osteodystrophy, while successful renal transplantation may alleviate the process.

renal rickets   A disorder of growing children with renal failure which is characterized by defective mineralization of the growth centers and may be associated with pain. There may also be accompanying skeletal disease such as diffuse demineralization, osteitis fibrosa, osteoporosis, osteomalacia, and osteosclerosis. Calcification of soft tissue may occur. Retarded growth and development are present. The renal failure leads to acquired resistance to vitamin D and its metabolites, and hyperparathyroidism may occur. Intestinal absorption of calcium is impaired. Impairment of local effects of vitamin D at the growth centers is not yet proved. See also RENAL OSTEODYSTROPHY.

renal tubular acidosis   See ACIDOSIS, RENAL DISTAL TUBULAR; ACIDOSIS, RENAL PROXIMAL TUBULAR; ACIDOSIS, RENAL TUBULAR.

renal vein thrombosis   A disorder characterized by the clinical manifestations of nephrotic syndrome associated with thrombotic obstruction of one or both renal veins. There are frequently associated pulmonary infarcts and other evidence of venous thrombosis. Thrombosis may develop in Hodgkin's disease, and in carcinoma of the lungs and pancreas. It also appears in amyloidosis or may develop in nephrotic patients with a hypercoagulemic state or in dehydrated infants or children. See also NEPHROTIC SYNDROME in Syndrome Glossary.

renal venous thrombosis   See RENAL VEIN THROMBOSIS.

retroperitoneal cysts   See under CYSTS.

retroperitoneal fibrosis, renal involvement with   A disease of unknown origin characterized by slow, progressive fibrosis in the retroperitoneal tissue and sometimes in the mediastinum. Clinical manifestations are obscure, particularly when the patient presents with oliguria or anuria. An intermittent flow of urine and a marked medial displacement of the ureters on x-ray examination are helpful in diagnosis. In addition, when the ureteric catheter is passed in retrograde fashion, considerable urinary flow may appear in a severely oliguric patient with a normal pelvic x-ray and normal urinalysis.

rickets, renal   See RENAL RICKETS.

Rickettsia prowazekii (typhus), *rickettsii* (Rocky Mountain spotted fever), *tsutsugamushi* (scrub typhus), and *diaporica* (also *Coxiella burnetti*; *Q fever*)   Similar renal symptoms occur in all four diseases. Proteinuria, microscopic hematuria, and cylindruria generally occur during the febrile phase. Oliguria and azotemia are common in severe cases. The lesions appear to be readily reversible.

ring kidney   See KIDNEY, FUSED.

Rocky Mountain spotted fever   See RICKETTSIA RICKETTSII.

rotation, renal, anomalies of   Congenital disturbances in the normal 90-degree medialward rotation of the renal mass as it ascends from the embryonic pelvis to the definitive lumbar position. Often therefore associated with renal aectopy, or renal fusion, or both, which inhibit rotation. Hypo-, hyper-, and counter-rotations are described.

salicylate toxicity   Early signs of toxicity are proteinuria, hematuria, and oliguria. Salicylates can induce respiratory alkalosis and potassium loss, compete with para-aminohippurate transport, increase renal tubular exfoliation, and produce uricosuria. Massive dosages may cause acute renal insufficiency.

sarcoidosis, renal involvement in   (also *Boeck's sarcoid, Besnier-Boeck-Schaumann disease*)   A granulomatous, inflammatory systemic reaction of unknown etiology, which may involve almost any organ. Hypercalcemia and hypercalciuria occur and are thought to be due to hypersensitivity to vitamin D. Damage to the kidney can occur through direct infiltration with sarcoid granuloma, or, more frequently, to nephrocalcinosis and nephrolithiasis secondary to hypercalciuria.

schistosomiasis   (also *bilharziasis*)   (See Figs. 72 and 73.) A widespread disorder of man and the most common source of hematuria. *Schistosoma haematobium*   This blood fluke (Trematoda class) is widely distributed in Africa, neighboring islands, the Middle East, in isolated foci in the Iberian peninsula, and in India, but is not found in the Western Hemisphere. Various snail species serve as intermediate hosts. Infection by the cercaria occurs through the alimentary tract, penetration of the skin, or more rarely, of mucous membranes.

Schistosomiasis is characterized by perivascular deposition of ova, which have high antigenic properties. Tissues react by producing sclerosing granulomas, leading to stenotic obstruction of vessels in the vicinity. *S. haematobium* predominantly involves the genitourinary system through obstruction of the vesical veins. Acute, subacute, or chronic lesions may cause ureteral or vesical obstruction. The bladder may become calcified. An association with bladder carcinoma is highly significant. Only a fraction of patients infested have symptoms of obvious morbidity. *S. mansoni* is distributed in Africa (where it occurs concomitantly with *S. haematobium*), Malagasy, northern South America, Puerto Rico, and the West Indies. Urinary tract infections may be identical with those caused by *S. haematobium*, although major sites of damage are intestinal or hepatic. In patients with hepatosplenomegaly a nephrotic syndrome may occur. Subendothelial accumulation of immune complexes has been reported. *S. japonicum* is confined to the Far East, Japan, China, and the Philippines. Urinary tract involvement is less common than with *S. haematobium* or *S. mansoni*, but similar pathologic effects may be seen. Widespread systemic involvement is common.

Schönlein-Henoch purpura nephritis (also *anaphylactoid purpura nephritis*) (See Fig. 74.) Nephritis is a frequent complication of anaphylactoid purpura. Most commonly the nephritis is mild and self-limiting, but a significant number of adults have serious involvement of the kidney. The course in children is milder, but rapid progressive renal disease or the nephrotic syndrome have been observed. The disease may reoccur in about 30 percent of patients, at which time renal involvement may develop. Microscopic hematuria without proteinuria or symptoms of functional impairment may persist for an extended period of time. Diagnostically, the presence of occult blood in the stool is useful when rash, joint, and abdominal pain are absent. The characteristic (though not specific), histologic lesion is focal and segmental necrotizing glomerulonephritis, accompanied by crescent formation. In the more severe cases, diffuse proliferative glomerulonephritis may be present.

scleroderma (also *primary systemic sclerosis*), **renal involvement in** Despite almost invariable renal vascular involvement, clinical manifestations of renal impairment are rare in scleroderma, although slight proteinuria occurs in approximately 15 percent of such patients. Severe intimal thickening in the interlobular and arcuate arteries results from increased amounts of loose connective tissue, which tends to be metachromatic. Arterioles often show fibrinoid necrosis. Glomerular lesions are uncommon, but interstitial fibrosis is usual. Whether the vascular lesions reflect or give rise to the hypertension often found in scleroderma is not clear. In rare instances, malignant hypertension may arise suddenly, followed by acute oliguric renal failure, progressing to death in uremia.

scrub typhus See RICKETTSIA TSUTSUGAMUSHI.

segmental hypoplasia See under HYPOPLASIA, RENAL.

self-induced hematuria See HEMATURIA, SELF-INDUCED.

self-induced proteinuria See under PROTEINURIA.

shock, gram-negative See ENDOTOXIN SHOCK in Syndrome Glossary.

sickle cell nephropathy Characteristic renal abnormalities occurring with the heterozygous sickle cell trait or, in sickle cell anemia, the homozygous condition. Most characteristic is hyposthenuria and hematuria, which may be microscopic, macroscopic, persistent, intermittent, or at times from one kidney only. Renal papillary necrosis is common with sickle cell anemia and may occur at times in sickle cell trait. Occasionally, minor problems in acidification, infarcts of the kidney, and the nephrotic syndrome have been observed (in sickle cell anemia). Chronic renal failure has been noted but is uncommon.

SLE See SYSTEMIC LUPUS ERYTHEMATOSUS.

Songo fever See EPIDEMIC HEMORRHAGIC FEVER.

sponge kidney, medullary A maldevelopment of the kidneys, usually present bilaterally and considered congenital in origin (a form of renal dysplasia or a transitional form of polycystic disease). Most patients are asymptomatic, but hematuria, renal colic, or pyuria may develop asymptomatically in association with minute calculi in the dilated collecting ducts. The condition occurs with a population frequency of 0.5 percent with a ratio of 2 males to 1 female. Longevity may be normal, but the condition may also lead to pyelonephritis. Renal tubular acidosis has been reported, and also unilateral or bilateral hypertrophy.

Stillweger's syndrome See Syndrome Glossary.

strangury Abnormal desire to micturate, characterized by passage of urine drop by drop, with pain and tenesmus.

streak abscesses See ABSCESSES, KIDNEY.

sublimate poisoning See MERCURY TOXICITY.

sulfonamide toxicity Hematuria, crystallization, tubular necrosis, oliguria, and anuria are among the renal signs and symptoms associated with an overdosage of sulfonamides, particularly of poorly soluble sulfonamide derivatives and especially in patients with acid or concentrated urine. There may be sulfonamide crystals in the urine or tubules and hemorrhagic inflammation of the mucosa of the renal pelvis and bladder. Hypersensitivity reactions can cause focal granulomatous or diffuse eosinophilic interstitial nephritis, with or without acute renal failure.

supernumerary kidney See KIDNEY, SUPERNUMERARY.

synpharyngitis See ACUTE BENIGN HEMORRHAGIC GLOMERULONEPHRITIS under GLOMERULONEPHRITIS.

syphilis, congenital, with nephrotic syndrome Nephrotic syndrome during the first months of life, caused by congenital syphilis. There are other evidences of syphilis, such as periostitis, snuffles, and positive serology in association with the cardinal findings of the nephrotic syndrome.

syphilitic nephritis See TREPONEMA PALLIDUM.

systemic lupus erythematosus (also *SLE; lupus nephritis*) (See Figs. 64 to 66.) A multisystemic syndrome with highly varied clinical and pathologic expression. Manifestations include arthralgias and arthritis, varied cutaneous eruptions, frequently with photosensitivity, alopecia, blood cytopenias (leukopenia, hemolytic anemia, thrombocytopenia), serositis (pleuritis and pericarditis), glomerulonephritis, and various neurovascular complications. Certain serologic phenomena are characteristic but not diagnostic of SLE. These include LE cell tests and a variety of antinuclear factor tests. The most specific serologic abnormality is the presence of anti-DNA antibodies measured by immunologic procedures. Serum complement levels are usually depressed with active disease.

Takayashu's syndrome See POLYARTERITIS; INFLAMMATION under ARTERIES, RENAL, ABNORMALITIES OF.

thrombosis, renal vein See RENAL VEIN THROMBOSIS.

thrombotic thrombocytopenic purpura (**TTP**) (also *Moschcowitz's syndrome; microangiopathy with thrombocytopenia*) A disease of unknown etiology characterized by widespread microthrombi and renal failure. Fever, thrombocytopenia with purpura, hemolysis and anemia, jaundice, and bizarre red blood cells are accompanied by fluctuating neurologic symptoms. The course of the disease is irregular, leading to variable clinical symptoms and pathologic lesions of different duration. Hyaline thrombi are particularly common in the kidney and myocardium. Endothelial cell proliferation in kidney arterioles and capillaries containing thrombi is conspicuous, sometimes resulting in masses of endothelial cells or glomera. Local absence of fibrinolytic activity at the site of the thrombi has also been described. Patients with severe forms of lupus erythematosus exhibit similar symptoms, but positive lupus erythematosus preparation and antinuclear factor have not been found in TTP. See also MICROANGIOPATHY, THROMBOTIC; HEMOLYTIC UREMIC SYNDROME in Syndrome Glossary; POSTPARTUM RENAL FAILURE.

toxemia of pregnancy Obsolete term. See PREECLAMPSIA AND ECLAMPSIA in Syndrome Glossary.

toxins See HYPERSENSITIVITY; POISONS AND TOXINS.

transplanation rejection crisis See Syndrome Glossary.

trauma, thermal See HYPOTHERMIA, RENAL TRAUMA DUE TO; HYPERTHERMIA, RENAL TRAUMA DUE TO.

Treponema pallidum The causative agent of syphilis. Infection with this microorganism (order Spirochaetales, family Treponemataceae) may yield three varieties of reaction in the kidney: the nephropathy of primary or secondary syphilis; the gummas and fibrogummatous reaction of tertiary syphilis; and the nephritis of congenital syphilis. Lesions may occasionally be morphologically indistinguishable from acute glomerulonephritis, and membranous nephropathy may be seen. The nephrotic syndrome may clear incompletely, and after a time, hematuria and hypertension with renal failure may develop, or the syndrome may disappear spontaneously and leave no residua.

tuberculosis, epididymal Any persistent chronic and nodular epididymitis may be indicative of tubercular infection, particularly if there is erosion to the skin and drainage.

tuberculosis, prostatic Prostatic tuberculosis is diagnosed by inference when any kind of prostatitis occurs in association with known renal tuberculosis and may be confirmed by x-ray and, if necessary, by biopsy.

tuberculosis, renal Infection of the kidneys with *Mycobacterium tuberculosis*. This is characterized clinically as a chronic urinary tract infection which does not respond to conventional chemotherapy. There is sterile pyuria, but no pyogenic bacteria can be recovered on urine culture. Symptoms may be very mild or absent in the early stages. Later, ulcerations and contractures of the bladder may give rise to frequency and hematuria. Renal pain is unusual. The radiologic picture of renal tuberculosis in more advanced stages shows a characteristic "moth-eaten" or "feathery" outline, due to the sloughing of the cavities produced by the tuberculous process. Calcifications of material in cavities may also occur, as well as cyst formation due to stricture at the neck of the calyx. Renal tuberculosis is secondary to tuberculous processes elsewhere in the body (primarily in the lungs) and may lie dormant for many years. Hemic types of tuberculosis, such as miliary tuberculosis, are often accompanied by seeding of the kidneys, with the appearance of tubercles in 25 to 20 percent of patients. A smaller percentage of the renal tubercular patients with blood-borne disease will also show tuberculous bone lesions.

tubular acidosis, type 1, type 2 See ACIDOSIS, RENAL DISTAL TUBULAR; ACIDOSIS, RENAL PROXIMAL TUBULAR.

tubular necrosis, acute See RENAL FAILURE, ACUTE ANURIC OR OLIGURIC in Syndrome Glossary.

tumors, extrarenal malignant See under TUMORS in Pathology Glossary. These tumors may present with hematuria and loin pain.

tumors, metastatic See under TUMORS in Pathology Glossary. These tumors may present with hematuria and loin pain.

tumors, renal benign See under TUMORS in Pathology Glossary. On rare occasions, capillary hemangiomas and other benign tumors may cause hematuria. Large tumors, particularly hamartomas, may be detected by radiography.

tumors, renal malignant See CARCINOMA, RENAL CELL; also WILMS' TUMOR.

type 1 and type 2 renal tubular acidosis See ACIDOSIS, RENAL DISTAL TUBULAR; ACIDOSIS, RENAL PROXIMAL TUBULAR.

typhus See RICKETTSIA PROWAZEKII.

tyrosinosis A relatively rare inborn error of metabolism in which tyrosine is imperfectly metabolized, and relatively large amounts are excreted in the urine.

tyrosinuria The excretion of abnormal amounts of tyrosine in the urine.

unilateral multicystic disease See KIDNEY, MULTICYSTIC; DYSPLASIA, RENAL.

urate nephropathy See INFARCTS, URIC ACID; also HYPERURICEMIC NEPHROPATHY.

uremia See Syndrome Glossary.

ureteropelvic junction obstruction, idiopathic A condition which is usually congenital and which may result from obstruction of the outlet of the renal pelvis by extrinsic fibrous bands, intrinsic stenosis, or abnormally high insertion of the ureter in the renal pelvis. These abnormalities may not necessarily cause hydronephrosis.

urgency Abnormal urination characterized by an exaggerated desire to urinate.

uricosuria The presence of uric acid in the urine.

urine, residual The urine remaining in the bladder after urination.

uropathy, obstructive A general expression used to describe structural changes in the urinary tract which impair outflow of urine. Depending on the severity and duration of the lesion, there may be dilatation proximal to the site of obstruction and hydroureter or hydronephrosis or both may develop.

vascular disease, hypertensive A disorder accompanying arterial hypertension and characterized by arteriolosclerosis and arteriosclerosis. The cerebral, retinal, and renal arterioles are primarily involved. Hypertensive heart disease is a frequent complication, as is premature atherosclerosis.

vascular reactivity The response of the systemic or pulmonary circulation or of local vascular beds to noxious stimuli or vasoactive agents. Increased vascular reactivity is generally found in patients with primary hypertension and in their relatives.

viruria The presence of viruses in the urine.

virus disease Renal manifestation may develop during the course of certain virus diseases, e.g., mumps. A causal relationship between viruses and renal disease has not been established.

virus disease, green monkey A rapidly fatal infectious disease of man, usually affecting animal handlers and investigators and involving both kidneys and liver.

von Gierke's disease See GLYCOGEN STORAGE DISEASE.

water drinking, compulsive (also *primary polydipsia; psychogenic polydipsia; potomania*) Usually seen in middle-aged women. It produces a sustained diuresis.

Wegener's granulomatosis See GRANULOMATOSIS, WEGENER'S.

Wilms' tumor (also *nephroblastoma, embryoma, adenomyosarcoma, blastomal tumor, malignant nephroma*) An embryonal malignancy of tubular epithelial cells and connective tissue organs occurring primarily in children. An abdominal mass is usually the presenting finding; hematuria is far less common.

Wilson's disease See COPPER STORAGE DISEASE.

xanthinuria and xanthine calculi Xanthine in the urine and the formation of xanthine calculi are rare disorders seen in childhood. The calculi are radioluscent, and the crystals are similar to uric acid crystals.

Syndromes

acute nephritic syndrome Sudden onset of hematuria (gross or microscopic), proteinuria, cylindruria, oliguria, edema, hypertension, and renal functional impairment, often leading to circulatory changes.

aldosteronism A syndrome resulting from increased secretion of aldosterone. Hypokalemia is generally found in the disorders associated with aldosteronism; hypertension, edema, or both are also frequent findings. Aldosteronism may be classified according to the pathologic state in the adrenal gland and level of activity of the renin-angiotensin system into (1) **primary**—aldosterone-producing adrenal adenoma, suppressed renin activity: (2) **secondary**—adrenal hyperplasia, increased renin activity; and (3) **idiopathic**—diffuse or nodular adrenal hyperplasia, suppressed renin activity.

Alport's syndrome See CHRONIC HEREDITARY NEPHRITIS under NEPHRITIS in Clinical Glossary.

Bartter's syndrome (also *juxtaglomerular hyperplasia with hyperaldosteronism; hypokalemic alkalosis and normal blood pressure*) A disorder of unknown etiology, characterized by hypokalemia and normal blood pressure, which may appear in early infancy and may be familial. All elements of the juxtaglomerular complex may show hyperplasia. Plasma renin and angiotensin concentrations are persistently elevated; aldosterone secretion is high.

Burnett's syndrome See MILK-ALKALI SYNDROME.

cephalopathia splanchnocystica See MICHEL'S SYNDROME.

cerebrohepatorenal syndrome See STILLWEGER'S SYNDROME.

de Toni-Debré-Fanconi syndrome See FANCONI SYNDROME, INFANTILE AND ADULT.

dialysis disequilibrium syndrome A symptom complex characterized by confusion, disorientation, headaches, muscle twitching, tremors, nausea, vomiting, and sometimes cardiac arrhythmias. It may develop during or following dialysis of a severely uremic patient. The syn-

drome is considered to be due to the development of a steep urea
gradient between plasma and brain tissue, with resultant increased
osmotic intracellular pressure and increased cerebrospinal fluid pressure.

endotoxin shock (also *gram-negative bacterial shock; renal failure due to
endotoxin shock; renal failure due to septic shock*) A syndrome
initiated by liberation of endotoxin from gram-negative bacteria.
Escherichia coli, the Klebsiella-Serratia group, Pseudomonas, Proteus,
and *Neisseria meningitidis* are the most common causative organisms.
Acute renal failure is a common complication. In addition to shock,
hepatic failure, respiratory disturbances, and myocardial dysfunction
also may occur. The mortality is high.

Fanconi syndrome, infantile and adult (also *de Toni-Debré-Fanconi syndrome, glucoaminophosphate diabetes*) A multiple functional defect
of the proximal tubular reabsorption of glucose, amino acids, and
phosphate. Resulting complications may be normoglycemic glucosuria,
generalized renal hyperaminoaciduria, hyperphosphaturic hypophosphatemia, proximal renal tubular acidosis with low serum bicarbonate
and hyperchloremia, and proteinuria of the tubular type. There is
usually a failure to concentrate the urine and (in children) vitamin-D
resistant rickets or osteomalacia growth retardation. Occasionally there
may be hypercalciuria and unidentified crystals in bone marrow cells.
This disorder is not fatal. The general condition of the patient remains
good, as long as secondary disturbances (e.g., hypokalemia, rickets) are
avoided by symptomatic treatment.

glomerulonephritis, rapidly progressive A syndrome, not a disease. As yet
no specific lesions have been definitely established, but in the so-called
idiopathic form, extracapillary proliferation is a main feature. The
clinical course is characterized by fulminant renal insufficiency and
hypertension.

glucoaminophosphate diabetes See FANCONI SYNDROME, INFANTILE AND
ADULT.

Goodpasture's syndrome See LUNG PURPURA WITH NEPHRITIS in Clinical
Glossary.

hemolytic uremic syndrome The simultaneous occurrence, after two or
three days of fever, diarrhea, and vomiting, of hemolytic anemia, renal
involvement, and thrombocytopenia, frequently in association with
neurologic disorders, mainly convulsions. Seldom are all of these signs
and symptoms found. The renal injury is manifested by oliguria, severe
uremia, hematuria, massive proteinuria (accompanied by hypoproteinemia), and, at times, by a fully developed nephrotic syndrome and

hypertension. The underlying anatomic lesion is called thrombotic microangiopathy.

hypertension syndrome, malignant Severe diastolic hypertension, usually associated with papilledema with retinal exudates and hemorrhages and failing renal function. Cardiac failure is common; hypertensive encephalopathy and intracerebral hematoma are the chief central nervous system complications, and episodes of bizarre abdominal pain sometimes occur. Headaches, weight loss, and progressively failing vision are the early symptoms, while those of uremia usually predominate in the later stages of the illness. The syndrome is the clinical expression of a diffuse, progressive, obstructive, and destructive arteriolar disease, which is most severe in the kidney but occurs throughout the body. It most often develops in the course of apparently benign hypertension but can occur de novo. It can complicate any of the secondary hypertensions, with the exception of aortic coarctation. Severe malignant hypertension is more common in blacks than in whites.

hypokalemic alkalosis and normal blood pressure See BARTTER'S SYNDROME.

Lowe's syndrome See OCULOCEREBRORENAL SYNDROME.

Michel's syndrome (also *cephalopathia splanchnocystica*) A familial syndrome characterized by bilateral cystic renal dysplasia and severe malformations of the central nervous system.

milk-alkali syndrome (also *Burnett's syndrome*) Impairment of renal excretory function attributable to the prolonged ingestion of calcium salts (or milk) and alkali, usually for relief of peptic ulcer pain. This condition shows a marked predilection for males. Chemical abnormalities commonly include hypercalcemia, alkalosis, and azotemia. Hypercalciuria and hypophosphatemia are usually absent, and serum alkaline phosphatase is normal. Calcinosis often occurs, chiefly in the corneas, conjunctivas, and kidneys. The renal insufficiency may be either acute and readily reversible or chronic and persistent despite correction of chemical abnormalities and reduction in calcium intake. Many patients with this syndrome have hyperparathyroidism.

nephrotic syndrome A condition characterized by persistent massive proteinuria, hypoalbuminemia, hypercholesterolemia, and edema. These are present in varying proportions, depending on the duration of proteinuria and the primary disease.

congenital nephrotic syndrome A familial (recessive) disorder characterized by appearance of the nephrotic syndrome in early infancy, often with other features such as hematuria, cylindruria, and hypertension. Progression to renal insufficiency is unresponsive to therapy, and death in uremia occurs usually before the age of 2 years. At birth or early in the course of the disease, the kidneys are normal by light microscopy. Later, in some cases, sequential cystic dilatations of renal proximal tubules (microcystic diseases) are apparent on nephron dissection.

Mechanical causes of nephrotic syndrome   Hemodynamic effects of pressure and flow on the venous system of the kidney from whatever cause (constrictive pericarditis, tricuspid disease, inferior vena caval thrombosis, or pressure on the inferior vena cava, renal venous thrombosis, and so on) can produce proteinuria. The commonest of these pathogenetic mechanisms is thrombosis of the renal vein. The proteinuria is usually severe and nonselective. This can lead to the nephrotic syndrome, which may be arrested in many cases if the cause of the hemodynamic process can be reversed early in the disorder. When onset is sudden, there is acute swelling of the kidneys, intractable pain, a mass in the loin, and transient hematuria. In other cases the onset is obscure, particularly when venous thrombosis spreads from the saphenous vein.

Radiologic techniques are vital for differential diagnosis. Amyloidosis is a common precursor of the conditions, as are abnormalities of the clotting mechanisms. If the condition is not treated early, prognosis is poor, and hypertension with progressive renal failure develops. In infants and children, the syndrome is often associated with dehydration.

The early histologic changes indicate inappropriately severe changes in the tubules and interstitium when compared with glomerular abnormalities, although diapedesis of the leukocytes through the glomerular capillaries is an important feature. Later, changes in the basement membrane develop. These cases may be mistakenly diagnosed as membranous nephropathy. See also RENAL VEIN THROMBOSIS in Clinical Glossary.

oculocerebrorenal syndrome (also *Lowe's syndrome*)   A congenital, sex-linked (hereditary) disease primarily seen in males and characterized by cataracts, glaucoma, or both, hypotonia, mental retardation, and subsequent development of a variety of biochemical abnormalities. There is generalized hyperaminoaciduria, proteinuria, and metabolic acidosis. X-ray and biochemical studies show hypophosphatemic rickets and defective mechanisms of renal acidification of urine. Death occurs as a result of renal failure or an intercurrent infection.

oliguric renal failure   See RENAL FAILURE, ACUTE ANURIC OR OLIGURIC.

preeclampsia and eclampsia (also *glomerular capillary endotheliosis, toxemia of pregnancy* [obsolete])   A syndrome characterized by hypertension, proteinuria, and usually edema, and due to pregnancy or the influence of a preceding pregnancy. Clinically it can occur after the twentieth week but usually appears after the thirtieth week of gestation. It may develop before this time with or without trophoblastic disease. It is predominantly a disorder of primigravidas, and its etiology is still not completely defined. It is dependent on the presence of placental tissue and regresses after delivery. The renal lesion consists mainly of swelling of the glomerular capillary endothelial cells, which is associated with deposition of fibrin aggregates; this in turn is associated with reduction of renal blood flow and glomerular filtration rate. In the severe form of the syndrome the associated defect of coagulation may progress to full-blown diffuse intravascular coagulation with infarction of the kidney, liver, and other organs. **Eclampsia** is the occurrence, in a patient with **preeclampsia,** of one or more convulsions, either prepartum or postpartum, not attributable to other cerebral conditions such as epilepsy or cerebral hemorrhage.

renal failure, acute anuric or oliguric A condition characterized by the abrupt onset of failure of the renal excretory function. By definition **anuric** means no urine output; in **oliguric** renal failure 24-hour urinary volumes are less than 400 ml. Occasionally renal failure with high urine output occurs (greater than 1000 ml per day). The syndrome may occur as a result of (1) obstruction of urinary outflow tract; (2) sustained decrease in glomerular filtration rate and renal plasma flow secondary to initial hypotension, decreased volume of extracellular fluid, or intravascular volume; (3) nephrotoxins (may be combined with [2]); (4) acute glomerular disease of any etiology; (5) acute renal vascular disease (embolus, thrombosis, vasculitis); (6) acute interstitial disease (infection, allergy); (7) crush injuries; (8) acute intravascular hemolysis; (9) renal cortical necrosis.

Most frequently, acute anuric or oliguric renal failure occurs as a sequela of hypotension following trauma, surgical shock, burns, and so on. In 50 percent of the cases it is difficult to determine the etiology. Reversible causes should be ruled out. The urine sediment is not diagnostic, since etiology is variable. Hematuria, proteinuria, and red cell casts are less frequent in (1), and (2) than in (3), (4), and (5). Diuresis with recovery of renal function after a period of oliguria is the rule in (2).

renal failure, acute polyuric (also *nonoliguric renal failure*) Acute renal failure associated with a decrease in glomerular filtration rate and renal plasma flow and the inability to excrete the wastes of protein metabolism, in the absence of oliguria. Usually the same etiological factors that produce acute oliguric renal failure are involved.

renal failure due to endotoxin shock See ENDOTOXIN SHOCK.

renal failure due to septic shock See ENDOTOXIN SHOCK.

renal failure, nonoliguric See RENAL FAILURE, ACUTE POLYURIC.

renal insufficiency, chronic A syndrome resulting from a multitude of pathologic processes which lead to derangements of renal excretory and regulatory functions. Chronic renal insufficiency develops over periods of months or years and ultimately leads to the uremic syndrome. Progression of renal insufficiency is characteristically associated with retention of end products of protein catabolism (i.e., azotemia) and with a multitude of biochemical abnormalities and clinical signs and symptoms including anemia.

salt-wasting nephritis A condition characterized by excess urinary excretion of sodium chloride leading to dehydration and hyponatremia. It is associated with chronic renal diseases involving distal nephrons, such as chronic pyelonephritis and medullary cystic disease.

Stillweger's syndrome (also *cerebrohepatorenal syndrome*) A familial form of renal dysplasia in the presence of nonspecific mental retardation and biliary stasis.

toxemia of pregnancy See PREECLAMPSIA AND ECLAMPSIA.

transplant rejection crises

    acute transplant rejection A phenomenon comparable to a first set rejection in experimental immunology. It may occur any time after transplantation but is rare before the first week or after 2 years and most commonly occurs during the first six months postoperative. The first manifestations are decrease in creatinine clearance and lymphocyturia and may be followed by pain over the transplanted kidney, malaise, fever, decreasing urinary output, weight gain, and hypertension. The kidney may be swollen and sometimes tender. This type of rejection is characterized pathologically by edema, interstitial hemorrhage, and vascular lesions. The prognosis is good, and the condition usually responds to increased dosages of immunosuppressive agents. **chronic transplant rejection** A condition characterized by a gradual decrease in function beginning several weeks to several months following transplantation and often preceded by several acute rejection episodes. There is usually no tenderness or swelling of the kidney, and the only symptoms are those referable to diminished excretory function. Pathologically there is interstitial fibrosis, narrowing of small blood vessels due to intimal proliferation, fragmentation of the internal elastic lamina, progressive hyalinization of glomeruli, focal interstitial infiltration of inflammatory cells, and dilatation and atrophy of tubules. Immunofluorescence studies often reveal deposits of IgM, IgG, complement, and fibrin in the walls of the small vessels and occasionally in the glomeruli. This type of rejection is usually slowly progressive and not responsive to increased dosages of adrenal cortical hormones. **hyperacute transplant rejection** A sudden, fulminant rejection, usually occurring within minutes of transplantation. Grossly the kidney is seen to become dark, swollen, and soft. Histologic studies reveal sequestration of platelets and polymorphonuclear leukocytes in the glomeruli and fibrin thrombi in both the glomeruli and the small blood vessels. If the kidney is not immediately removed, the process proceeds to cortical necrosis and interstitial hemorrhage and edema. This type of rejection is mediated by circulating antibodies to components of the kidney endothelium. Deposition of antibody is rapidly followed by activation of complement, release of leukotactic and vasoactive substances, and subsequent destruction of small vessels and glomeruli. There is no known therapy for this lesion.

uremia A symptom complex characterized by multiple metabolic and physiologic alterations which result from renal insufficiency. Uremia may develop acutely or gradually, over periods of several months to several years, with progression to chronic renal insufficiency. The uremic syndrome is due to diffuse parenchymal disease. Uremia does not necessarily cause electrolyte imbalance. The substance or substances responsible for the symptoms of uremia have not been identified; however, phenols, guanidine, and guanidine-like compounds have been implicated. Whatever the substance or substances responsible for uremic symptoms, dialysis removes them and causes the uremia to subside. Two major groups of symptoms and signs are present in uremia: those due to impaired excretory and regulatory function of the kidney and those due to involvement of other organs and systems. Thus in addition to manifestations of impaired renal function (azotemia, acidosis, hyponatremia, hypocalcemia, edema, oliguria, hypokalemia or hyperkalemia, and hyperphosphatemia) there are also gastrointestinal, cardiovascular, neuromuscular, hemopoietic, pulmonary, skeletal, and skin abnormalities present in uremia.

vasopressin, inappropriate secretion of Excess secretion of vasopressin or vasopressin-like substances resulting in water retention (often to the point of intoxication), hyponatremia and hypoosmolality of the plasma, urine-plasma osmolality ratios persistently greater than 1.0, and a tendency to excessive excretion of sodium. Adrenal and renal function are usually normal. The most common cause is oat cell bronchogenic carcinoma, but the syndrome can result from a variety of other diseases, including pulmonary tuberculosis, various types of central nervous system lesions, myxedema, and acute intermittent porphyria.

Radiology

abdominal survey film   A radiogram of the abdomen, usually obtained in the course of intravenous pyelography prior to the injection of contrast medium.

angiography   X-ray visualization of a vessel after injection of a contrast medium. The vessel can be a vein (**phlebography**), an artery (**arteriography**), or a lymph vessel (**lymphangiography**).
  intravenous angiography   Angiography following introduction of the contrast medium through the venous system. The term is usually synonymous with **intravenous aortography,** in which the contrast medium is injected into the venous system and the filming of the abdomen is delayed until the contrast medium has reached the aorta and its branches.   **selective angiography**   Angiography in which the contrast medium is injected into a chosen artery or vein. In selective renal arteriography a catheter is introduced into a renal artery. In selective renal vein catheterization the catheter is introduced directly into a vein, usually for the purpose of collecting blood to determine levels of renin. This technique is also used for phlebography.

aortography   Angiography of the aorta.   **intravenous aortography**   See under ANGIOGRAPHY.   **translumbar aortography**   Aortography in which contrast medium is introduced into the abdominal aorta from the back, the patient lying prone on the examining table.

arteriography   Angiography of an artery.

blunting of the calyx   See CLUBBING OF THE CALYX.
body-section roentgenography   See TOMOGRAPHY.
branched calculus   See STAGHORN CALCULUS.

caliectasis   Dilatation of a calyx. Loss of cupping (see CLUBBING OF THE CALYX) is not a necessary accompaniment. Thus caliectasis may be apparent only in serial studies, in which changes in calyx size can be noted. See also HYDROCALYX.
calyceal clubbing   See CLUBBING OF THE CALYX.
calyx   See CLUBBING OF THE CALYX; CUPPING OF THE CALYX.

cavography, inferior vena   X-ray study of the inferior vena cava opacified by contrast medium.

cineradiography   Motion picture roentgenography used in nephrology primarily to demonstrate vesicoureteral reflux.

clubbing of the calyx   Loss of the calyceal cup due to back pressure, scarring, or loss of papilla.

contrast medium   A chemical substance which is introduced into the body to render one or several organs opaque to x-rays.

crescent sign (also *Dunbar's crescent*)   Curvilinear collection of contrast material in the parenchyma of the kidney during intravenous pyelography, representing compressed collecting ducts, as seen in hydronephrosis.

cupping of the calyx   Normal invagination of the calyx by the pyramid.

cystography   X-ray visualization of the urinary bladder following injection of contrast medium. The contrast medium may be introduced through a catheter, or the bladder may be visualized as part of the excretion urogram.

delayed nephrogram   See NEPHROGRAM.

delayed urogram   See EXCRETION UROGRAM.

drip infusion technique   A technique of opacification of the urinary tract by contrast medium, based on the introduction of a large amount of contrast medium by continuous intravenous infusion. It is used to render the collecting system opaque in the presence of decreased kidney function.

dromedary hump   Bulging of the lateral outline of the left kidney, possibly related to pressure from the spleen. This is a normal variation.

Dunbar's crescent   See CRESCENT SIGN.

excretion urogram   Roentgenologic image of the urinary tract opacified by intravenously administered contrast medium.

hydrocalyx   Localized caliectasis.

inferior vena cavography   See CAVOGRAPHY, INFERIOR VENA.

intravenous pyelogram (*IVP*)   Pyelogram obtained by the intravenous injection of contrast medium. See also EXCRETION UROGRAM.

IVP   See INTRAVENOUS PYELOGRAM; EXCRETION UROGRAM.

laminagraphy   See TOMOGRAPHY.

lymphangiography   Angiography of a lymph vessel.

nephrogram   Roentgenologic image of renal parenchyma opacified during excretory urography. Delay in the appearance of the nephrogram may occur in prerenal or postrenal obstructive disease.

phlebography Angiography of a vein.

pyelocaliectasis Dilatation of the kidney pelvis and calyces.

pyelogram Roentgenologic image of the kidney and ureter.

pyelolymphatic backflow A type of pyelorenal backflow. The contrast medium is seen draining medially to the periaortic lymph nodes through one or more lymphatic channels. This most likely represents lymphatic drainage of pyelosinus backflow.

pyelorenal backflow See PYELOLYMPHATIC BACKFLOW; PYELOSINUS BACK-FLOW; PYELOTUBULAR BACKFLOW; PYELOVENOUS BACKFLOW.

pyelosinus backflow A type of pyelorenal backflow, most likely due to rupture of the tip of a fornix of a calyx. The contrast medium is seen extending either medially or laterally from the fornix of the calyx in an irregular fashion or alongside the infundibula, and sometimes reaching medially around the renal pelvis and inferiorly along the proximal ureter.

pyelotubular backflow A type of pyelorenal backflow. The contrast material is seen in the collecting ducts, evidenced as brushlike lines of increased density extending from the calyx into the corresponding papilla. This most likely represents retrograde flow of the contrast material from the calyx.

pyelovenous backflow A type of pyelorenal backflow. The contrast material is seen in the venous system. Recent observations suggest that this radiologic picture is usually produced by rupture of a calyceal fornix into the sinus (**fornix-sinus reflux**) or into the lymphatic system (**pyelolymphatic reflux**) without actual extension from the renal pelvis into the large, superficial renal veins in the minor calyces at the base of the pyramids.

renal pseudotumor Radiologically demonstrated renal mass which may consist of normal renal tissue, fat, or blood clot.

renal scan The plane projection of radioactivity recorded by scanners or gamma camera following administration of a nucleide which is taken up by the kidney.

renogram A time record of the radioactivity measured externally over the kidneys following intravenous injection of a nucleide which is taken up and excreted by the kidney.

retrograde radiography Radiography in which the contrast medium is injected into the renal pelvis through a ureteral catheter positioned in the pelvis or as high up the ureter as possible.

ring sign Radiologic sign of papillary necrosis.

selective angiography See under ANGIOGRAPHY.

sinus fibrolipomatosis sign See RENAL PSEUDOTUMOR.

spider-leg deformity Stretching and narrowing of calyces and infundibula by an intrarenal mass or masses as seen with neoplasms, cysts, and fibrolipomatosis.

staghorn calculus (also *branched calculus*) A renal calculus in the shape of a calyx or even forming a cast of the pelvis and calyces.

timed IVP An excretory urogram in which pictures are taken at 30 seconds and at 1, 2, 3, 5, and 15 minutes to determine the difference in time of opacification of one kidney as compared with the other and variations in the concentration of dye in the urinary tract.

tomography (also *laminagraphy; body-section roentgenography*) A radiographic technique which permits sectional or plane views of an organ at a specific level. During exposure the x-ray tube is given a curvilinear motion synchronous with the recording plate but in the opposite direction. This has the effect of blurring the film except for the selected plane.

urethrography X-ray study of the urethra after injection of contrast medium by either a forward or a retrograde method.

vesicoureteral reflux Reflux of urine or contrast material from the bladder into the ureter.

II

Criteria for the Diagnosis of Selected Renal Disorders

Criteria for Diagnosis

ACIDOSIS, RENAL DISTAL TUBULAR
Definite

1. Metabolic acidosis, hypokalemia, hyperchloremia, and low plasma bicarbonate concentration.
2. Alkaline urine that persists at any level of plasma bicarbonate.
3. In infants and children, symptoms of retarded growth and dehydration.
4. In adults, symptoms of bone disease and renal calcification.
5. Absence of other tubular defects.
6. Family history of the disease.

ACIDOSIS, RENAL PROXIMAL TUBULAR
Definite

1. Low plasma bicarbonate concentration.
2. Alkaline urine that becomes acid if the extracellular bicarbonate level is reduced below the patient's maximum reabsorptive limit.
3. In the absence of bicarbonate in the urine, essentially normal titrable acid, ammonia formation, and urinary pH.
4. Retarded growth that improves strikingly with alkaline therapy.
5. Possible calciuria.
6. Absence of bone disease and renal calcification.

AMYLOIDOSIS, RENAL
Definite

1. Persistent proteinuria.
2. Characteristic renal electron microscopic histopathologic findings and/or tissue staining for amyloid (see Pathology Glossary).

Probable

1. Presence of pertinent antecedent or coexisting disease.
2. Proteinuria or concentration defect.
3. Tissue diagnosis of amyloidosis in other organ(s), e.g., rectal biopsy.

Possible

1. Presence of pertinent antecedent or coexisting disease.
2. Hypertension.
3. No renal symptomatology or findings.
4. Tissue diagnosis of amyloidosis in other organ(s), e.g., rectal biopsy.

ANALGESIC NEPHROPATHY (Fig. 55)

Definite

1. History of ingestion of more than 2 kg of mixed analgesic compounds.
2. Impaired renal function.
3. Histologic or radiographic evidence of papillary necrosis.
4. Chronic interstitial nephritis in cortical biopsies.
5. Positive ferric chloride test in urine or sulfhemoglobinemia or methemo-globinemia.

Probable

1. History of excessive analgesic ingestion or demonstration of methemo-globin or sulfhemoglobin.
2. Interstitial nephritis or papillary necrosis.
3. Abnormal renal function or urinalysis.
4. No evidence of other causes of renal abnormalities.

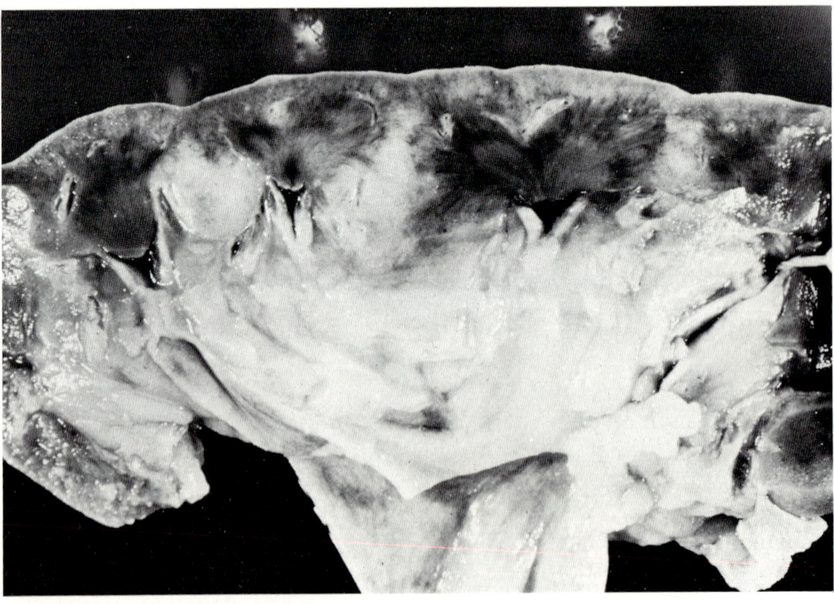

Fig. 55. Papillary necrosis in phenacetin nephropathy with interstitial nephritis and scarring of cortex. (Courtesy of M. Susin.)

Possible

1. Interstitial nephritis or papillary necrosis.
2. Abnormal renal function or urinalysis.
3. Analgesic ingestion of less than 2 kg.

CYSTIC DISEASE, MEDULLARY (Figs. 56 to 58)
Definite

1. Insidious onset of anemia, azotemia, and hyposthenuria with or without salt wasting, combined with a relatively normal urinary sediment and no proteinuria.
2. Family history of chronic renal insufficiency.
3. Characteristic histologic changes (see Clinical Glossary) without glomerular lesions. Proximal and distal tubules as well as collecting ducts are dilated, and cysts of varying sizes are seen predominantly at the corticomedullary junction. Tubular basement membranes are greatly thickened, and there is a diffuse interstitial cellular exudate and fibrosis.

Probable

1. Insidious onset of anemia, azotemia, and hyposthenuria with or without salt wasting, combined with a relatively normal urinary sediment and no proteinuria.
2. Family history of chronic renal insufficiency.

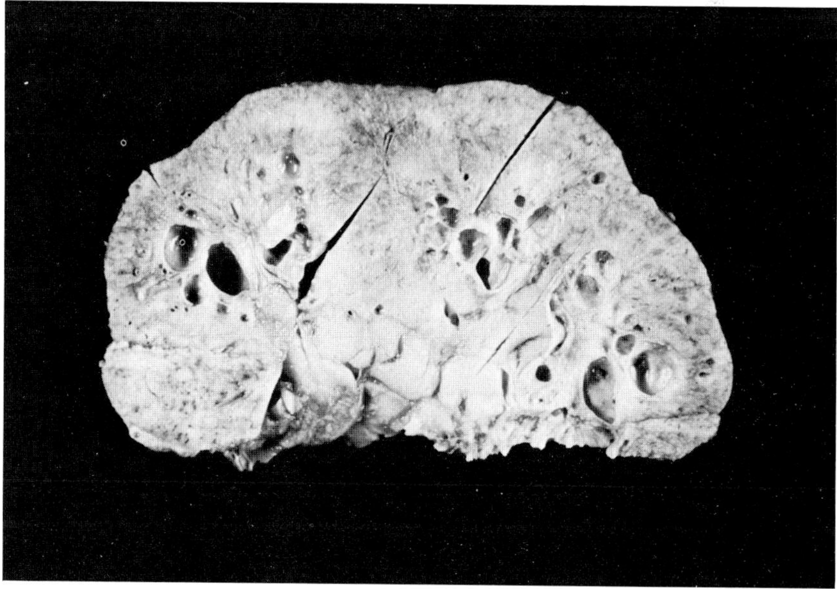

Fig. 56.   Gross specimen of a medullary cystic kidney. (Courtesy of M. Susin.)

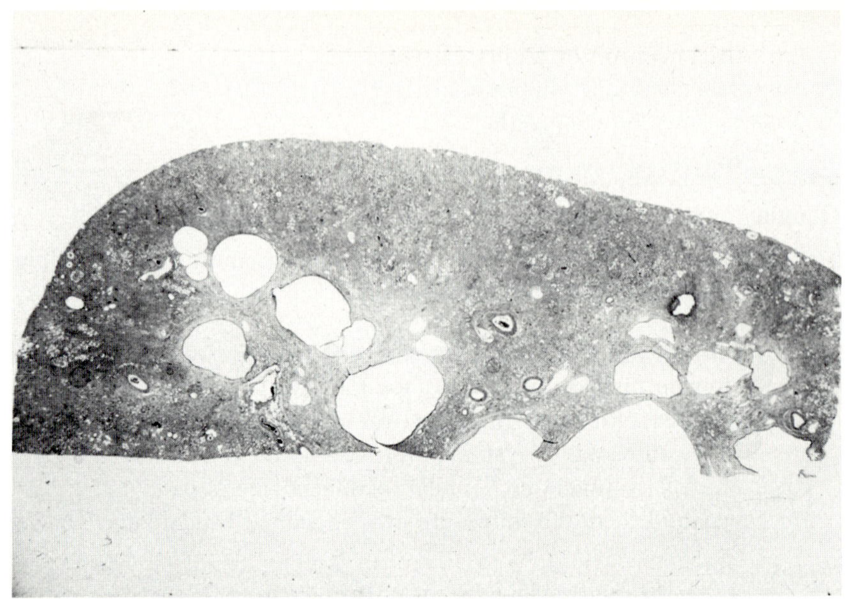

Fig. 57. Microscopic study of cystic kidney in Figure 56, showing cystic areas in the medulla and contracted cortex. (Courtesy of M. Susin.)

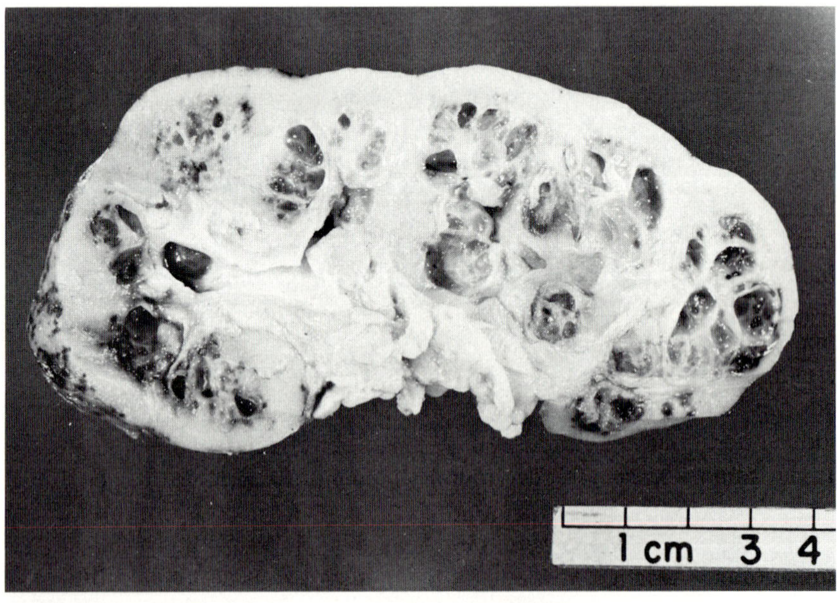

Fig. 58. Widespread cysts in a medullary cystic kidney. (Courtesy of M. Susin.)

3. Characteristic histologic changes with some partially or completely
   hyalinized glomeruli and some periglomerular fibrosis.

Possible

Hyposthenuria unresponsive to vasopressin and associated with azotemia,
with no ascertainable cause.

CYSTINURIA
Definite

1. Clinical signs of renal calculus.
2. Radiopaque renal calculi.
3. Characteristic calculi demonstrated to contain cystine.
4. More than 200 mg cystine in urine per 24 hours.

Probable

1. Clinical signs of renal calculus.
2. More than 200 mg cystine in urine per 24 hours, or positive Brand or
   Sullivan test on urine.

Possible

1. Clinical signs of renal calculus, especially when multiple.
2. Cystine crystals in urinary sediment.

DIABETES INSIPIDUS
Definite

1. Failure to increase the urine osmolality above 600 mOsm/kg following
   24 hours' dehydration indicates a severe defect in the urine concentrating mechanism. In true diabetes insipidus this defect can be corrected
   by ADH. Occasional patients with compulsive water-drinking show a
   similar response. In nephrogenic diabetes insipidus the urine osmolarity
   fails to rise in spite of ADH administration.
2. Decreased serum arginine vasopressin on biologic assay or immunoassay.

DIABETIC GLOMERULOSCLEROSIS (Figs. 59 and 60)
Definite

1. Diabetes mellitus.
2. Nephrotic syndrome.
3. Renal insufficiency.
4. Capillary microaneurysms in fundi.
5. Nodular glomerulosclerosis seen on renal biopsy.

Probable

1. Diabetes mellitus.
2. Proteinuria.

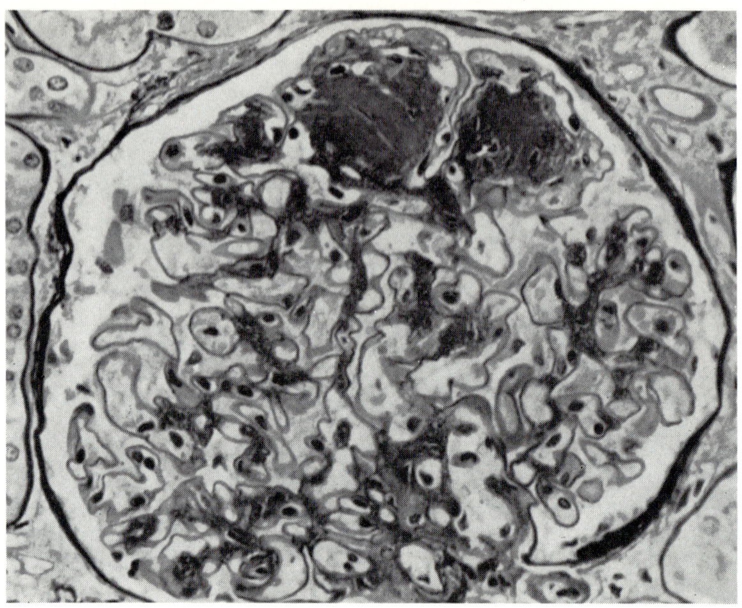

Fig. 59. Two characteristic nodules with patent peripheral capillaries in a glomerulus from a patient with nodular diabetic glomerulosclerosis. The nodules are lined by crisp basement membranes. There is only minimal deposition of PAS-positive material elsewhere in the mesangium. PAS. (From P. Kimmelstiel, Diabetic Nephropathy, in Becker [1].)

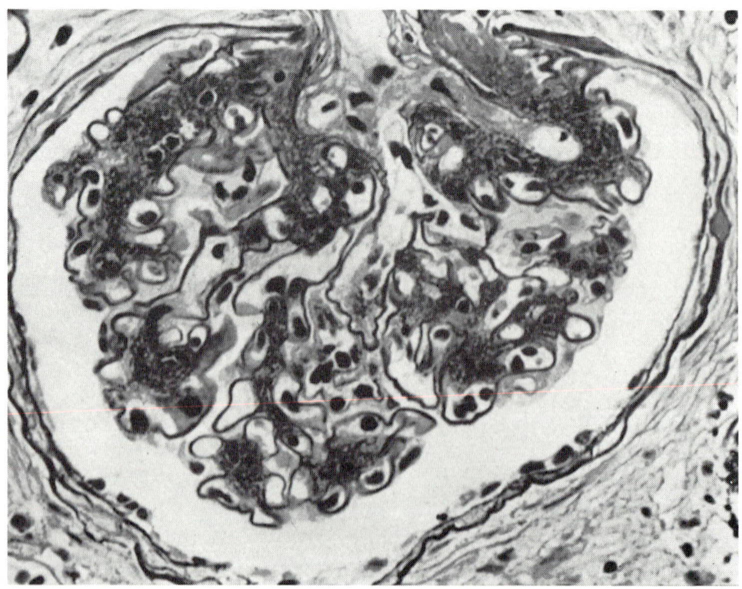

Fig. 60. Advanced diffuse intercapillary glomerulosclerosis. Glomerulus showing fine fibrillar mesangial deposit and a patent peripheral capillary with crisp basement membranes. PAS. (From P. Kimmelstiel, Diabetic Nephropathy, in Becker [1].)

3. Capillary microaneurysms in fundi.
4. On renal biopsy, diffuse glomerulosclerosis with or without exudative lesions.

Possible

1. Diabetes mellitus.
2. Proteinuria.
3. No evidence of pyelonephritis or other renal disease.

DIABETIC RENAL MICROANGIOPATHY

Definite

Unequivocal diagnosis can be made only by kidney biopsy revealing characteristic histologic features.

Probable

1. No evidence of other disease that might cause urine abnormalities.
2. Diagnosis of diabetes mellitus established and, in growth onset diabetes, of several years' duration.
3. Urine protein 1+ on two occasions or more plus any two of the following: edema, hypertension, BUN more than 20, or creatinine more than 1.2.
4. Small to large numbers of casts and usually no excess red blood cells.

Possible

1. No evidence of other disease that might cause urine abnormalities.
2. Diagnosis of diabetes mellitus established and, in growth onset diabetes, of several years' duration.
3. Urine protein 1+ on two occasions or more.
4. Small to large numbers of casts, and usually no excess red blood cells.

ENDOCARDITIS, SUBACUTE BACTERIAL, associated with NEPHRITIS

Definite

1. Auscultatory evidence of acquired or congenital heart disease.
2. Positive blood culture.
3. Proteinuria, usually mild but occasionally severe, especially early in the untreated phase of the disease.
4. Microhematuria often in "showers" (intermittent).
5. Focal glomerular involvement characterized by intracapillary thrombosis with or without capillary necrosis or dense sclerotic areas often obstructing capillaries. No immunohistologic abnormalities.

or

Diffuse (or focal) glomerulonephritis. In this form serum complement activity is depressed and immune glomerular deposits may be present.

Probable

1. Clinical manifestations of heart disease, acquired or congenital, with bloodstream infection.
2. Microscopic or macroscopic hematuria.

ENDOTOXIN SHOCK

Definite

1. Onset of chills, fever, and shock following manipulation of urinary tract or in the presence of severe localized infection due to gram-negative bacteria.
2. Positive blood culture for gram-negative bacterial species, with evidence of hypotension and onset of renal failure.

Probable

1. Acute or chronic urinary tract infection with sudden onset of shock and renal failure.
2. Shock and renal failure associated with peritonitis due to rupture of viscus.
3. Shock and renal failure following septic abortion.
4. Shock and renal failure associated with suppuration of biliary tract.
5. Shock and renal failure associated with meningococcal meningitis.
6. Shock and renal failure associated with body burns infected with gram-negative bacteria.
7. Shock and renal failure associated with urinary obstruction in elderly, especially males.
8. Shock and renal failure with chills and fever in patients receiving corticosteroids or immunosuppressive therapy.
9. Shock and renal failure in patients with chills and fever following surgery on intestinal tract, biliary tract, or urinary tract.
10. Postpartum chills and fever with shock and renal failure.

GLOMERULONEPHRITIS, ACUTE POSTSTREPTOCOCCAL (Fig. 61)

Definite

1. Sudden onset of hematuria and proteinuria.
2. Positive culture for group A streptococci from lesions in mucous membranes or on body surface.
3. Significant increase in serum antistreptolysin titer (ASO) or other streptococcal antibodies (e.g., antihyaluronidase).
4. Edema.
5. Blood urea nitrogen above normal.
6. Hypertension.
7. Decreased serum complement.
8. Characteristic histologic findings on electron microscopy and immunofluorescence.

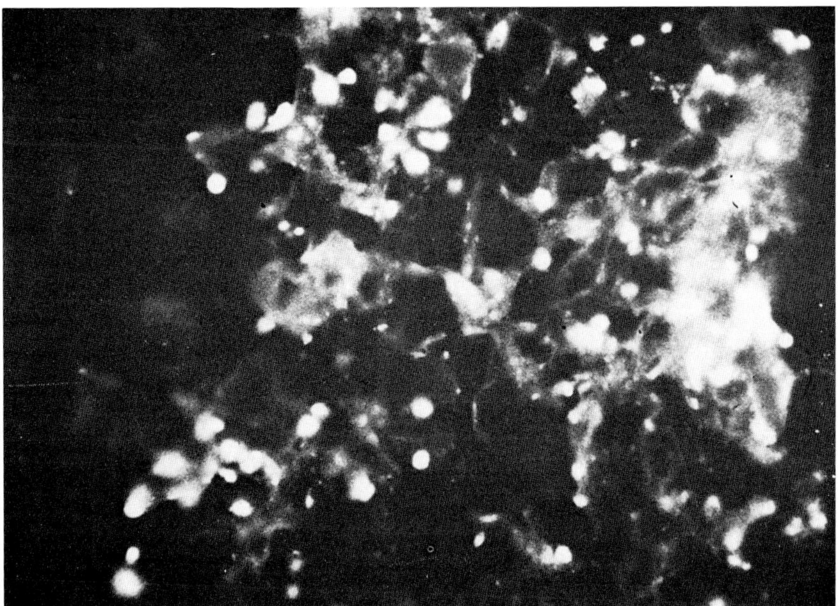

Fig. 61. Fluorescein-tagged antihuman IgG showing large number of "humps" of antigen-antibody complex in a patient with acute glomerulonephritis. (From Becker and Churg [2].)

Probable

1. Sudden onset of hematuria and proteinuria.
2. History of previous respiratory infection, recent positive culture for Group A streptococci, or significant increase in antistreptococcal antibodies.
3. Any one of the following:
   a. Edema.
   b. Hypertension.
   c. Blood urea nitrogen above normal.
   d. Decreased serum complement.
   e. Characteristic histologic findings on electron microscopy and immunofluorescence.

Possible

1. History of sudden onset of hematuria and/or proteinuria without any of the above criteria.
2. History of mucous membrane or body surface infection.

INFARCTED KIDNEY
Definite

Demonstration of the obstruction by arteriography or surgical visualization.

Probable

1. Sudden flank pain in a patient with vascular, especially cardiac, disease.
2. Nonfunction or greatly reduced function on the symptomatic side as revealed by radioactive hippuran studies.
3. Hematuria, gross or microscopic.
4. Normal pyelogram by retrograde method.
5. Later, a shrunken kidney or portion thereof.

Possible

1. Sudden proteinuria or hematuria in a patient with cardiovascular disease.
2. Rapidly developing hypertension.
3. Rising serum glutamic oxaloacetic transaminase, lactic dehydrogenase, or alkaline phosphatase.

LEPTOSPIRAL NEPHRITIS

Definite

1. Presence of acute febrile illness.
2. Proteinuria and/or hematuria.
3. Petechial hemorrhages.
4. Muscle pains and backaches.
5. Recovery of appropriate leptospira by laboratory animal inoculation and/or culture with the patient's blood or urine.

Probable

1. Presence of acute febrile illness.
2. Proteinuria and/or hematuria.
3. Increasing titers, in patient's serum, of specific antibodies to appropriate leptospiral organism.

Possible

1. Febrile illness.
2. Hematuria and/or proteinuria.
3. Sojourn in epidemic or endemic area.
4. History of possible or definite exposure to or contact with infected animals or waters contaminated with urine from infected animals.

LIPOID NEPHROSIS

Definite

1. Massive proteinuria (in infants and children, greater than 40 mg/m^2 per hour; in adults, greater than 0.2 gm/kg per day).
2. Selective proteinuria.
3. Reduction of serum albumin.
4. Spontaneous recovery or rapid disappearance of proteinuria with steroids.
5. No hypertension.

6. No red blood cells or red blood cell casts in urinary sediment.
7. No evidence of other systemic disease.
8. No azotemia.
9. Histologic lesion confirmed by electron microscopy (See FOOT PROCESS LOSS in Pathology Glossary).

Probable

1. Massive proteinuria (in infants and children, greater than 40 mg/m² per hour; in adults, greater than 0.2 gm/kg per day).
2. Selective proteinuria.
3. Reduction of serum albumin.
4. Transient azotemia, disappearing with diuresis.
5. Transient hypertension, disappearing with diuresis.
6. Less rapid response to steroids.
7. Occasional increase in red blood cells in urine (see FOOT PROCESS LOSS in Pathology Glossary), but no red blood cell casts.
8. No evidence of other systemic disease.
9. Histologic findings confirmed by silver methenamine stain.

Possible

1. Massive proteinuria whenever tested (especially in childhood).
2. Selective proteinuria or specific electron microscopic findings.
3. Azotemia, disappearing with diuresis.
4. Hypertension, disappearing with diuresis.
5. Occasional increase in red blood cells in urine (see FOOT PROCESS LOSS in Pathology Glossary), but no red blood cell casts.
6. Either response or lack of response to steroids.
7. Silver methenamine stains normal, but minimal proliferation present.

LUNG PURPURA with NEPHRITIS
(also GOODPASTURE'S SYNDROME) (Figs. 62 and 63)

Definite

1. Hemoptysis.
2. Dyspnea.
3. Characteristic radiographic pulmonary opacities.
4. Iron deficiency anemia.
5. Proteinuria and excess of red blood cells and red blood cell casts in urinary sediment.
6. Characteristic linear pattern of immunofluorescent deposits along glomerular capillary basement membranes in renal biopsy.
7. Rapid deterioration in renal function.

Probable

1. Hemoptysis or dyspnea accompanied by radiographic pulmonary abnormalities consistent with hemorrhage into alveoli.

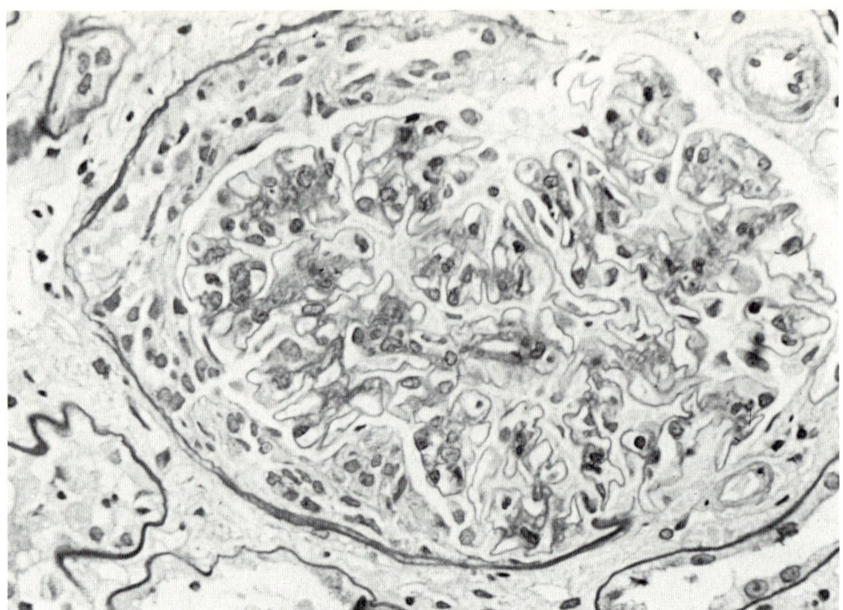

Fig. 62. Glomerulonephritis with extracapillary proliferation. Large crescents form in the glomerular (Bowman's) capsular space, while there is comparatively little activity in the capillaries and mesangium. Clinically there is rapidly progressive glomerulonephritis which on occasion is accompanied by the nephrotic syndrome. (From Becker and Churg [2].)

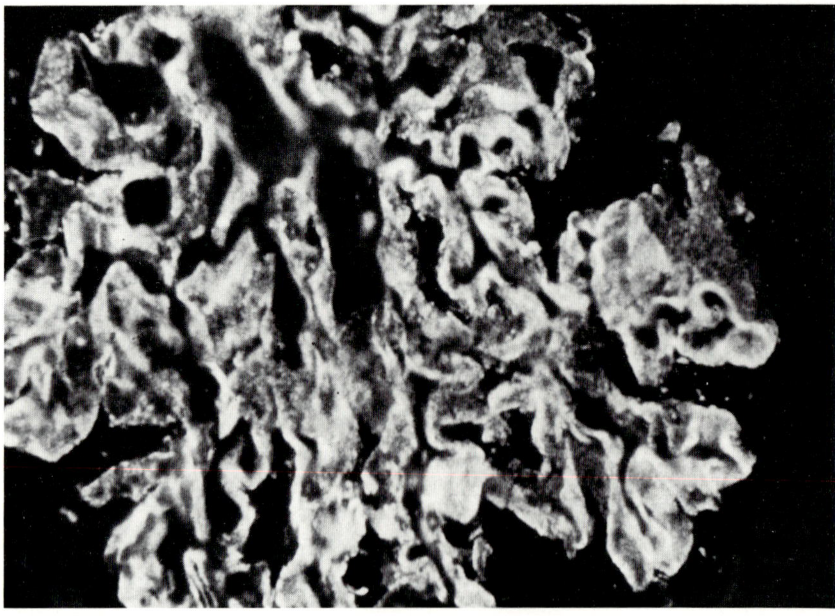

Fig. 63. Fluorescein-tagged antihuman complement as seen in lung purpura with nephritis. (Courtesy of C. Becker.)

2. Proteinuria and excess red blood cells in urinary sediment.
3. Focal or diffuse proliferative glomerulonephritis without definite evidence of fibrinoid necrosis.
4. Rapid deterioration in renal function.

Possible

1. Proteinuria and excess red blood cells in urinary sediment.
2. Focal or diffuse proliferative glomerulonephritis without evidence of fibrinoid necrosis.
3. Radiographic pulmonary abnormalities consistent with hemorrhage into alveoli without hemoptysis or dyspnea.

LUPUS NEPHRITIS (Figs. 64 to 66)

Definite

1. Clinical picture of systemic lupus nephritis (SLE).
2. Clinical findings of renal involvement.
3. Decreased complement and presence of antinuclear antibodies in serum.
4. Renal histologic features consistent with SLE (see Clinical Glossary), including presence of hematoxylin bodies.

Probable

1. Clinical picture not diagnostic for SLE.
2. Clinical findings of renal involvement.
3. Decreased serum complement.
4. Renal histologic features suggestive of lupus nephritis without hematoxylin bodies.

Possible

1. Clinical picture not diagnostic for SLE.
2. Clinical findings of renal involvement.
3. Decreased serum complement.
4. Renal histologic features not diagnostic.

MEMBRANOUS NEPHROPATHY (Figs. 67 and 68)

Definite

1. Prolonged massive proteinuria (greater than 0.2 gm/kg per day).
2. No evidence of generalized disease processes such as diabetes, clotting defects, or mechanical increase in venous pressure (renal venous thrombosis), nor any past history of these conditions.
3. Exclusion of above generalized disease processes by radiography and appropriate biochemical and coagulation studies.
4. No response of proteinuria to steroid therapy.
5. Characteristic electron microscopic changes (see MEMBRANOUS TRANSFORMATION in Pathology Glossary).

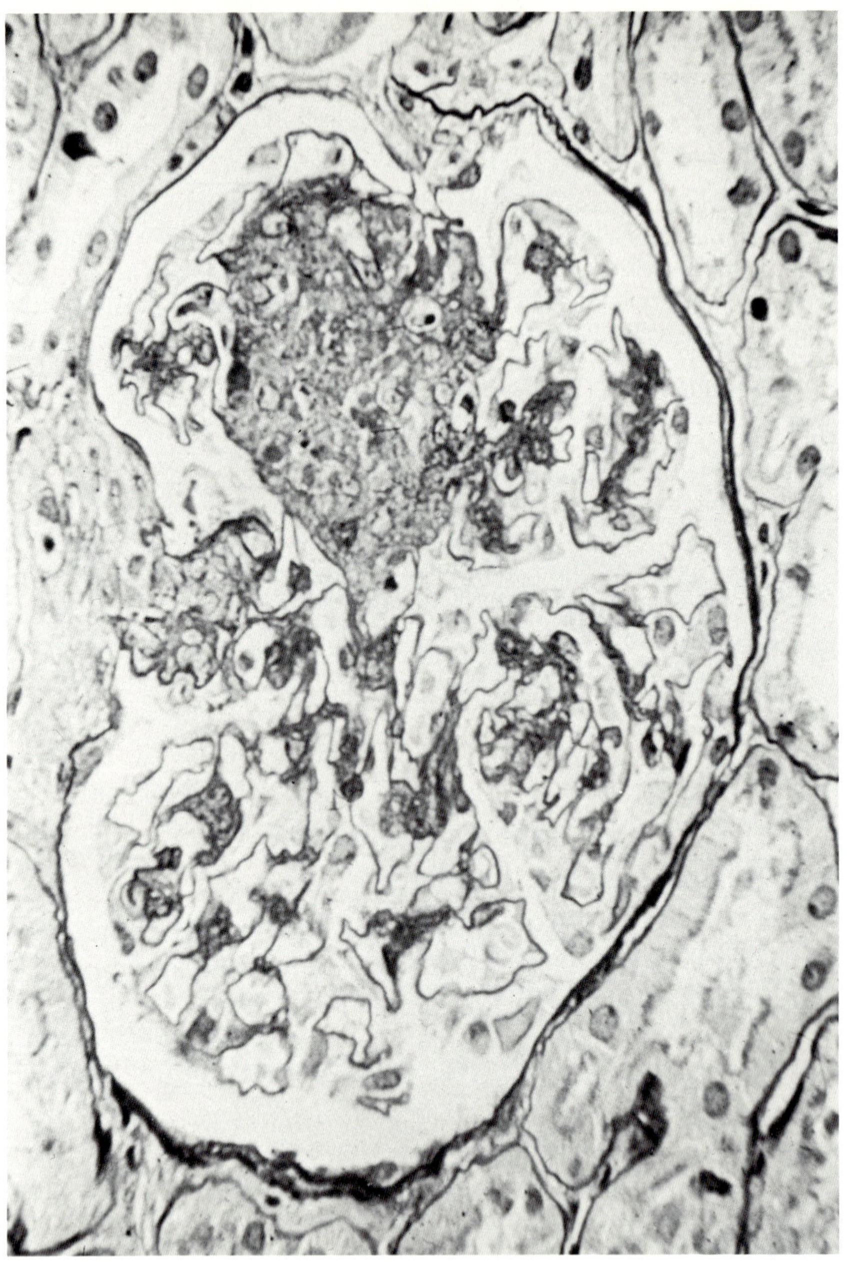

Fig. 64. A case of focal lupus nephritis in which part of the glomerulus is converted into a dense nodule with a moderate number of proliferated cells. (From Becker and Churg [2].)

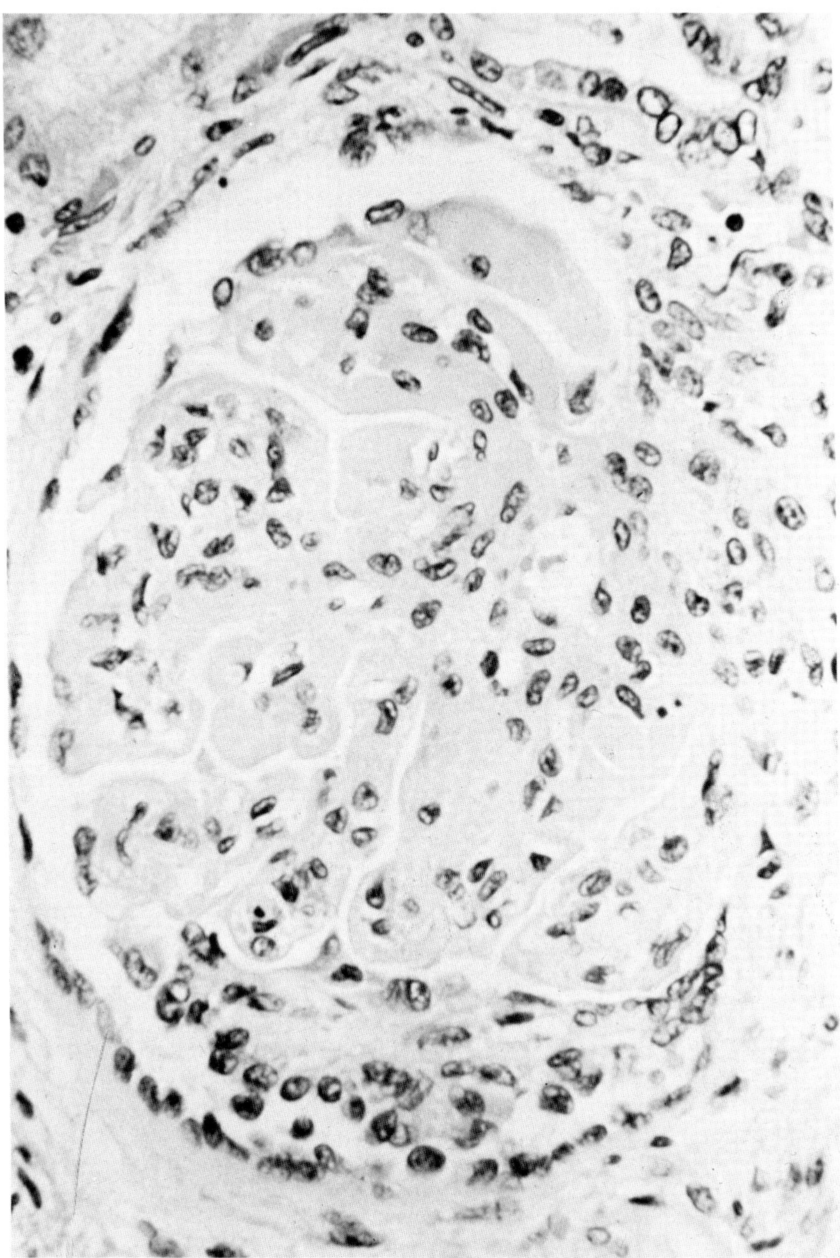

Fig. 65. While not absolutely specific, the eosinophilic areas in this glomerulus, some in the form of wire loops, are strongly suggestive of lupus nephritis. (From Becker and Churg [2].)

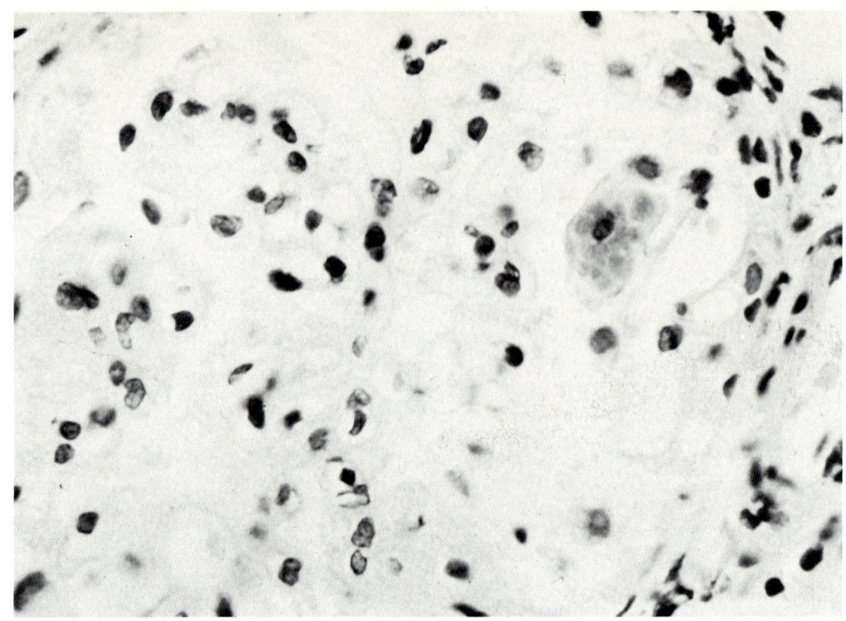

Fig. 66. A hematoxylin body in a glomerulus in lupus nephritis. A fairly large aggregate of light to dark purplish structures is seen at center right. Although this is a pathognomonic finding in lupus nephritis, it is seen in only about 5 percent of biopsies. (From Becker and Churg [2].)

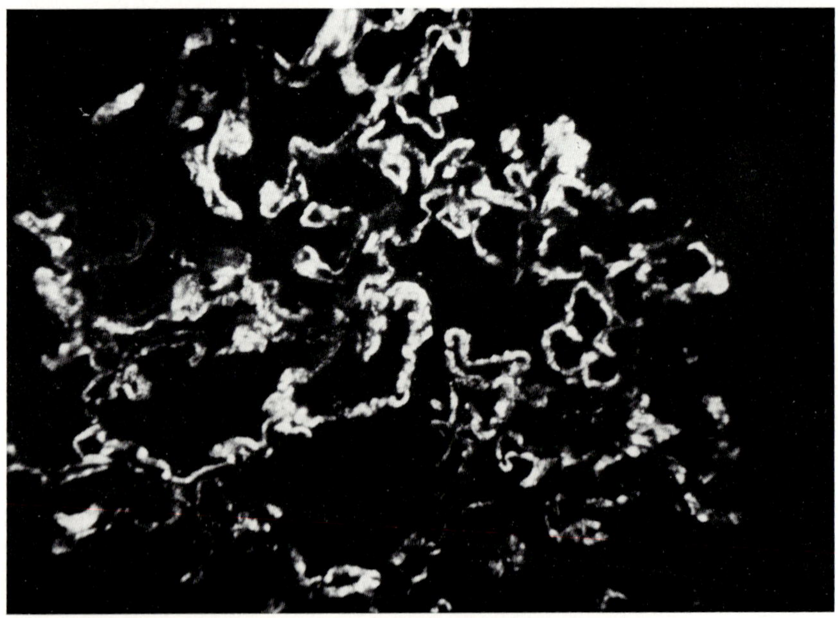

Fig. 67. Immunofluorescence miscroscopy and a stain for gamma globulin (IgG) reveal diffuse, finely granular deposits along the capillary walls. (From Becker and Churg [2].)

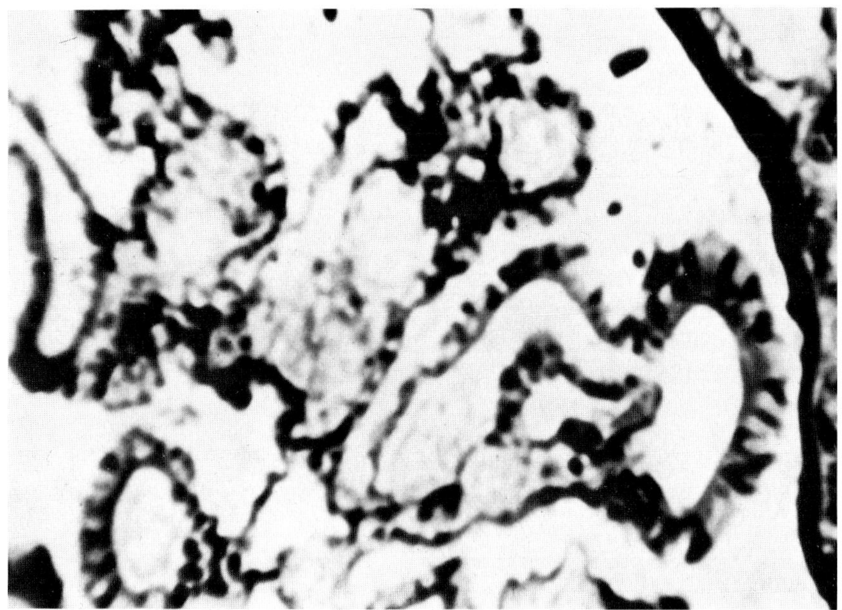

Fig. 68. In advanced membranous nephropathy silver methenamine stain reveals distinct projections (spikes) covering most of the capillary surfaces. (From Becker and Churg [2].)

6. Typical staining seen on fluorescence microscopy (see MEMBRANOUS TRANSFORMATION in Pathology Glossary).
7. Characteristic changes seen by light microscopy with silver methenamine stain.

Probable

1. Massive proteinuria.
2. Typical basement membrane changes seen on light microscopy with silver or other mechanical methenamine.
3. No history of venous thrombosis, clotting defects, diabetes, or proteinuria.
4. Failure of response to steroid therapy.

Possible

1. Heavy proteinuria whenever examined.
2. Diffuse uniform basement membrane changes seen on light microscopy, with negative stains for amyloid.
3. No history of diabetes or other mechanical causes.
4. Negative response to steroids.

MERCURY TOXICITY
Definite

1. History of exposure to mercury.
2. Demonstration of excess of mercury in body fluids or tissue.
3. Acute renal failure, nephrotic syndrome, or specific tubular defects.
4. Renal biopsy showing proximal tubular necrosis.

Probable

1. History of mercury exposure.
2. Compatible clinical renal syndrome.
3. Absence of other causative factors in history.
4. Absence of evidence of other disease by renal biopsy.

Possible

1. History of exposure to mercury.
2. Compatible clinical renal syndrome.

NEPHRITIS, HEREDITARY, CHRONIC
Definite

1. Abnormal urinary sediment with erythrocytes, leukocytes, and casts.
2. Nerve deafness.
3. Demonstrated involvement of more than one family member by 1 and/ or 2 above.
4. Normal serum complement.
5. Renal biopsy showing glomerulonephritis, interstitial nephritis, and renal foam cells (see INTERSTITIAL INFILTRATES in Pathology Glossary).

Probable

1. Abnormal urinary sediment with erythrocytes, leukocytes, and casts.
2. Possible family history of nerve deafness.
3. Positive family history for renal disease without definite involvement of more than one family member.
4. Normal serum complement.
5. Renal biopsy showing glomerulonephritis, interstitial nephritis, and renal foam cells.

Possible

1. Abnormal urinary sediment with erythrocytes, leukocytes, and casts.
2. Positive family history.
3. Renal biopsy showing glomerulonephritis and interstitial nephritis.

NEPHROTIC SYNDROME, MECHANICAL CAUSES OF
Definite

1. Proteinuria greater than 0.3 mg/kg per day or 3 gm per 24 hours.
2. Radiologic renal evidence of venous obstructive lesions.

3. Clinical findings of thrombosis elsewhere.
4. Loin pain, tenderness, and swelling when onset is sudden.
5. Transient microscopic hematuria when onset is sudden.
6. Renal biopsy findings as described in Syndrome Glossary.

Probable

1. Proteinuria greater than 0.3 mg/kg per day or 3 gm per 24 hours.
2. Suggestive renal radiologic studies.
3. Suggestive history of thromboembolic disorders.
4. Typical histologic features of membranous nephropathy.
5. Clinical evidence of amyloidosis.
6. In infants and children, acute dehydration.

Possible

1. Proteinuria greater than 0.3 mg/kg per day or 3 gm per 24 hours.
2. Suggestive history of thromboembolic disorders.
3. Clinical evidence of amyloidosis.
4. Membranous nephropathy.

POLYCYSTIC RENAL DISEASE

Definite

1. Palpable kidneys with irregular surface.
2. X-ray evidence of cysts.
3. Positive family history.

Probable

Positive family history with enlarged kidneys and any or all of the following:
    a. Proteinuria.
    b. Hematuria.
    c. Recurrent urinary tract infection.
    d. Raised blood pressure.
    e. Impaired kidney function.
    f. Loin pain.

Possible

As under Probable, but in the absence of a positive family history and/or palpable kidneys.

PREECLAMPSIA AND ECLAMPSIA (Fig. 69)

Definite

1. No evidence of previous hypertensive or renal parenchymal disease.
2. Raised uric acid in the face of normal BUN or creatinine for that stage of pregnancy.

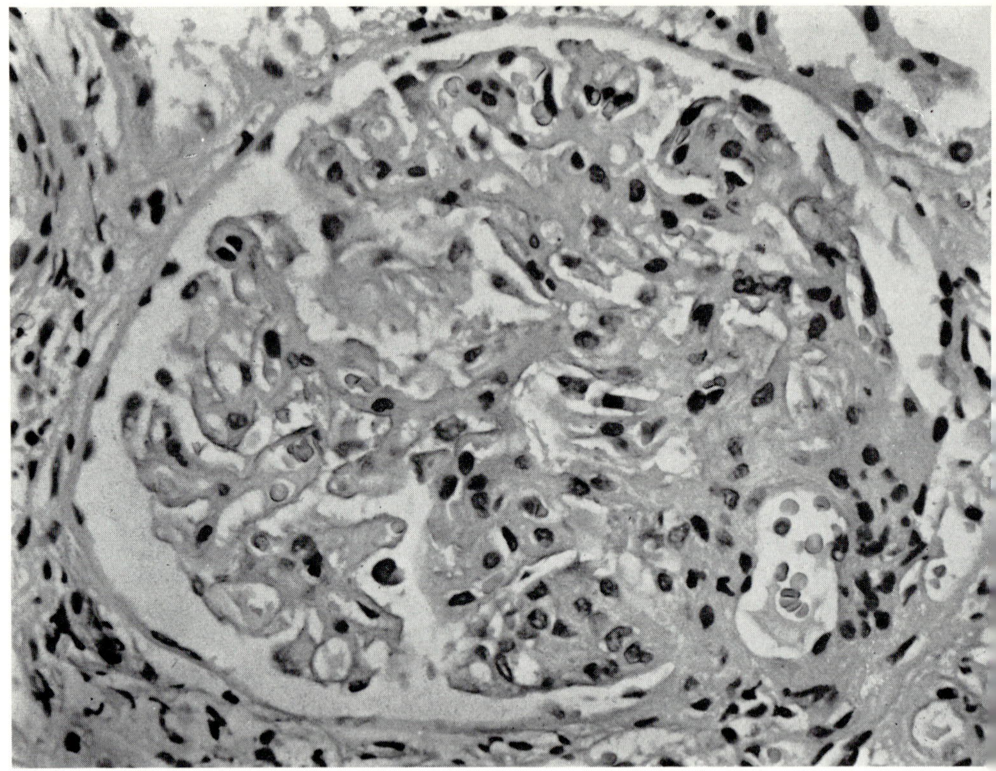

Fig. 69. In the more severe forms of preeclampsia the glomerular capillary wall has a smudgy appearance as a result of the abundant deposition of fibrinoid material. Note the large juxtaglomerular apparatus, a common finding in preeclampsia, and the sclerotic changes in the arteriole (right lower corner). H&E. (From C. L. Pirani and V. E. Pollak, Renal Involvement in Toxemia of Pregnancy, in Becker [1].)

3. Persistent or intermittent hypertension ($>$120/90 mm Hg) and/or edema and/or proteinuria.
4. Ophthalmologic changes consisting of retinal edema and/or papilledema and changing segmental arteriolar spasm.
5. Renal biopsy seldom performed except for differentiation from preexisting renal disease.

Probable

1. No evidence of previous hypertensive or renal parenchymal disease.
2. Persistent or intermittent hypertension ($>$120/90 mm Hg) and/or edema and/or proteinuria.
3. Raised uric acid, BUN, and creatinine. This may indicate preexisting renal disease, severe preeclampsia, or a combination of the two.

Possible

Hypertension and/or edema and/or proteinuria.

PYELONEPHRITIS, ACUTE NONOBSTRUCTIVE (Fig. 70)
Definite

Significant bacteriuria associated with loin pain, fever, and other symptoms referable to the upper urinary tract.

PYELONEPHRITIS, ASYMPTOMATIC
Definite

1. Positive ureteric urine culture.
2. Positive renal biopsy culture (rarely found).
3. Positive Fairley test.

Probable

1. Bacteriuria.
2. Rise of serum antibody titer to infecting strain of *E. coli*.
3. Urinary sediment abnormalities.

Possible

1. Pyuria.
2. Defect of urinary concentrating ability.
3. Increased urinary enzyme excretion, e.g., catalase.

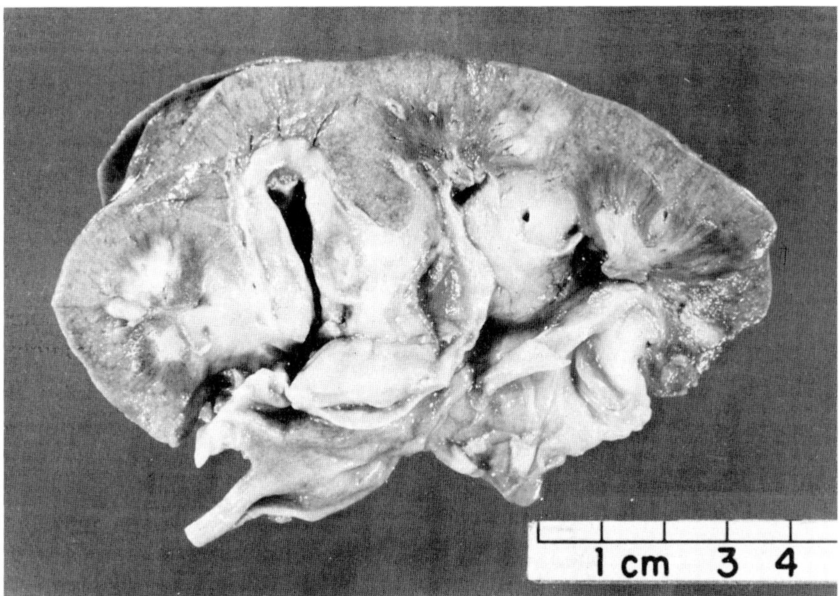

Fig. 70.   Papillary necrosis in acute pyelonephritis. (Courtesy of M. Susin.)

RADIATION NEPHRITIS (Fig. 71)

Definite

1. Previous history of exposure of kidneys (one or both) to ionizing radiation in a dose of at least 2300 rads administered over a period of 6 weeks or less.
2. Development of proteinuria and/or high blood pressure after a latent interval of several months.
3. On renal biopsy, histologic evidence of radiation nephritis consisting of severe vascular damage with or without interstitial fibrosis.

Probable

1. Previous history of exposure of kidneys (one or both) to ionizing radiation in a dose of at least 2300 rads administered over a period of 6 weeks or less.
2. Development of proteinuria and/or high blood pressure after a latent interval of several months.

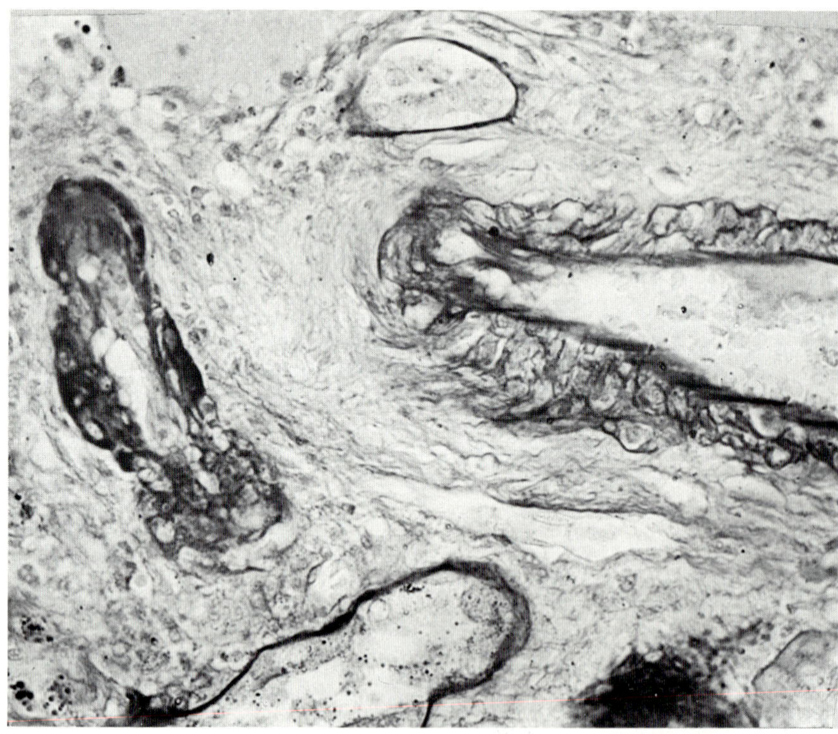

Fig. 71. Artery and arteriole from a patient with acute radiation nephritis. The artery is normal. The arteriole shows a hyalin change in the muscle. Note the atropic tubules. PAS. (From R. W. Luxton and S. B. de C. Baker, Radiation Nephritis, in Becker [1].)

Possible

Evidence of parenchymatous renal disease with a history of exposure to ionizing radiation.

RENAL FAILURE, ACUTE ANURIC or OLIGURIC (also ACUTE TUBULAR NECROSIS)

Definite

1. Urine volume of less than 400 ml per 24 hours (nonoliguric renal failure may occur).
2. Increase in serum creatinine concentration.

Probable

1. Urine sodium concentration greater than 40 mEq/liter, osmolality of urine differing no more than 50 mOsm/kg from that of plasma in a patient with urine volume of less than 400 ml per 24 hours.
2. Failure of urine volume to increase significantly following an intravenous dose of 150 mg ethacrynic acid or 80 mg furosemide.

RENAL INSUFFICIENCY, ACUTE NONOBSTRUCTIVE (OLIGURIC or ANURIC)

Definite

1. Acute reduction of urinary output (usually less than 400 ml per 24 hours).
2. Increasing serum creatinine concentration in the absence of severe dehydration and/or severe sodium depletion.
3. In the presence of tubular necrosis with oliguria, a lower than normal U/P ratio of urea and osmolality.

$$U_{urea}/P_{urea} < 10 \qquad U_{osmol}/P_{osmol} < 1.2$$

Probable

1. Acute reduction of urinary output.
2. Increase of BUN.

Possible

Acute reduction of urinary output in the presence of predisposing cause.

RENAL INSUFFICIENCY, ACUTE POLYURIC

Definite

1. Rising serum creatinine in the face of normal or increased urinary output.
2. Reduced U/P urea and osmolality ratios.
3. Presence of precipitating factors such as urinary tract obstruction and anesthetics (methoxyflurane).
4. No evidence of previous episode of oliguric or anuric renal insufficiency.

Probable

1. Rising serum creatinine in the face of normal or increased urinary output.
2. Reduced U/P urea and osmolality ratios.
3. No evidence of previous episode of oliguric or anuric renal insufficiency.

Possible

Rising serum creatinine in the face of normal or increased urinary ouput.

RENAL OSTEODYSTROPHY
Definite

1. Chronic renal insufficiency.
2. Osteodystrophic changes shown by x-ray.
3. Positive bone biopsy.
4. No other metabolic, congenital, or hereditary bone disease.

Probable

1. Chronic renal insufficiency.
2. Osteodystrophic changes shown by x-ray.
3. No other metabolic, congenital, or hereditary bone disease.

RENAL RICKETS
Definite

1. Chronic renal insufficiency.
2. Osteodystrophic changes shown by x-ray.
3. Positive bone biopsy.
4. Growth disturbances in children.
5. No other metabolic, congenital, or hereditary bone disease.

Probable

1. Chronic renal insufficiency.
2. Osteodystrophic changes shown by x-ray.
3. No other metabolic, congenital, or hereditary bone disease.

RENAL SCHISTOSOMIASIS (Figs. 72 and 73)
Definite

1. Recovery of characteristic ova ($140 \times 60\ \mu$). These have a conspicuous terminal spine. Ova may be found in the urine or stool, especially after physical activity, and by rectal or bladder wall biopsy.
2. Cystoscopic demonstration of papules, "sandy patches," and areas of fibrosis.
3. White blood cell casts, red blood cell casts, or waxy or granular casts in the urine at each repeated examination.

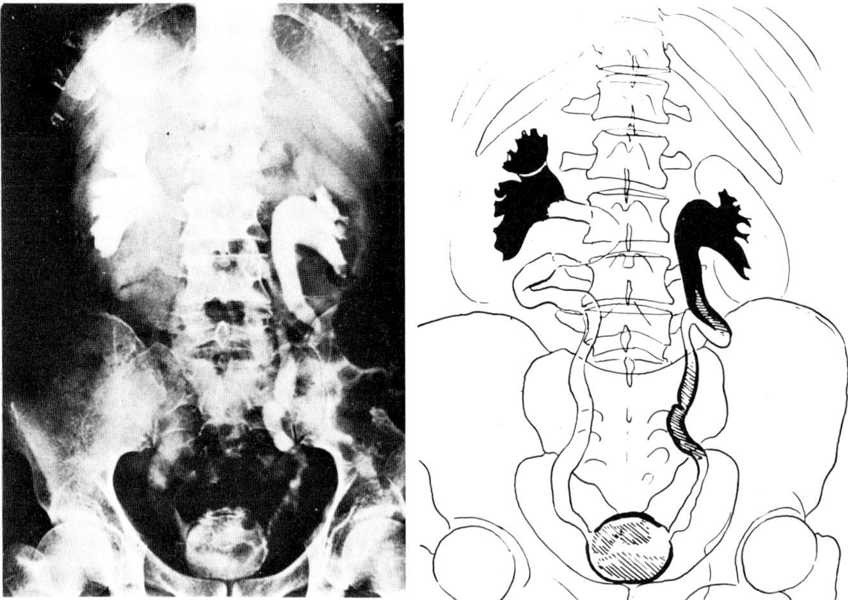

Fig. 72. Haematobium schistosomiasis is characterized by obstruction to the urinary outflow tract, particularly at the vesicoureteral junction as seen on radiologic examination. Granulomatous lesions of the bladder may also be seen, and calcified schistosoma eggs are frequently noted. (Courtesy of E. L. Becker.)

Probable

1. Positive bilharzial complement fixation test with rising titer.
2. Hematuria.
3. Normal cystoscopic examination.

Possible

1. Recovery of ova in urine.
2. Hematuria.

RENOVASCULAR HYPERTENSION

Definite

1. Diastolic blood pressure above 90 mm Hg.
2. Stenosis of main or branch renal artery on arteriogram, usually with greater than 50 percent reduction of luminal diameter and with evidence of collateral circulation.
3. Greater than 2:1 ratio of renal vein renin activity of ischemic kidney to uninvolved kidney.
4. Positive divided renal function test, based on excessive sodium and water reabsorption by the ischemic kidney:

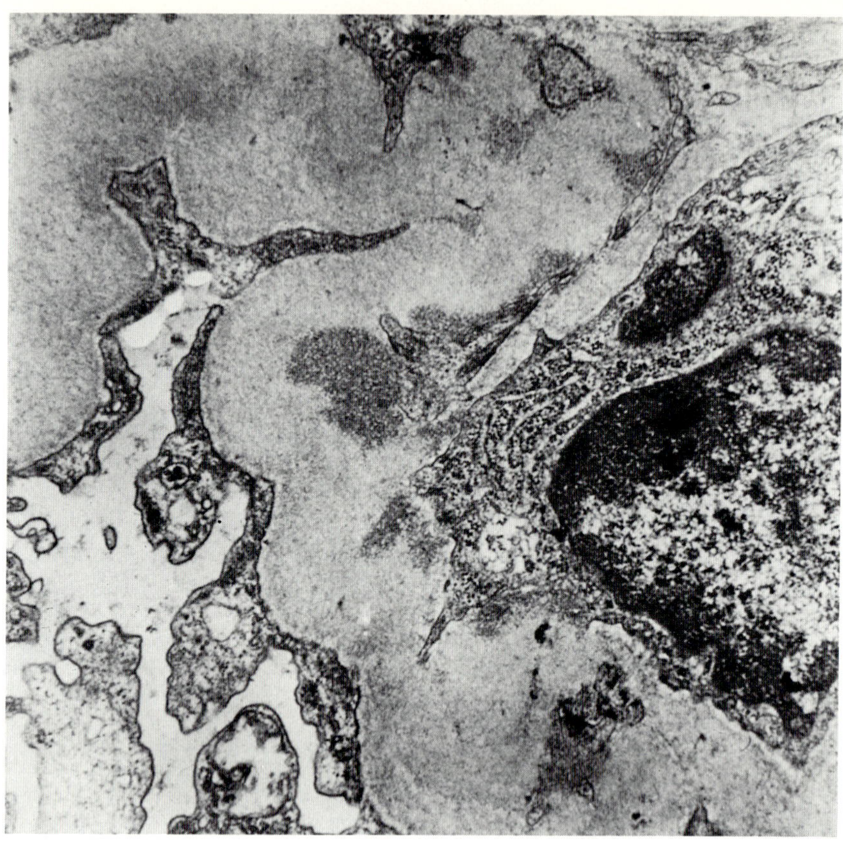

Fig. 73. In Mansoni schistosomiasis a true nephritis with nephrotic syndrome has been reported on occasion. The electronmicroscopic findings reveal a subendothelial accumulation of antigen-antibody complexes. (Courtesy of E. L. Becker.)

HOWARD TEST—At least 40 percent reduction in urine volume from the ischemic kidney with either a 15 percent reduction in urine sodium concentration or a 50 percent increase in urine creatinine concentration on the same side.

STAMEY TEST—MAIN ARTERY LESION. 66 percent reduction in urine flow from the ischemic kidney and greater than 100 percent increase in urine paraamino hippuric acid (PAH) or creatinine concentration on the same side.

STAMEY TEST—BRANCH ARTERY LESION. 50 percent reduction in urine flow from the ischemic kidney and greater than 20 percent increase in urine PAH or creatinine concentration on the same side.

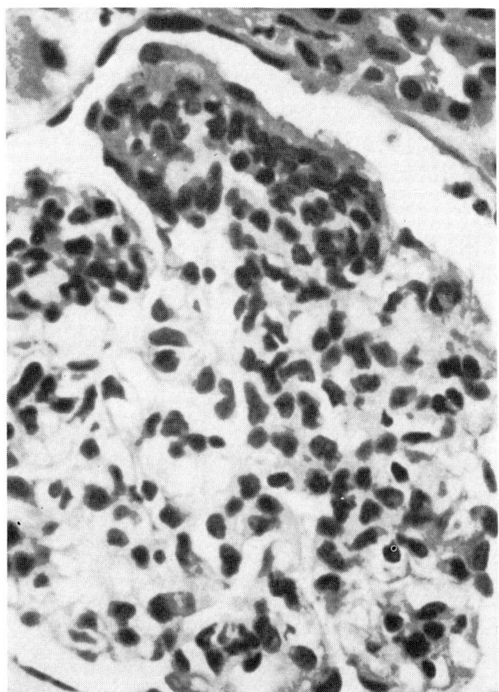

Fig. 74. Focal proliferative glomerular lesion in a patient with Schönlein-Henoch purpura. The lesion was associated with purpura, microscopic hematuria, and proteinuria. H&E. (From J. D. Blainey, J. Hardwicke, and R. Lanningan, Focal Glomeruloncphritis, in Becker [1].)

Probable

1. Diastolic blood pressure above 90 mm Hg.
2. On intravenous pyelogram, delay in appearance time and/or late hyperconcentration of contrast material by the ischemic kidney.

Possible

1. Diastolic blood pressure above 90 mm Hg.
2. Abdominal or flank bruit.
3. Demonstrable vascular occlusive disease outside of the kidney.
4. On intravenous pyelogram, disparity in size of kidneys.
5. Unilateral abnormality in radioisotope renogram.
6. Increased peripheral vein renin activity.

SCHÖNLEIN-HENOCH PURPURA (Fig. 74)

Definite

1. No evidence of other disease that might cause hematuria or other urinary abnormalities.

2. Skin manifestations: purpura rash, usually on buttocks and lower extremities.
3. Gastrointestinal symptoms: colicky pain with occult blood in stool.
4. Edema and pain in joints of lower extremities.
5. No abnormality in clotting mechanism or platelets.
6. Normal or elevated serum complement levels.
7. Hematuria and/or proteinuria occasionally severe, leading to the nephrotic syndrome.
8. Typical glomerular histologic findings: focal and segmental endothelial proliferation with positive immunohistologic findings on kidney biopsy.
9. Typical skin biopsy findings: perivascular infiltrates with polymorphonuclear cells and eosinophils.

Possible

1. No other disease that might cause urinary abnormalities.
2. Indefinite purpuric skin rash without typical skin biopsy but with wheals and skin necrosis.
3. Mild proteinuria (<1 gm/24 hours).
4. 2 to 10 RBC/HPF.
5. Focal and segmental endothelial proliferation with positive immunohistologic findings on kidney biopsy.
6. Occult blood in stool with or without abdominal symptoms.
7. Typical histologic findings on renal biopsy.

SPONGE KIDNEY, MEDULLARY

Definite

Roentgenography only can provide diagnosis. Urography is more reliable than retrograde pyelography, and findings are limited to renal medulla.

WITHOUT CALCULI. With the contrast the collecting tubules of single or multiple renal pyramids are seen as linear striations or small cystic cavities 1–5 mm in size. The papillae and minor calyces are enlarged.

WITH CALCULI. Numerous clusters of small calcifications localized to the pyramids within the cystic dilatations described above. A form of nephrocalcinosis.

TUBERCULOSIS, RENAL

Definite

Repeated positive cultural evidence of *M. tuberculosis* from the urine or renal tissue.

Probable

1. Radiologic signs characteristic of renal tuberculosis.
2. Presence or history of pulmonary tuberculosis.
3. Pyuria.

Possible

1. Hematuria, pyuria, mild proteinuria, or lowered specific gravity of urine.
2. Renal pain or dysuria.
3. Presence or history of pulmonary tuberculosis.

UROPATHY, OBSTRUCTIVE

Definite

Demonstration of a structural lesion interfering with the free flow of urine. This is accomplished by cystoscopy, intravenous urography, or retrograde pyelography.

III

Laboratory Procedures Aiding Diagnosis

Examination of the Urine

Examination of the urine is of paramount importance in the evaluation of a patient suspected of having renal disease.

Since the first voided morning specimen of urine is usually concentrated, it is the one most likely to reveal abnormalities, particularly on microscopic examination. The morning specimen is usually satisfactory for routine examination, but analyses of properly preserved 24-hour samples will give more accurate quantitative measurements of protein and other constituents. The urine sample is examined preferably within thirty minutes after it is passed, but if necessary it may be stored under refrigeration. (See discussion of collection techniques under Diagnosis of Urinary Tract Infection, pp. 223–224.) Both color and odor are significant in a gross inspection of urine. Discoloration may be due to medication or to the presence of blood or blood clots. A cloudy urine may indicate mucus, pus, or both. The odor may be ammoniacal because of bacterial action on urea, disease states, or the presence of amines such as asparagine.

URINALYSIS

All routine urinalyses should include a measurement of specific gravity or, preferably, of osmolality. The latter may be measured by determining the freezing point depression. This is frequently impracticable for the routine physician's office. At the present time, however, the estimation of refractive index is a relatively simple and rapid procedure performed with the clinical hand refractometer and requiring only a single drop of urine. The readings are translated into specific gravity or osmolality by means of conversion tables or charts.

The pH of the urine varies throughout the day and also should be measured in all urine specimens.

Evaluation of proteinuria is of primary importance in urinalysis, since fixed and reproducible proteinuria always signifies renal disease and must be investigated. Proteinuria may be a sign of altered glomerular filtration but also may be due to failure or inadequate function of tubular cells in reabsorbing filtered proteins. There are numerous techniques available to measure proteinuria, including electrophoresis, immunodiffusion, dipsticks, and various chemical methods.

Glucose and other reducing substances must also be measured, and this can be done by dipsticks, Tes-Tape, or both. Examination for occult blood and ketonuria should also be done routinely.

THE URINARY SEDIMENT

In health the urine contains small numbers of cells and other formed elements from the genitourinary tract: casts and epithelial cells from the nephron; epithelial cells from the pelves, ureters, bladder, and urethra; and mucous threads and spermatozoa. A few erythrocytes and leukocytes apparently reach the urine by diapedesis from any part of the urinary tract.

In renal parenchymal disease the urine usually contains increased numbers of cells and casts discharged from an organ which is otherwise accessible only by biopsy or at operation. The urinary sediment provides information useful for both diagnosis and prognosis. In some instances, even of advanced parenchymal renal lesions, however, the urinary sediment may appear normal.

Preparation of the Sediment

The rules of collecting and handling urine specified under Diagnosis of Urinary Tract Infection (pp. 223–224) apply when the urinary sediment is to be examined. The urine should be a clean catch, well mixed and freshly voided. The first morning specimen, examined soon after it is passed, is most suitable for sediment analysis, because it is concentrated and the formed elements are less likely to be lysed or distorted. If the examination must be delayed for a short period, the urine may be stored in a refrigerator for an hour or so, but a number of cells and casts may be destroyed thus. Urine can also be preserved by addition of formalin or preservative tablets, but these may interfere with chemical analysis. If a preservative is used, the urine should first be divided into two portions, one for microscopic examination of sediment, to which the preservative is added, and one for chemical analysis, to which nothing is added.

When a lesion is suspected in the lower genitourinary tract, it is advisable to collect three successive specimens during voiding. If abnormalities such as leukocytes are more obvious in the earlier specimens, the underlying lesions may be in the prostate or seminal vesicles, for example.

So that separate microscopic examinations of different urine specimens may be compared with each other, always use the same technique when examining the sediment. In a chemically clean, conical centrifuge tube, spin a constant volume (15 ml) of the first voided urine at a constant rate (2000 rpm) for a fixed time (5 minutes) (if the rate is slower than 2000 rpm, spin for somewhat longer). Quickly invert the centrifuge tube and allow the supernatant urine to escape, then stand the tube upright. This will leave a small amount of urine with the solid sediment, if any, in the conical tip of the tube. With a small glass pipet and bulb, or by stirring with a clean rod, make sure that the "button" of urinary sediment is resuspended in the residual fluid.

Caution

With the pipet place one drop of the suspension on an absolutely clean slide. Stain with methylene blue, if desired. Cover with a clean thin cover slip. Examine while still wet.

If the sediment is particularly heavy, it may be impossible to resuspend it in the small amount of urine normally remaining after the tube is inverted. More urine should be left in the tube, and this should be recorded when reporting results.

When there is gross blood or pus in the urine, a drop of the well-mixed specimen should be examined *undiluted*. Casts are found only with difficulty in such urines and should be looked for with special care, before and after gentle centrifugation.

Heavy deposits of phosphates in neutral or alkaline urine, or of urates in acid urine, may obscure formed elements in the sediment. Phosphates can be dissolved by adding one drop of 2% acetic acid to the sediment, and urates can be dissolved by gently warming the original tube of urine to 55°F but not above.

Use of Microscope

With the standard light microscope, always use subdued light; rack the condenser down and close the diaphragm. Hyaline casts and other partially transparent solid elements may be obscured by excessively bright light. Examine the wet film with the low-power objective first; use the higher magnification later if necessary.

Many of the formed elements of the urine are somewhat refractile, notably hyaline casts, erythrocytes, and leukocytes. To see these, keep varying the fine focus of the microscope during examination of the urine.

A drop of 2% acetic acid added to the sediment lyses erythrocytes and helps to delineate the nuclei of leukocytes. This may be valuable particularly in distinguishing small epithelial cells and leukocytes. A drop of Brodie's stain added to the sediment also helps to delineate the formed elements.

A rough quantitation of the contents of the sediment may be obtained by counting at least ten fields and averaging the number of individual elements seen per high-power field.

Oval or round fat bodies look dark and opaque in subdued transmitted light but with increased illumination may appear lighter and highly refractile. Many contain doubly refractile cholesterol esters which may be identified by polarized light. To produce such light, two Polaroid lenses or plastic sheets are used. One is inserted beneath the condenser so that the light (which has to be increased for this examination) is transmitted through it. The other is placed over the eyepiece and is rotated until the field is black, indicating extinction of the polarized transmitted light by maximal crossing of the axes of polarization. The degree of rotation of the lens is critical and should be carefully adjusted. At the critical point doubly refractile lipids appear as brilliant, yellowish white small dots or "hot cross buns," (the so-called maltese crosses), the crosses being dark. (See Figs. 1-12 and 1-13.) Fat in the urine which is not doubly refractile does not give this appearance but can be identified with Sudan III stains.

Constituents of Urinary Sediment

Some erythrocytes, leukocytes, and casts are excreted in health, but they are seen only occasionally in urinary sediments examined by the standardized technique just described. Two to three red blood cells, four to five leukocytes per high-power field, and occasional hyaline casts are accepted as normal. Casts always originate in the renal tubules, but red and white cells may originate anywhere in the urinary tract. Large numbers of erythrocytes, leukocytes, and casts may appear in the urine of healthy subjects who perform strenuous exercise or who are exposed to severe cold. Except under such conditions these abnormal constituents always indicate renal disease (Figs. 1-1 to 1-9).

Many exogenous substances may contaminate the urinary sediment and will cause confusion if not recognized for what they are. Fragments of cotton or other fibers, oil droplets from lubricants, bacteria or yeasts from unclean receptacles, and starch granules are quite common. Vaginal secretions, including bacilli and trichomonads, may also appear in the urine (see Fig. 1-14).

Occasionally during diarrhea or in the presence of a rectovesical fistula the urine may be grossly contaminated with fecal material. The intestinal flagellate *Giardia lamblia* is sometimes seen as a result of fecal contamination.

Bacteria, Ova, Spermatozoa, Parasites, Cells, and Cellular Material

When bacteria are seen in the unstained or Gram-stained sediment from a fresh, clean-voided, properly collected urine specimen, there is probably infection of the genitourinary tract.

Epithelial cells arise from the urinary tract and may occur in the urine in large numbers but generally are of little significance. Occasionally the large cells of vaginal epithelium are also present. Spermatozoa commonly appear in the urine of adult males. Ova or parasites may be found in the urine in infestations such as schistosomiasis.

In infections due to fungi, these fungi may at times be recognized in the urinary sediment; for example, filamentous basophilic mycelia in moniliasis and round organisms with a thick gelatinous capsule in cryptococcosis (torulosis).

Hemosiderin is found in the urine in association with conditions producing hemoglobinuria. It is also seen in hemochromatosis. Hemosiderin

[Continued on p. 212]

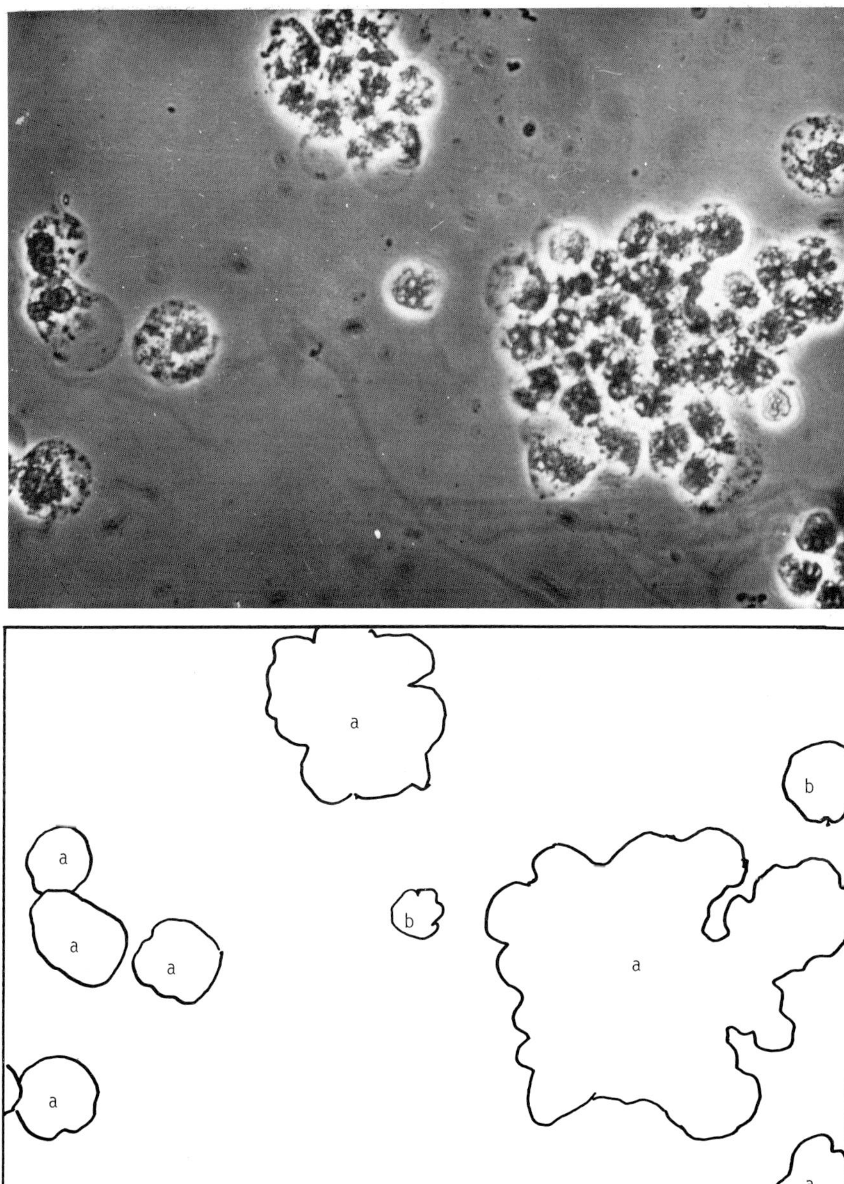

Fig. 1-1. The presence of white blood cells in the sediment is evidence of inflammation somewhere in the urinary tract. Here we have white blood cell clumps (*a*) and white blood cells (*b*) from a patient with urinary tract infection. Note increase in number of white blood cells, severe vacuolation of the cytoplasm, and presence of bacteria.

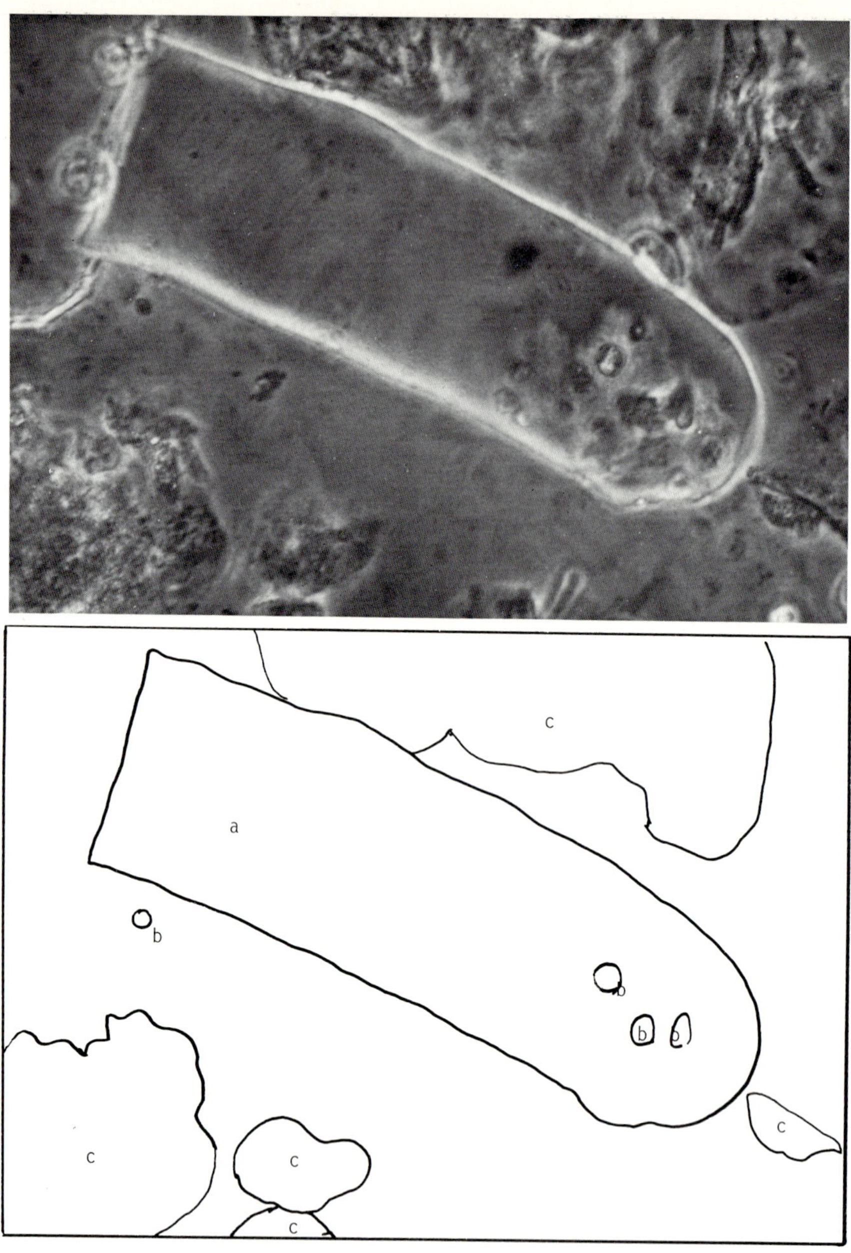

Fig. 1-2. Broad waxy cast (*a*) in urine from a patient under treatment with steroids for lupus nephritis. *b*, red blood cell; *c*, vaginal epithelial cell.

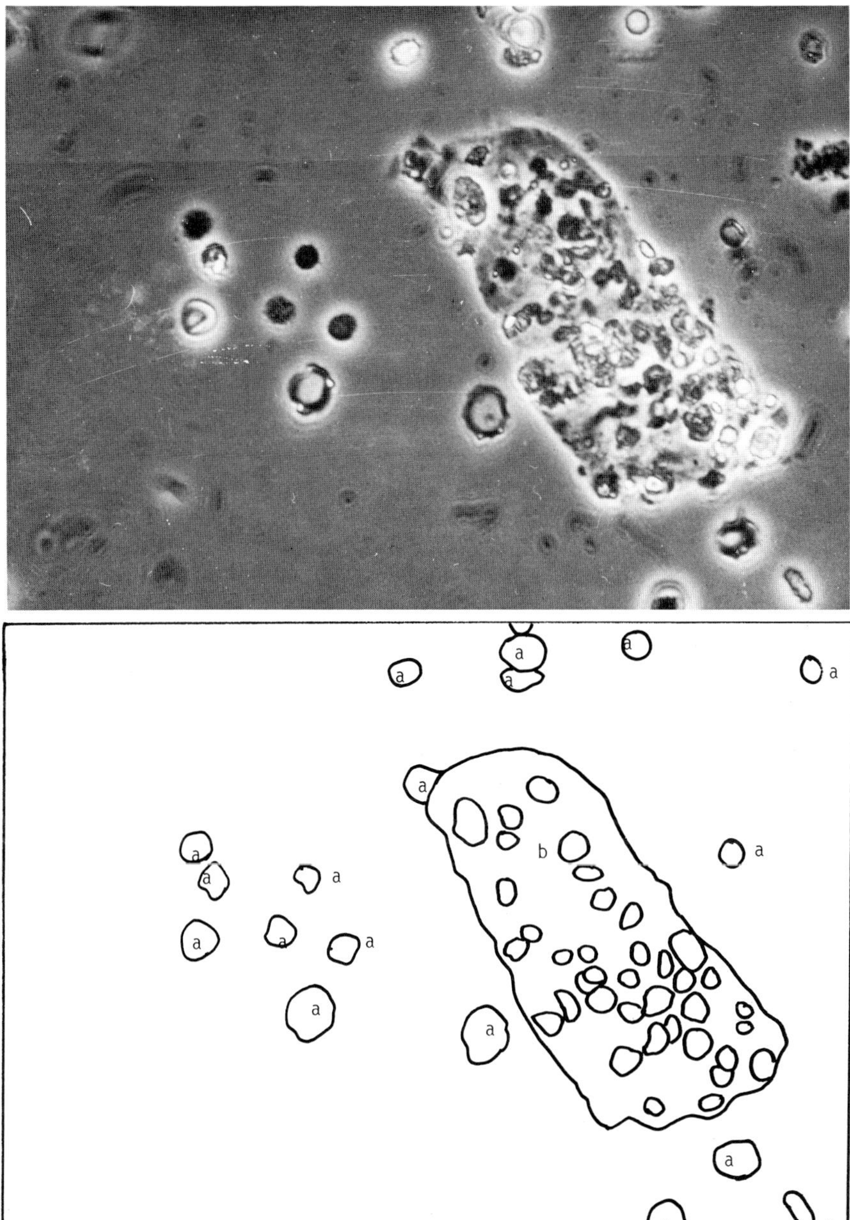

Fig. 1-3. Many red blood cells (*a*) and broad red blood cell cast (*b*) from urine of a patient with acute glomerulonephritis.

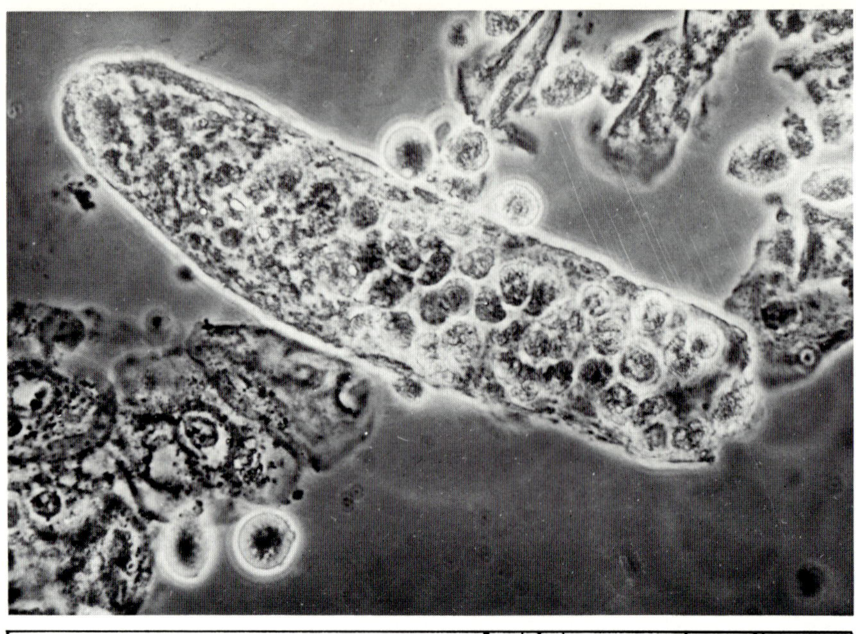

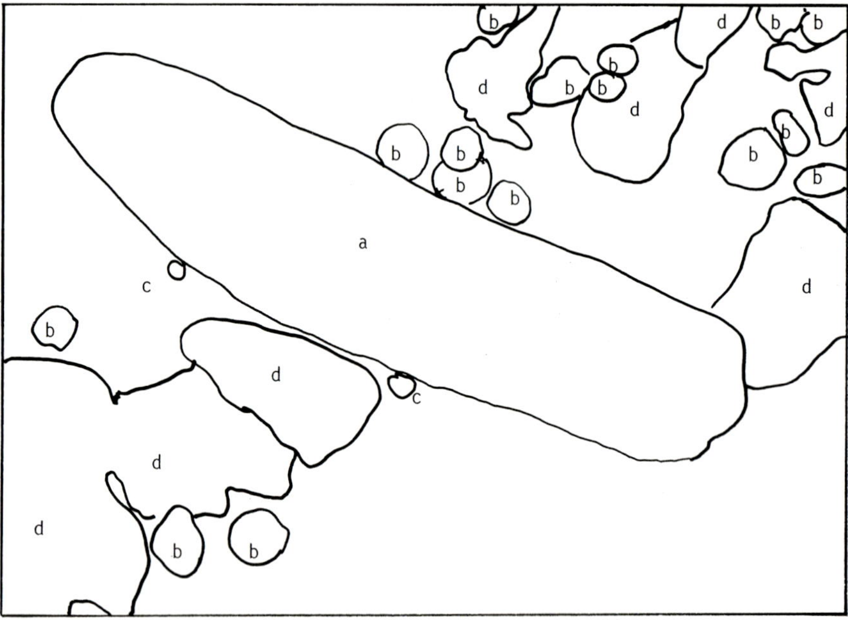

Fig. 1-4. White blood cell cast (*a*) from a patient with interstitial nephritis. Segmented nuclei can be seen in the cells enmeshed in the cast as well as in leukocytes (*b*) outside the cast. The presence of a white blood cell cast in the sediment is evidence of inflammation in the kidney. *c*, red blood cell; *d*, vaginal epithelial cell.

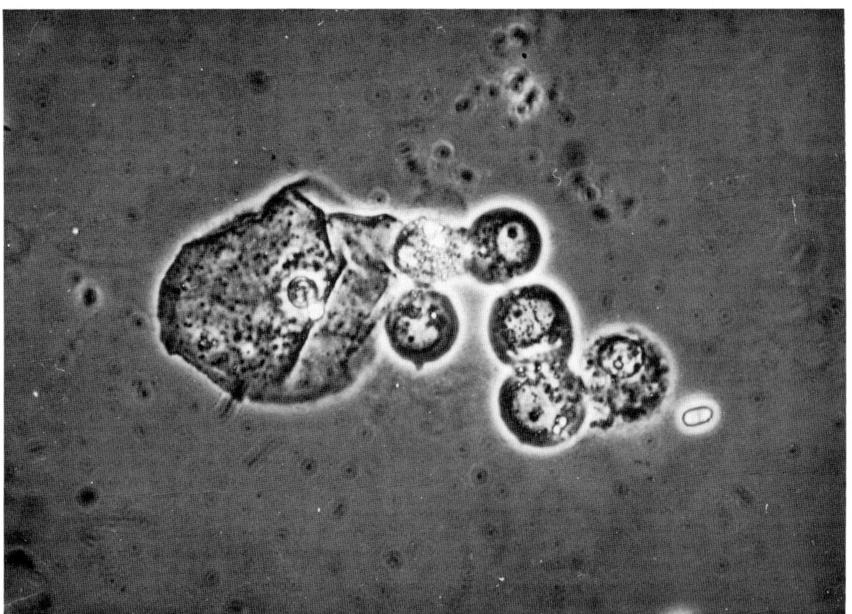

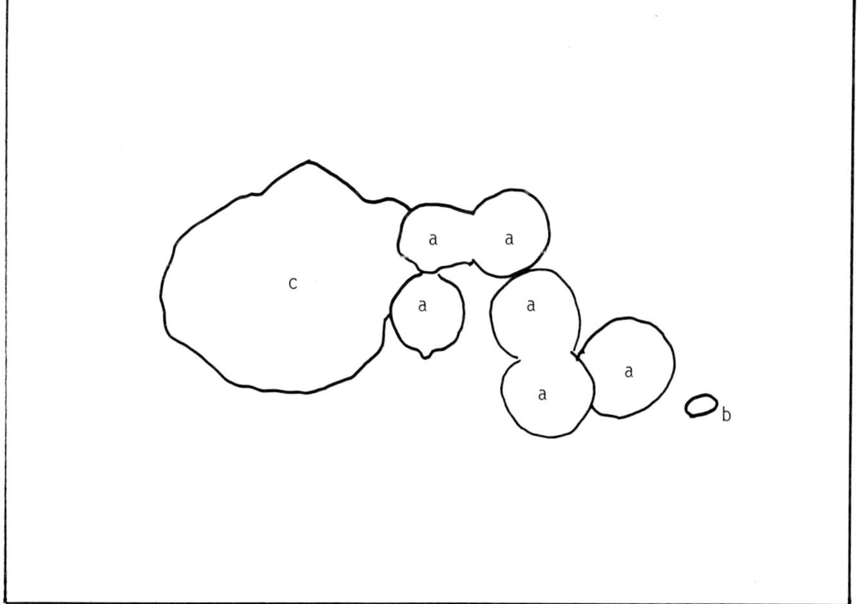

Fig. 1-5. Renal epithelial cells (*a*) from a patient with chronic glomerulone-phritis. These cells probably come from the distal convolutions of the tubules as evidenced by the high nuclear-cytoplasmic ratio. Shiny bubbles in the renal epithelial cells indicate presence of fat. *b*, red blood cell; *c*, vaginal epithelial cell.

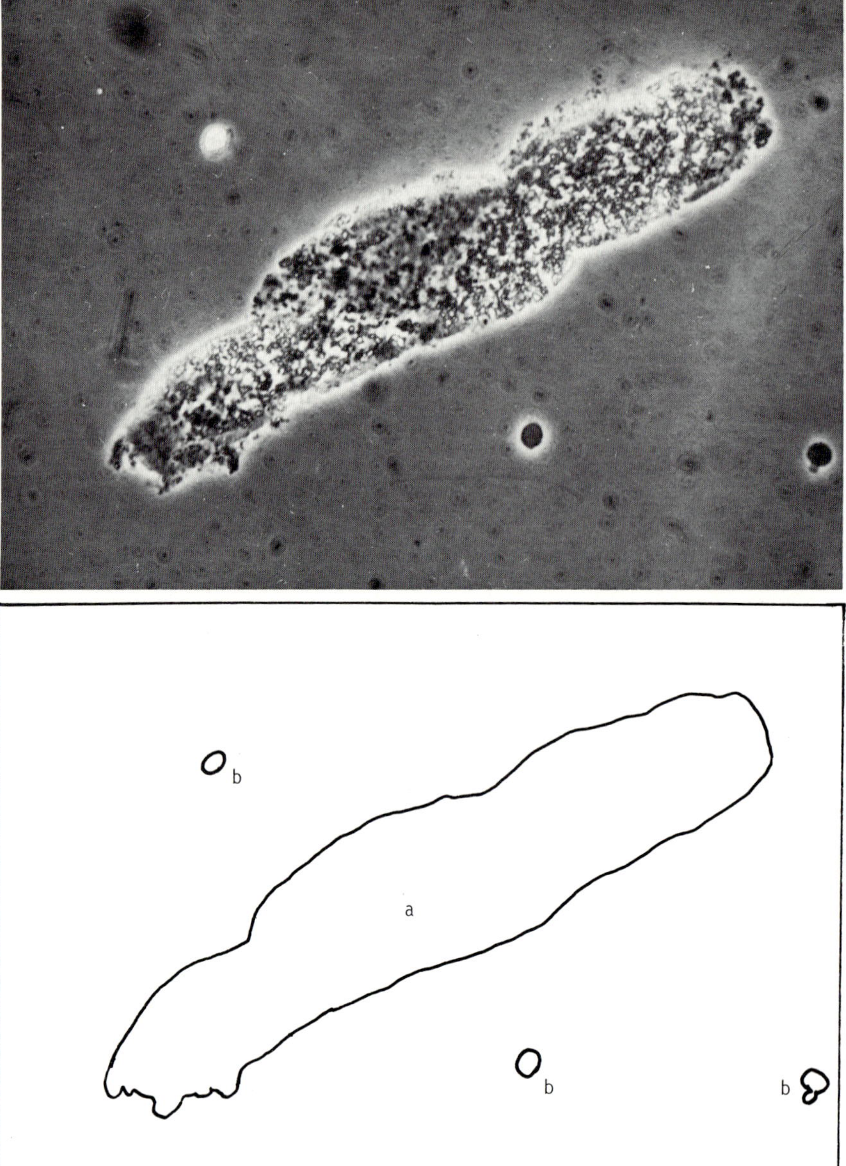

Fig. 1-6. A granular cast (*a*) and a few red blood cells (*b*) from a patient with chronic glomerulonephritis.

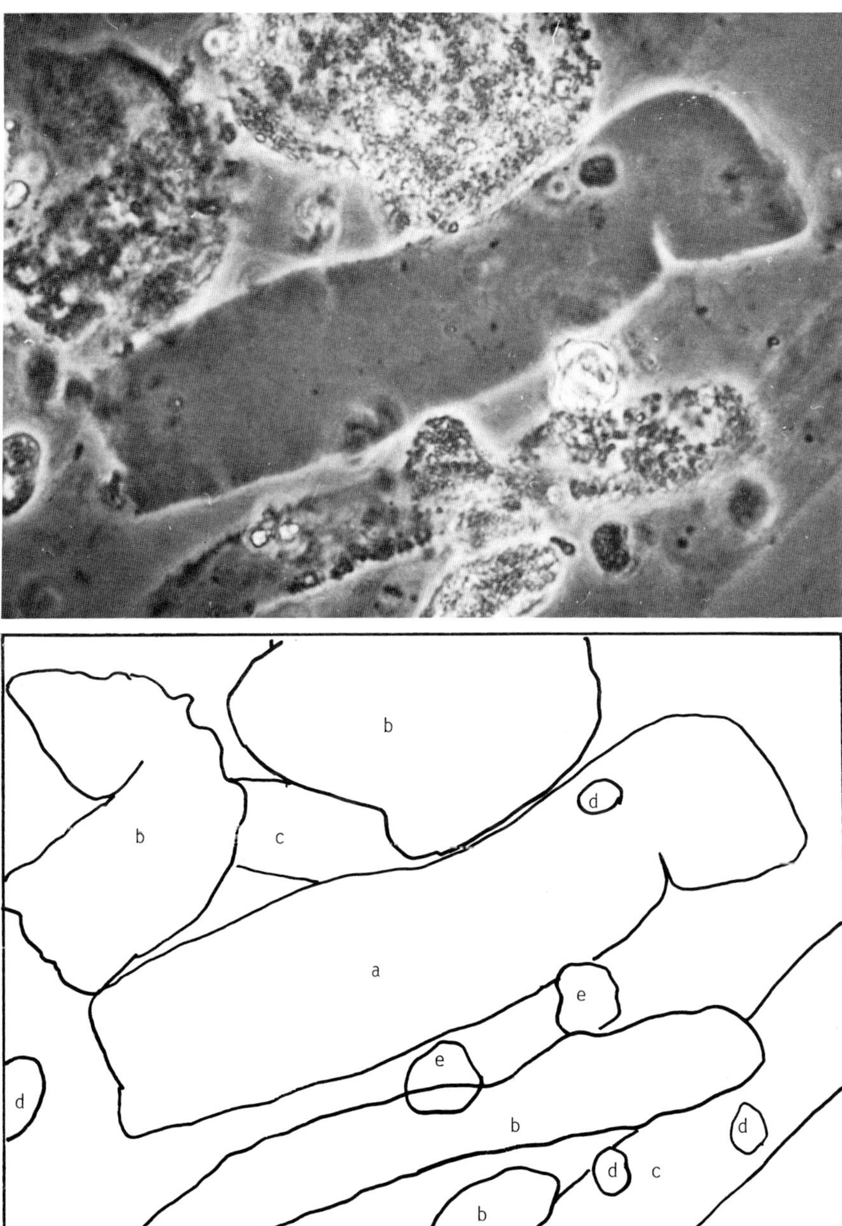

Fig. 1-7.   A broad waxy cast (*a*) and many granular casts (*b*) from a patient with chronic renal failure. Broad casts ("renal failure casts") are identified by squared ends and one or more notches or breaks in the side of the cast. *c*, hyaline cast; *d*, white blood cell; *e*, small renal epithelial cell.

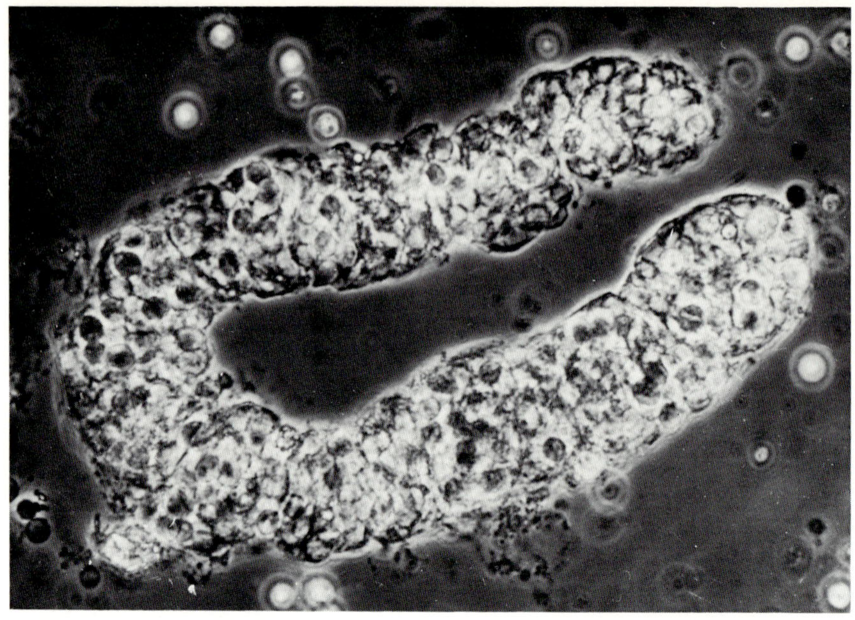

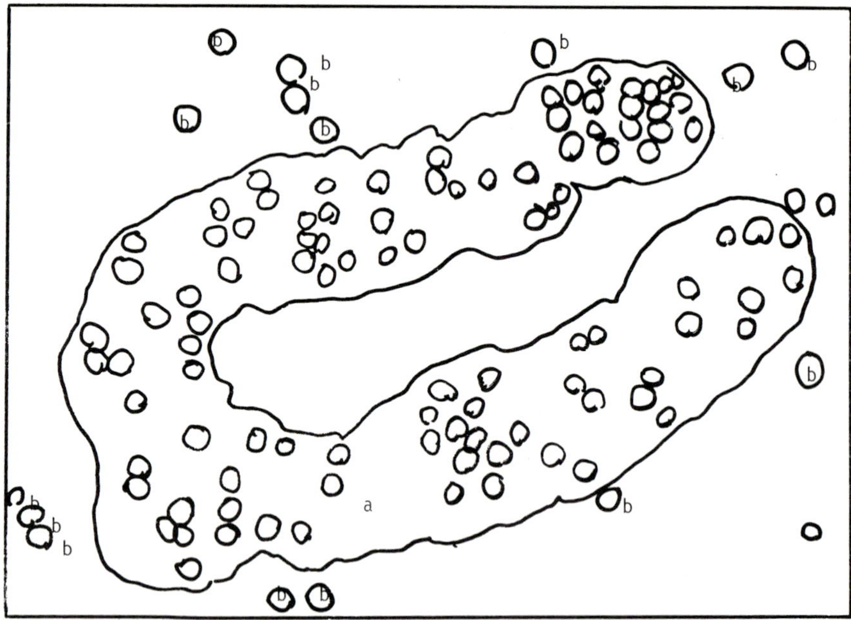

Fig. 1-8. A red blood cell cast (*a*) and many red blood cells (*b*) in urine from a patient with acute glomerulonephritis. This is an excellent example of the Tamm-Horsfall mucoprotein matrix of casts whose "hair net" quality traps the cells.

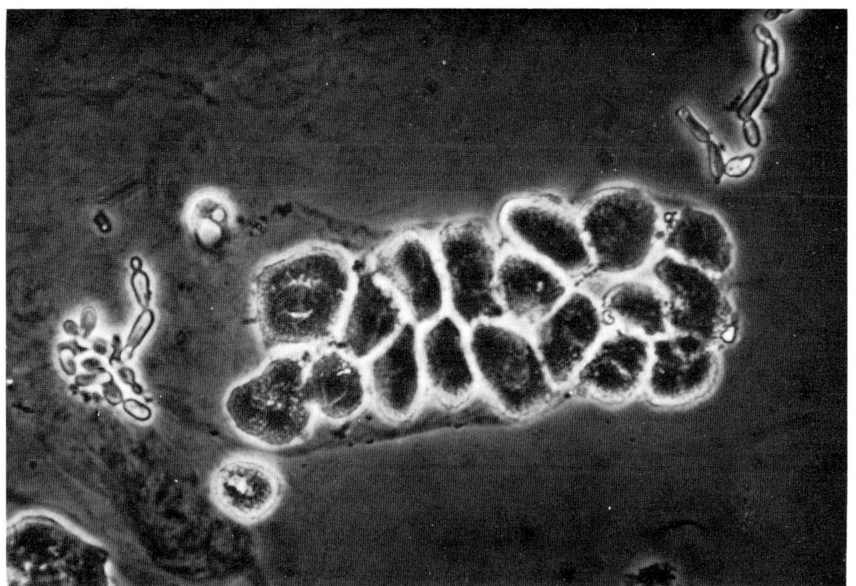

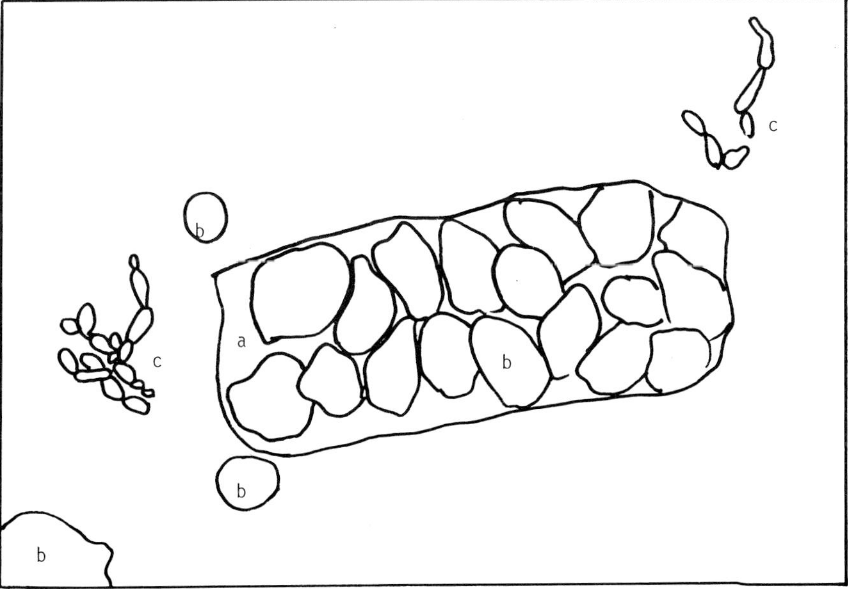

Fig. 1-9. A broad epithelial cell cast (*a*). The cells in the cast exemplify the cuboidal character of the tubular epithelial cells (*b*). *c*, yeast cells.

may be visible as clumps of golden brown granules, occurring either free or in epithelial cells or casts. With a Prussian blue stain the granules appear blue, and they are black when ferrous sulfide is formed after the sediment has been exposed to 30% aqueous ammonium sulfide.

Red Blood Cells and Red Blood Cell Casts

Red blood cells are normally biconcave discs, but in the urine erythrocytes may be globular, crenated, or shrunken. In health, occasional red blood cells are found in the urine, presumably entering it by diapedesis, but the persistent finding of even small numbers of erythrocytes should be thoroughly investigated.

Red blood cells from a patient with hematuria may not be seen under the microscope if they have been lysed by hypotonic or alkaline urine. When hemoglobin is found in the urine and no erythrocytes are seen microscopically, the origin of the hemoglobin should be determined. Under the microscope, red cells may be confused with many structures, including fat droplets, yeasts, and degenerated epithelial cells. Unlike most of these other structures, red cells are lysed in 2% acetic acid.

Hematuria varies from gross clots and obvious blood staining to amounts detectable only by microscopy or chemical tests. Bleeding without severe proteinuria, casts, or other evidence of kidney disease most often originates in the lower portion of the genitourinary tract, and massive hematuria is perhaps more common in surgical conditions such as tumor or lithiasis.

Hematuria is a cardinal feature of glomerulonephritis and is often gross (see Fig. 1-15). The urine has a characteristic smoky appearance due to the red cells, which are crenated. Red cell casts are frequently present.

Red cell casts always indicate renal parenchymal disease and should be looked for diligently, particularly when there are red cells in the urine. The red cells may be distinct or may be incorporated into a homogeneous mass, but they characteristically have an orange-red color.

Subacute bacterial endocarditis often causes intermittent showers of red blood cells in the urine. When this diagnosis is being considered, the urine should be examined for red blood cells daily or even more frequently.

Leukocytes and White Blood Cell Casts

Leukocytes may come from anywhere in the genitourinary tract. White cell casts always come from the kidney. Both leukocytes and leukocyte casts are found in inflammatory disorders of the kidney such as pyelonephritis and in the noninfective inflammatory diseases of the kidney like lupus nephritis. However, whenever they are found, one or more quantitative urine cultures must be made.

As white cell casts can be formed only in the renal tubules, their presence in the urine indicates that at least some leukocytes have come from the kidney. However, as urinary tract infection commonly complicates renal parenchymal disease, leukocytes from the kidney and from the lower urinary tract may be found together.

When pus is visible to the naked eye, or when leukocytes exceed about fifty per high-power field, genitourinary tract infection almost certainly exists. Clumping of leukocytes in the urine also suggests infection. Such urine should be cultured quantitatively, repeatedly if necessary. If pathogenic bacteria are not found, a diagnosis of systemic lupus erythematosus or tuberculous infection should be considered. It should be remembered that finding leukocytes in the urine is not diagnostic of urinary tract infection, because white cells may appear in any inflammatory process in the renal parenchyma.

Conversely, leukocytes are not always present in the urine when significant urinary tract infection is shown by persistent bacteriuria. In cases of chronic pyelonephritis it may be necessary to make repeated examinations of the urine before abnormal formed elements are seen or before pathogenic bacteria can be cultured.

Hyaline, Granular, and Other Casts

Hyaline casts (Fig. 1-10) are formed in the tubules from Tamm-Horsfall mucoprotein. Their appearance in the urine depends on the urine flow rate, urine pH, and degree of proteinuria. They are clear cylinders characterized by slight refractility and are best recognized in dim light. Hyaline casts dissolve readily in alkaline solutions.

Casts may be distinguished from other contaminants like mucus fibers or crystals by their regular parallel walls and squared ends. As they are formed in various tubules, casts vary in diameter. Broad casts come from collecting tubules. In large numbers they indicate the end-stage kidney and consequently a grave prognosis. Occasional hyaline casts are present in normal urine and do not necessarily indicate renal parenchymal damage.

Hyaline casts may incorporate formed elements and become erythrocyte, leukocyte, or epithelial casts. As the cellular elements degenerate, the casts become coarsely granular, finely granular, and finally waxy, and indicate renal parenchymal damage (Fig. 1-11).

Fats in the Urine

Oval fat bodies are degenerated fat-filled tubular cells shed into the urine (Fig. 1-12). Their predominant lipid is cholesterol ester and they are easily seen by polarized light (Fig. 1-13). With normal subdued illumination they are dark and may appear refractile. Urinary fat which is not refractile may be identified by staining with Sudan III.

Fatty casts indicate tubular fatty change. Urinary fatty casts and oval fat bodies are found frequently in the nephrotic syndrome, whatever its cause, and also occur in diabetic nephropathy.

Chyluria may occur when the upper abdominal and thoracic lymph

[Continued on p. 219]

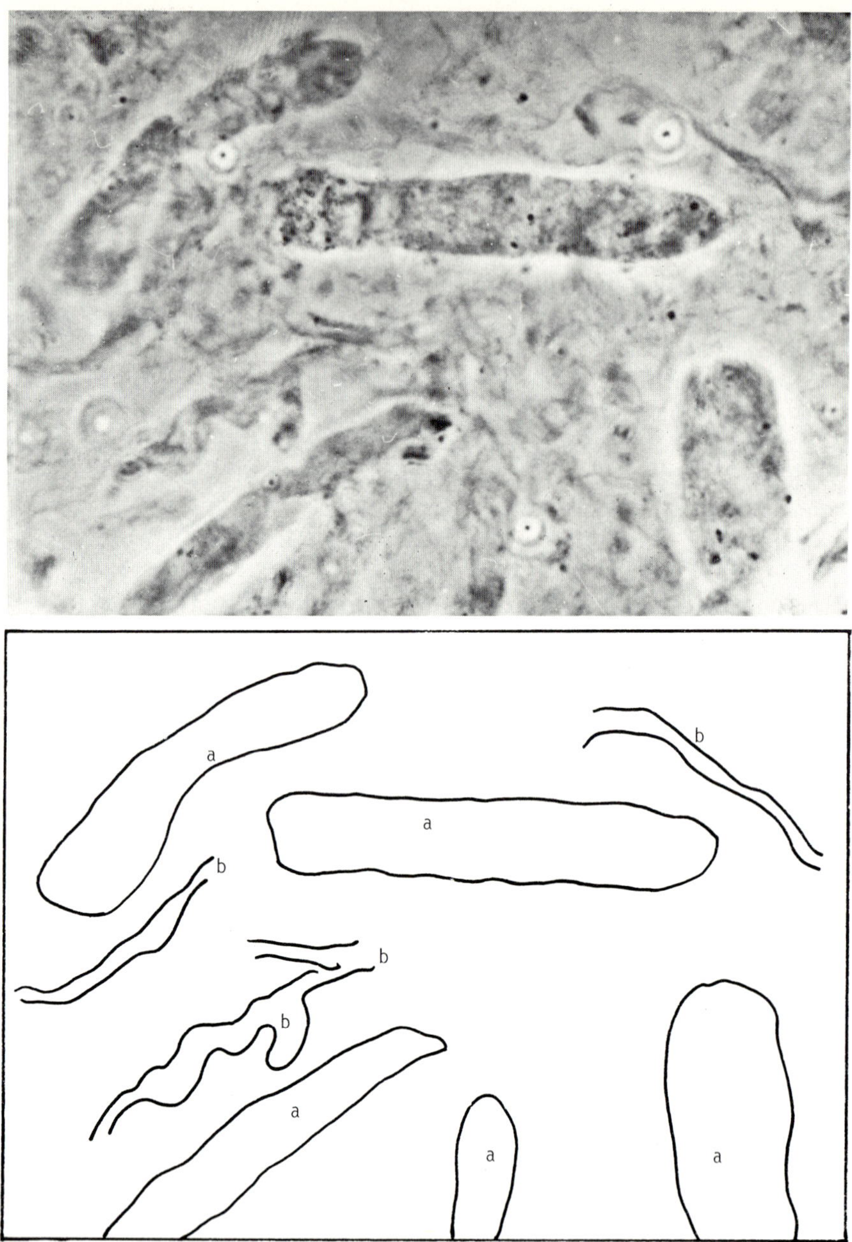

Fig. 1-10. Numerous hyaline casts (*a*) in urine from a patient recovering from postoperative shock. Without phase-contrast microscopy these casts would be very difficult to see. *b*, mucus threads.

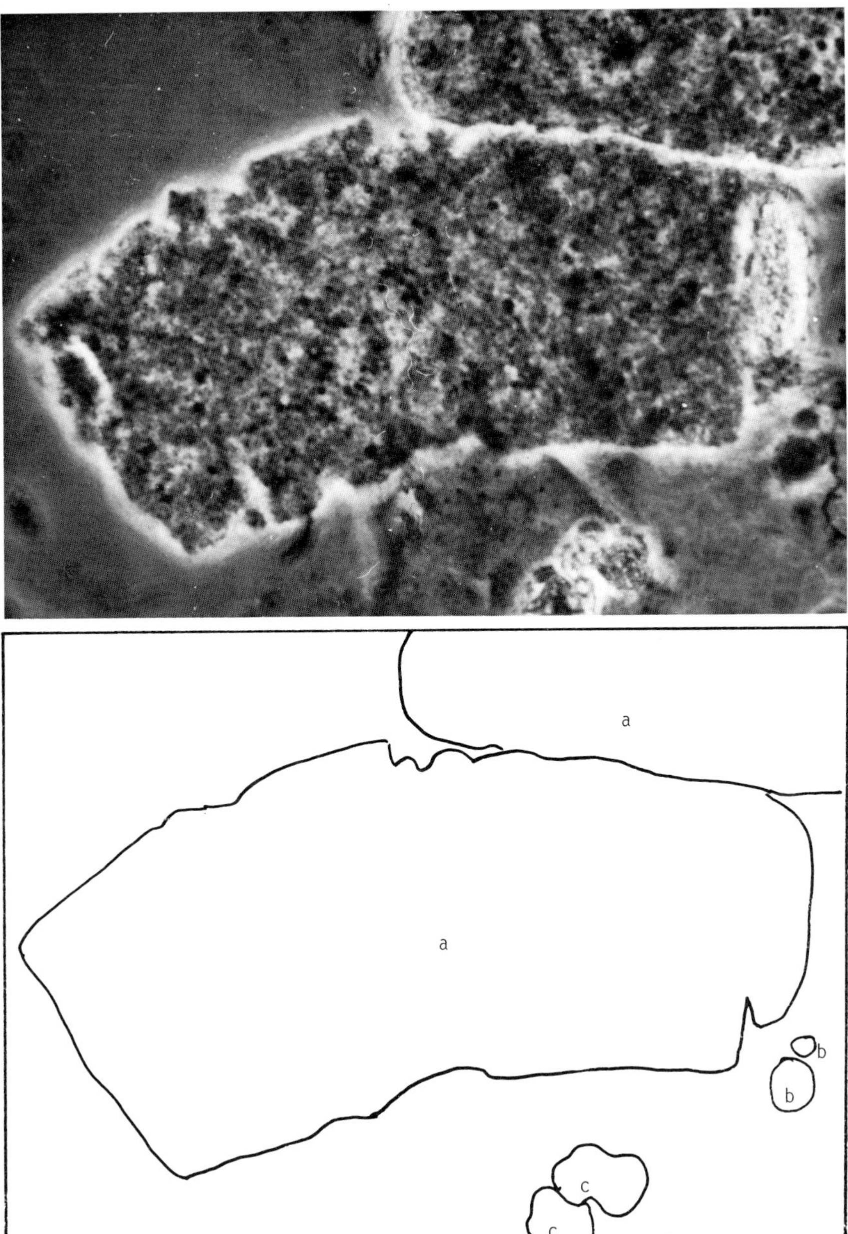

Fig. 1-11. A broad granular cast (*a*) from urine of a patient who had acute renal failure after treatment with amphotericin. *b*, red blood cell; *c*, white blood cell.

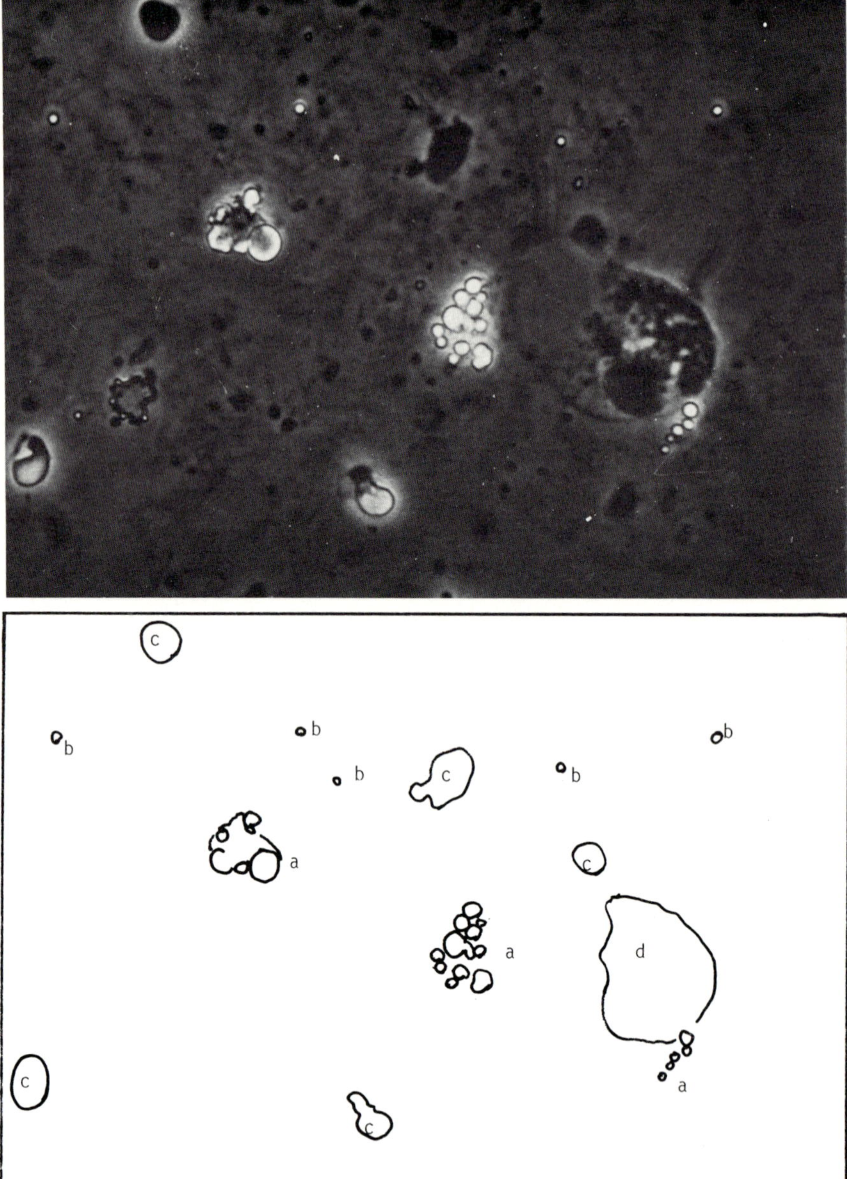

Fig. 1-12A. Oval fat bodies (*a*) (including cholesterol ester crystals, *b*) and red blood cells (*c*) from a patient with nephrotic syndrome and lupus nephritis.

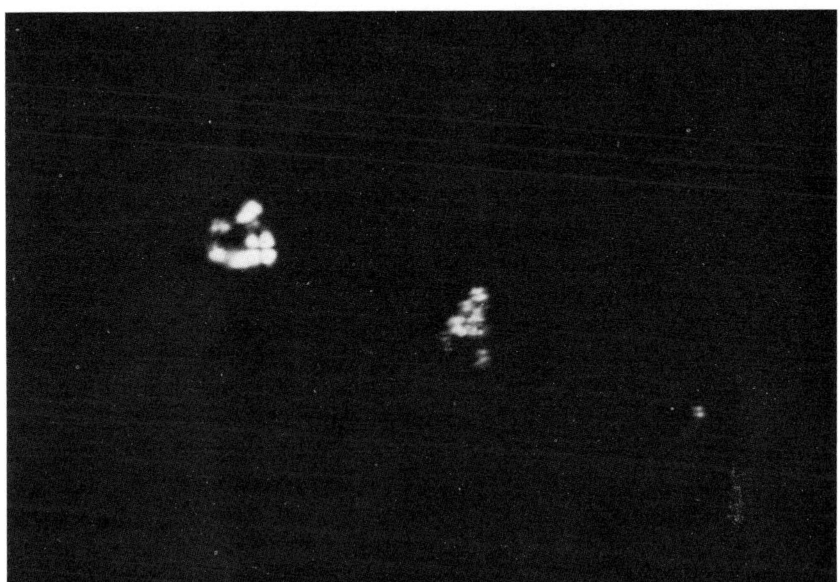

Fig. 1-12B. Same field, polarized view, with maltese crosses.

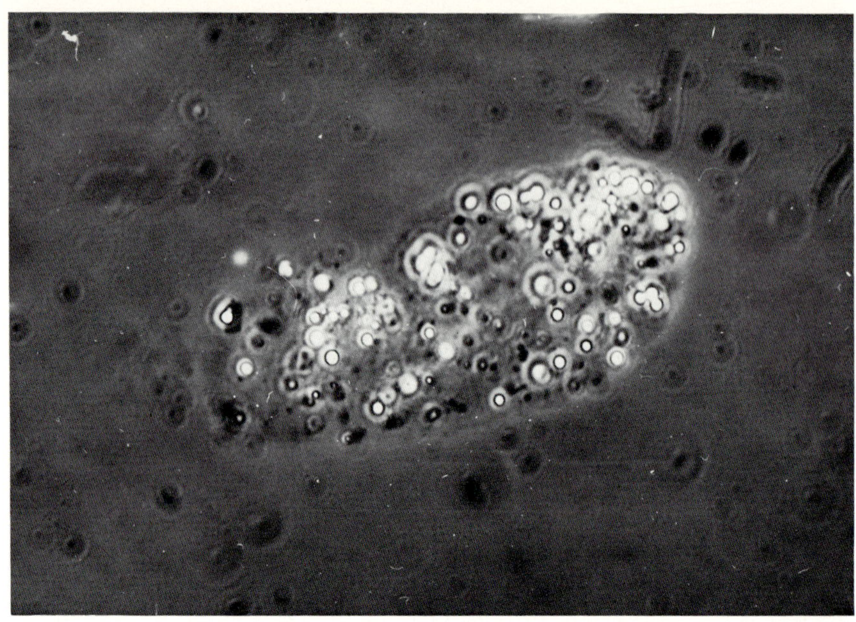

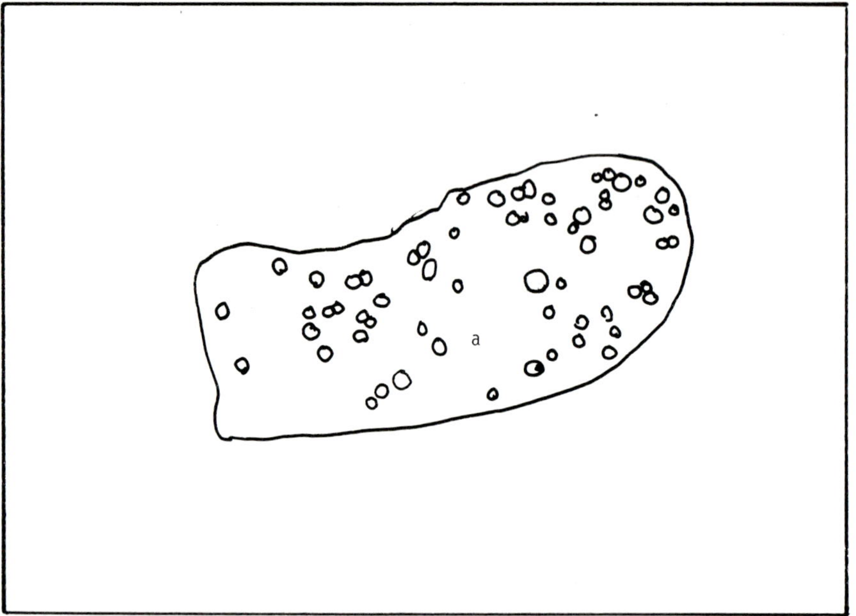

Fig. 1-13A. Same patient as in Figure 1-12. Here the oval fat body is caught up in the hyaline cast matrix (*a*).

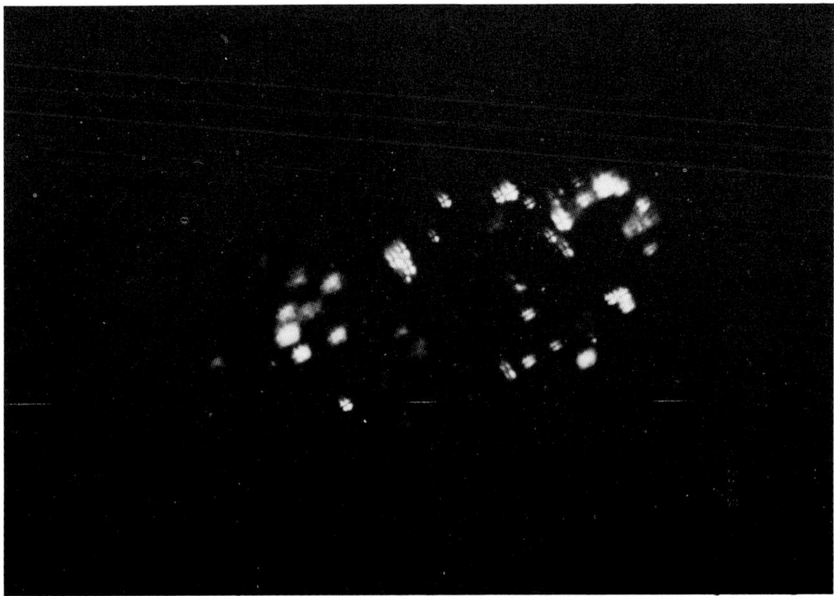

Fig. 1-13B. Same field, polarized view, with maltese crosses.

flow is obstructed, if the lymphatics rupture and leak into the renal pelvis. The urine looks milky and contains chyle and protein.

Crystals

Except in certain special circumstances, the finding of crystals in the urine has relatively little clinical value. Many crystals appear in both acid and alkaline urine. Those listed below are grouped according to the type of urine in which they are found predominantly.

In alkaline urine:
    ammonium urates ("thorn apples")
    triple (ammonium magnesium) phosphates ("coffin lids")
    calcium carbonates ("dumbbells")
    calcium phosphates (amorphous or wedge-shaped crystals)
In acid urine:
    uric acid crystals (red rhombic prisms)
    sodium urates (amorphous brown clumps, or needles and fan-shaped
       clusters)
    calcium oxalates ("envelopes")

Any of these may be significant if found persistently in patients with renal lithiasis.

In certain metabolic diseases and drug intoxications characteristic crystals may appear. Sulfonamides produce sheaves of crystals varying according to

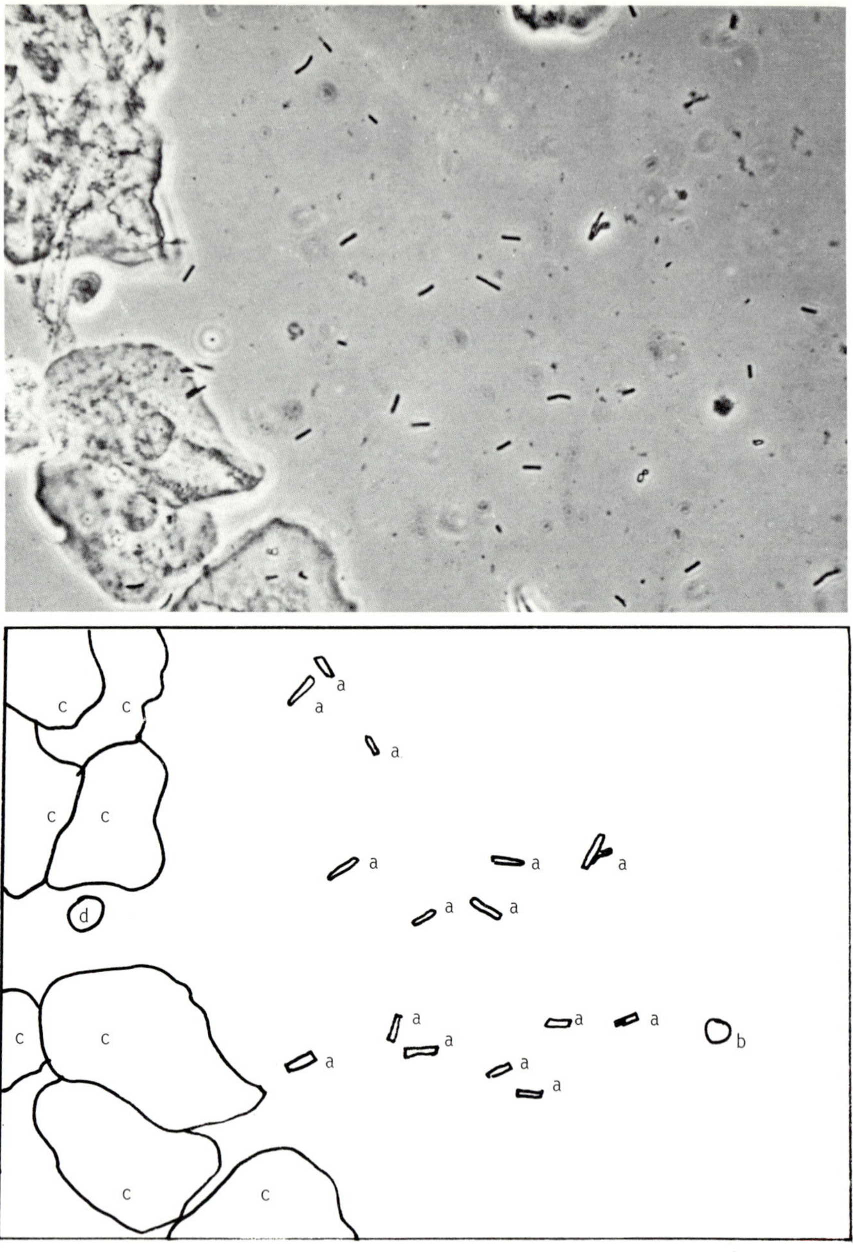

Fig. 1-14. Numerous bacterial rods and vaginal epithelial cells due to contamination of the urine by vaginal discharge. *a*, bacteria; *b*, red blood cell; *c*, vaginal epithelial cell; *d*, red blood cell.

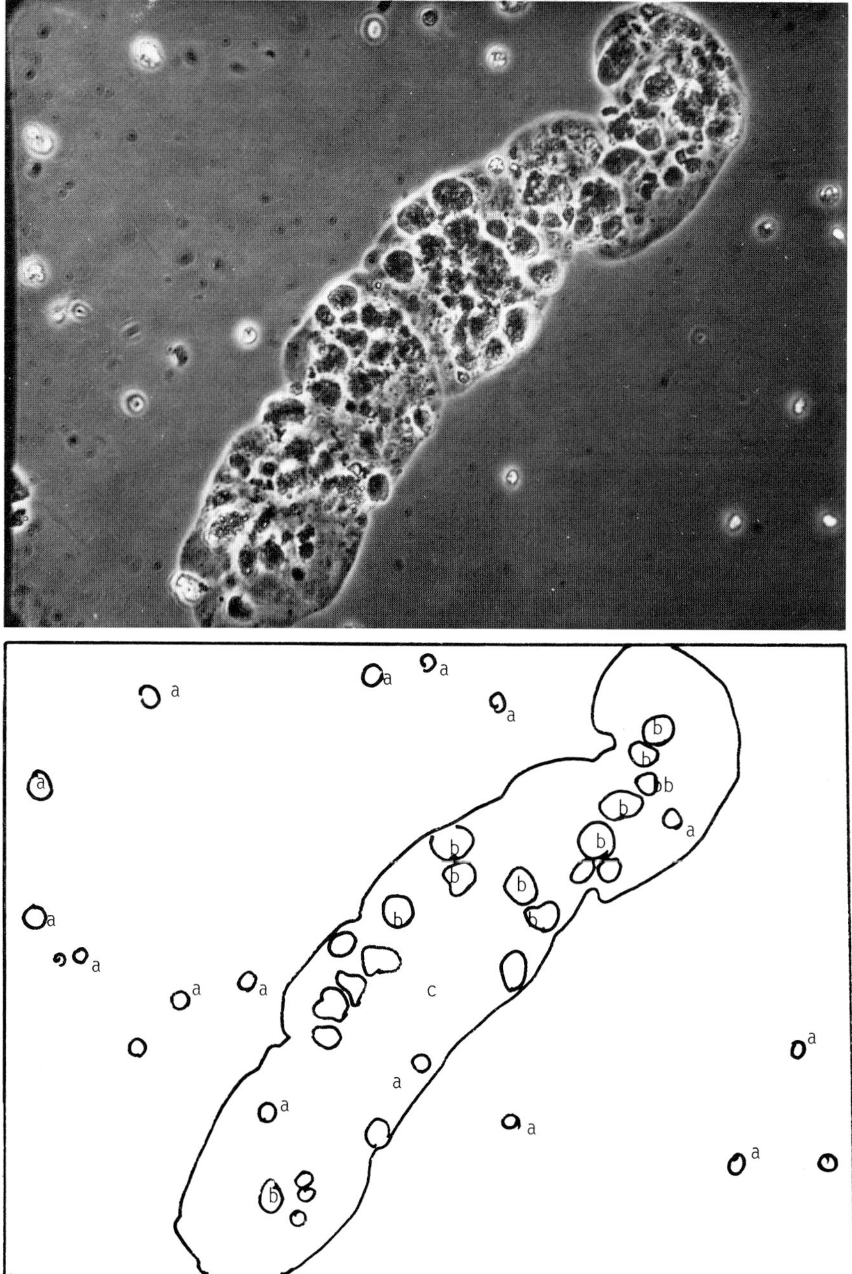

Fig. 1-15. A mixed white blood cell and red blood cell cast in urine from a patient with acute glomerulonephritis. *a*, red blood cell; *b*, white blood cell; *c*, mixed cellular cast.

the chemical constitution of the drug. Characteristic hexagonal crystals of cystine appear in the urine of patients with cystinosis when the pH of the fresh specimen is acid. They dissolve in dilute hydrochloric acid. Other amino acids, particularly leucine and tyrosine, may appear in the urine as crystals when there is massive aminoaciduria such as occurs with hepatic necrosis.

Phase-Contrast Examination of the Urinary Sediment

The phase-contrast method is far superior to any other microscopic examination of the urinary sediment for both the beginner and the expert in urinalysis. Since there are many makes of instruments available and each instrument is organized differently, it is necessary here simply to refer the reader to the directions given by the manufacturers.

2   Diagnosis of Urinary Tract Infection

Urinary tract infection is among the commonest bacterial infections encountered in medicine. It is frequently asymptomatic, and symptoms may or may not be related to the site, or may exist without actual infection.

The isolation of bacteria from the urine may be central to the diagnosis of urinary tract infection. Because contamination is frequent in voided specimens, careful collection techniques are of the utmost importance. Collection techniques used for the individual patient differ from those used in population studies.

Population Studies

In epidemiologic studies a clean voided urine specimen is used. Bacterial counts in excess of 100,000 colonies per milliliter in two consecutive specimens convey a high probability that organisms are present within the bladder urine.

Clinical Studies

INFANTS AND TODDLERS. If a single freshly voided specimen contains more than 10,000 colonies per milliliter, suprapubic aspiration should be done. This technique is facilitated by the intraabdominal position of the bladder.

CHILDREN AND ADULTS. Contamination with vaginal organisms is the greatest problem. The following points should be observed in collecting specimens:

1. The periurethral area and perineum should be cleaned carefully, preferably with soap (three washes), and dried with a sterile swab (in the male the foreskin must be retracted).
2. A vaginal tampon should be used.
3. In females it is important that the labia be spread by the patient during voiding.
4. In the diagnosis of urethritis the first part of the stream should be collected separately.
5. In the diagnosis of prostatitis a postprostatic massage specimen should be obtained.

6. It is important that a wide-mouthed container be used.
7. If the patient cannot cooperate, or where doubt exists, percutaneous aspiration of the bladder should be carried out.

When these precautions are used, and pure growth of identical organisms is obtained in successive specimens, infection is likely to exist irrespective of the count, particularly if white blood cells are present in excess. A count of 10^5 organisms per milliliter should not be used as the absolute criterion of infection.

Meticulous urethral catheterization is an acceptable technique for patients for whom the other methods of collection are not possible. In such cases antibacterial agents may be given to cover the procedure.

HANDLING OF THE URINE SPECIMEN

After the specimen is obtained by the above procedures, the urine must be cultured immediately or kept at 4°C. This latter procedure is extremely important, because urine is a good culture medium for bacteria, and if it stands, is stored, or is transported at room temperature for any length of time, a falsely high bacterial count will be obtained due to multiplication of bacteria.

If the specimen must be carried to the laboratory, it should be transported in a precooled box at a temperature of 4° to 6°C. There are devices which, when prefrozen, can be placed in the box and will keep the specimen cool for 24 hours. The difficulty may be obviated by use of the recently developed dip slide method (see Microculture Technique, p. 226).

LABORATORY PROCEDURES

The following two methods are based on visualization of bacteria.

Wet Spread

(See Urinary Sediment.) Both bacteria and white blood cells are significant in the diagnosis of urinary tract infection.

Gram-Stained Smear

A large drop of well-mixed urine, such as that delivered by a medicine dropper, is placed on a slide, air dried, heat fixed, and Gram stained. The preparation is examined with the oil immersion objective, and bacteria are sought. Observation of several bacteria in 90 percent of the fields examined is the equivalent of approximately 10^5 organisms per milliliter of urine.

Although both of these methods are simple and can be used in the physician's office, it should be realized that there is only an 80 percent correlation between these methods and the culture procedures described below.

Screening Tests

The only acceptable screening techniques are bacteriologic and depend upon culture of organisms. Of these the most practical is the dip slide technique (p. 226).

Culture Methods

The first two methods described here are the standard procedures used in the culture of urine. The third method, employing dip slides, is practical as a screening technique.

The Pour Plate Method

The pour plate method is the most accurate one. Pour plates are prepared in the following manner:

1. Sterile 0.9% sodium chloride solution (9.9 ml) is delivered to each of three sterile, 20- by 150-mm, screwcapped culture tubes labeled 10^2, 10^4, and 10^6, respectively.
2. Urine (0.1 ml) is transferred (1.0 ml sterile serologic pipet) to the 10^2 tube. With the cap screwed firmly in place, the tube is inverted three to five times to obtain thorough mixing.
3. One milliliter is transferred to an empty, sterile, 100- by 15-mm Petri dish labeled 10^2, and 0.1 ml is transferred to the 10^4 saline dilution tube.
4. Operations 2 and 3 are repeated with the 10^4 tube and then with the 10^6 tube.
5. Sterile nutrient agar (12 to 15 ml) at 56°C is added (by means of a sterile pipet) to each Petri dish, and mixing is obtained by swirling.
6. When cool, the plates are inverted and incubated overnight at 37°C. The dilution yielding 75 to 150 colonies is used for making the count recorded for the specimen.

A simplified pour plate method requires two Petri dishes, one test tube containing 9.9 ml of sterile broth or neutral buffer, and two sterile pipets. Into the first pipet 0.6 ml of urine is drawn, of which 0.5 ml is added to one Petri dish and 0.1 ml to the sterile broth. The second pipet is used to mix the contents of the tube and to remove 0.1 ml of the 1:100 dilution of the original urine and add it to the second Petri dish.

Molten agar at 56°C is poured into each plate and mixed with the contents. Incubation time is 24 hours, after which the colonies are counted. The plate that contains 75 to 150 colonies is used for the recorded count. If one is unable to count colonies on second plate, the urine contains over 100,000 organisms per milliliter.

At the same time a blood agar plate and an eosin–methylene blue agar plate are inoculated to assist in the identification of the organisms.

The Semiquantitative Streak Method

The materials necessary for the semiquantitative streak method are a sterile blood agar plate, an eosin–methylene blue agar plate or MacConkey's agar plate, and a 0.001-cc standardized platinum loop.

The 0.001-cc loop is dipped into the urine and is then streaked across the blood agar plate, which is incubated for 24 hours at 37°C, and the colonies present on the blood agar plate are then counted. If 100 or more organisms are present this is equal to 10^5 organisms per milliliter and is indicative of significant bacteriuria. (See Fig. 2-1.)

The inhibitory agar plate is also inoculated with a loopful of urine to assist in identification of the organisms. Gram-negative organisms will grow preferentially on this plate.

There are 0.01-ml loops available, but they should not be used because the volume they deliver varies greatly.

Microculture Technique

The dip slide technique employs glass microscope slides, each coated with a different medium. The slides are momentarily dipped into the urine specimen, and the excess urine is allowed to run off on to a piece of filter paper. In such a manner between 0.01 and 0.02 ml of urine is taken up by each slide. The slides are then incubated in a capped vial at 37°C for 24 hours, after which time they are examined for growth. There appears to be a good correlation between this technique and the standard loop method. The limited growth of the isolated colonies on the dip slides presents some difficulties; however, this technique may be useful as a screening procedure in the diagnostic laboratory.

Identification of Organisms

Once significant bacteriuria has been demonstrated, the causative organism must be identified. Identification is dependent on the metabolic requirement and fermentation reactions of the various bacteria.

Sensitivity Tests

For routine use these are very satisfactory ways of determining the choice of drugs.

Antibiogram Studies

Failure to respond to antibacterial therapy may be due to inadequate concentration of the therapeutic agent. In these instances, more accurate determination of the susceptibility of the organism may be helpful.

Antibiotic profiles are readily obtained by the single high concentration disc method. It should be stressed that the mere presence of a clear zone around the disc does not indicate that the organism is sensitive to the therapeutic level of the antibiotic; it is necessary to express the size of the zone in millimeters. Comparison with the tube dilution method shows good correlation.

PREPARATION OF AGAR PLATE FOR ANTIBIOGRAM. Appropriate commercial material is available in most countries. The agar should be poured into a sterile Petri dish to the stipulated depth. The plates may be stored under refrigeration for approximately five days. Prior to use they should be allowed to reach room temperature.

THE PREPARATION OF INOCULUM. This should be done in accordance with the manufacturer's instructions.

INOCULATION OF AGAR PLATES. This is critical to the accuracy of the technique.

APPLICATION OF DISCS. Discs are applied either with a commercial dispenser or manually, using aseptic precautions. They are deposited with their centers at least 30 mm apart and are gently pressed with a sterile needle, forceps, or applicator stick so that they make complete contact with the surface of the agar plate. The plates are incubated at 37°C for approximately 18 hours.

EXAMINATION OF PLATES. Only zones showing complete inhibition as determined by gross visual inspection are to be measured to the nearest millimeter. If only isolated colonies grow, the inoculum is too light, and the test must be repeated.

Detection of Bacterial Variants

Recent developments concerning the role of L-forms and mycoplasma in persistent and recurrent infections of the urinary tract make it mandatory to culture urine for these agents when clinical findings point to them.

L-forms, protoplasts, and spheroplasts are any bacteria which for any of many reasons have lost the ability to form an intact rigid cell wall. Under proper conditions they may revert to the classic parent bacterial forms. Mycoplasma, a separate genus of microorganisms, do not revert to classic bacterial forms but have other features in common with L-forms, including inability to build an intact cell wall. Because of this cell wall deficiency, both the L-form and mycoplasma demonstrate the following characteristics:

1. Osmotic fragility requiring cultivation in hypertonic broth
2. Filterability through a bacteriologic filter
3. Gram-negative staining and intense staining with Giemsa
4. Severe pleomorphism (Fig. 2-2)

CULTURE PROCEDURES. To determine the presence of classic bacterial forms, the clean-catch midstream urine is mixed well and cultured according to any of the previously mentioned laboratory procedures. Approximately 5 ml of the urine is mixed with a similar amount of 20 percent sucrose in order to stabilize the L-forms. The urine-sucrose mixture is poured through a 0.5-μ Millipore filter. The L-forms, because of their

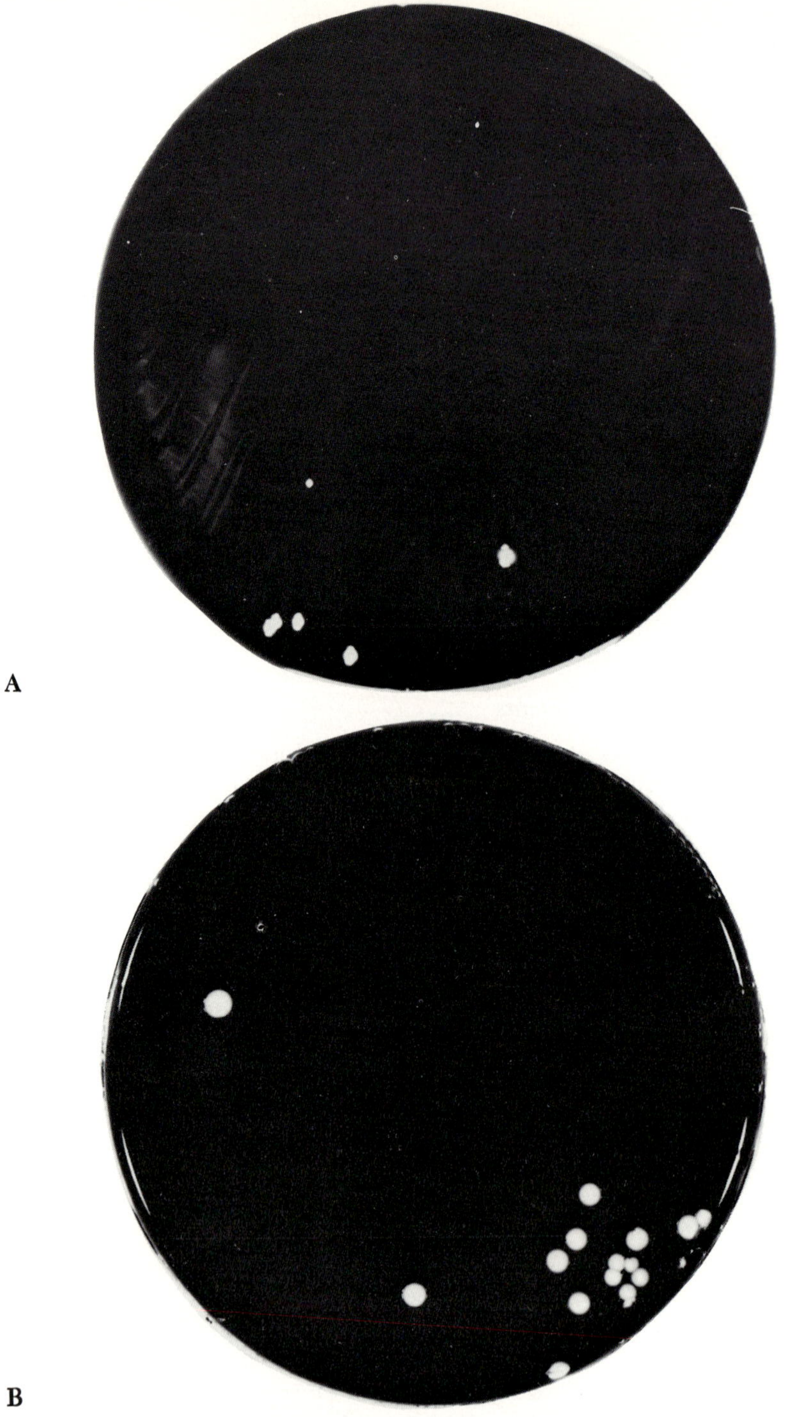

Fig. 2-1. Standardized platinum loop (0.001 ml), streaked blood agar plates incubated at 37°C, for 18 hours. A. Approximately 5×10^3 organisms per milliliter urine. B. Approximately 5×10^4 organisms per milliliter urine. C. Approximately 5×10^5 organisms per milliliter urine. D. Approximately 5×10^6 organisms per milliliter urine.

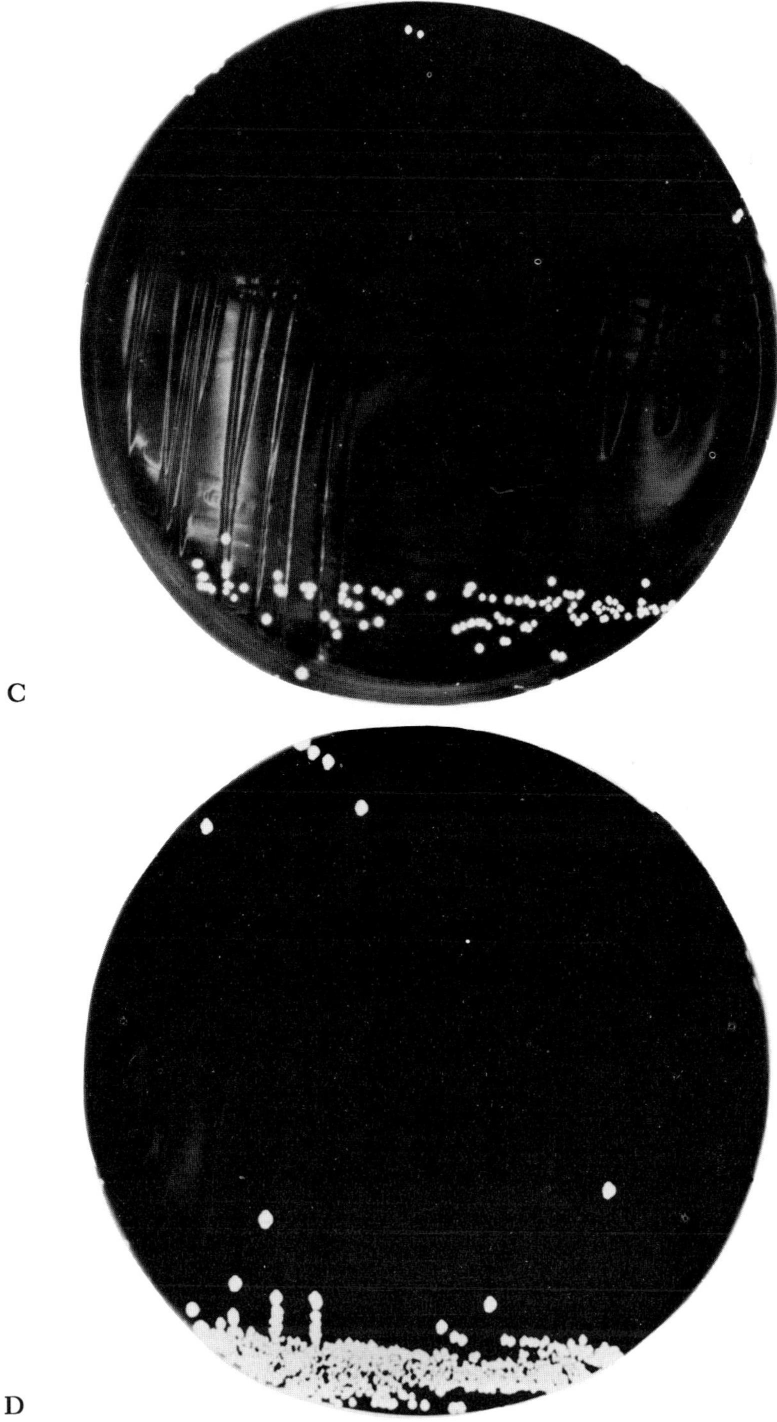

C
D

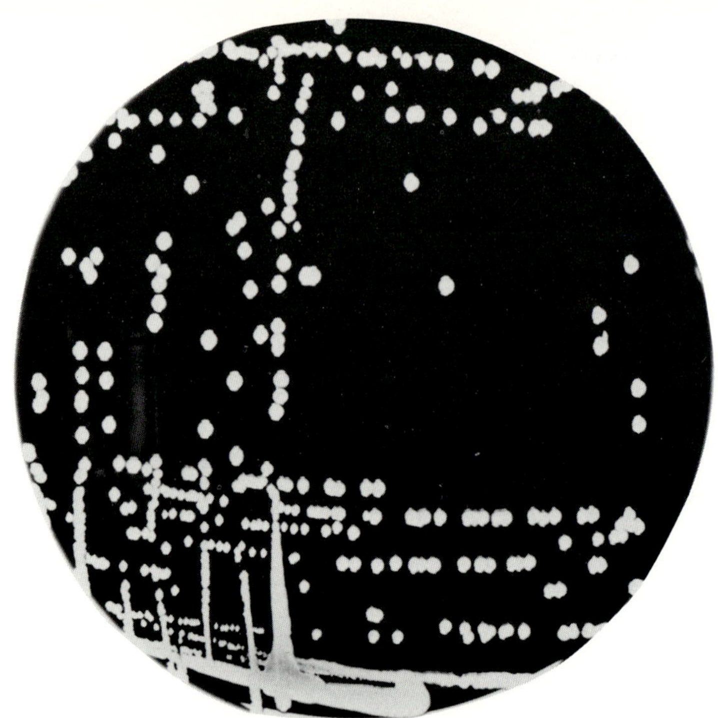

E

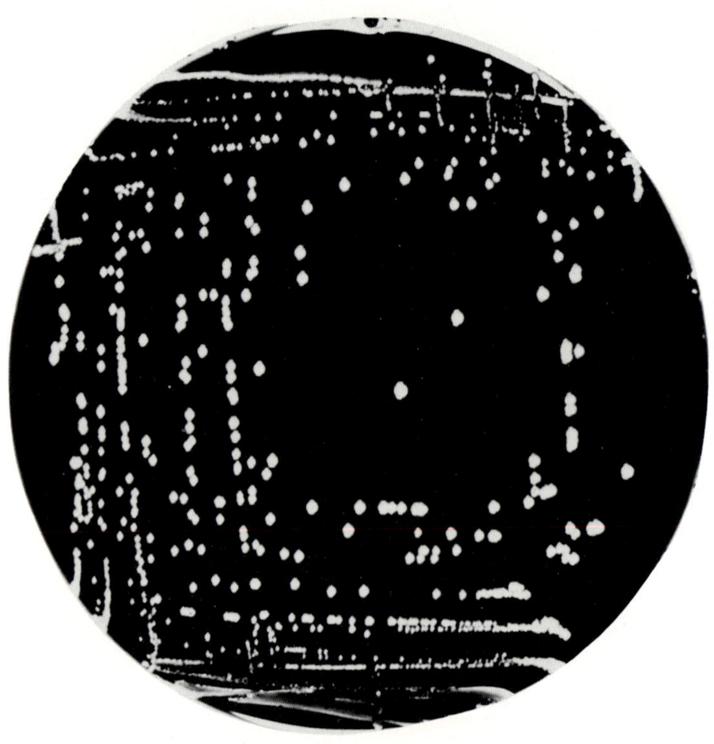

F

Fig. 2-1 *(Continued)*.   E. Approximately 5×10^7 organisms per milliliter urine. F. Approximately 5×10^8 organisms per milliliter urine.

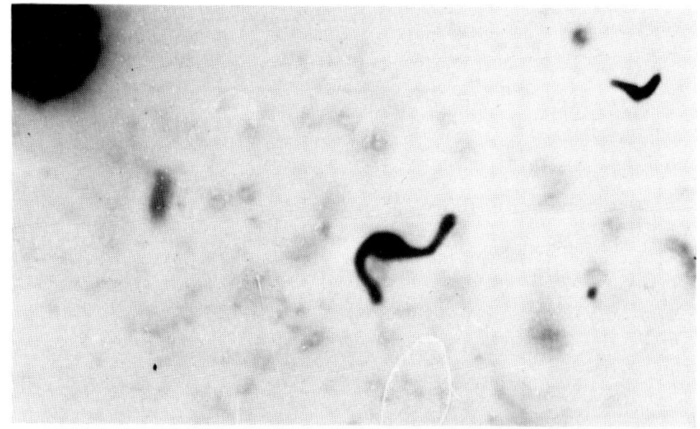

Fig. 2-2. L-form, Giemsa stain. Total magnification ×3000.

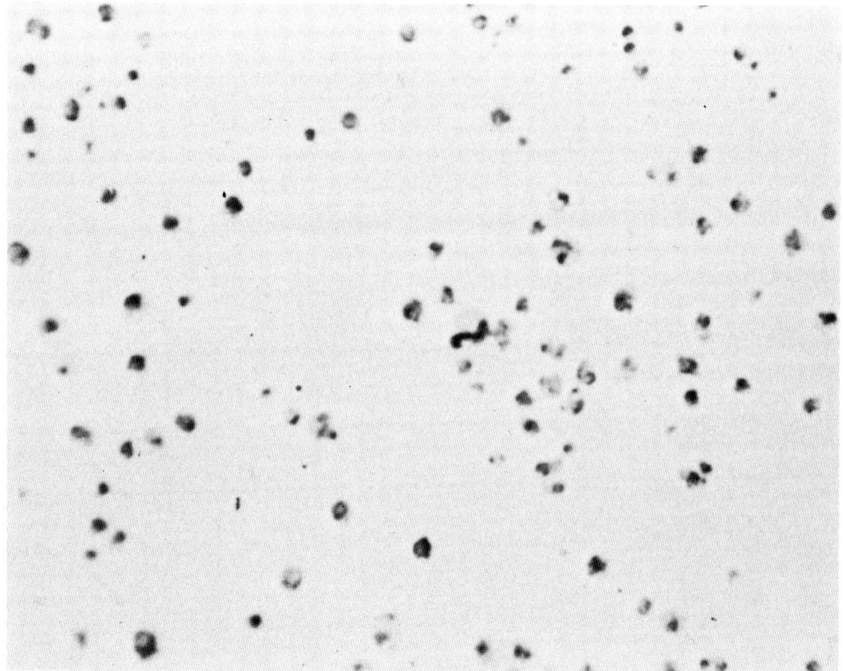

Fig. 2-3. L-form colonies. Total magnification ×60.

plasticity, will pass through the filter. The filtrate, collected in a sterile 15-ml screw cap centrifuge tube, is centrifuged at 5000 rpm for 5 minutes. The sediment, along with approximately 3 ml of filtrate, is removed with a sterile, cotton-plugged, Pasteur pipet. Several drops of the filtrate are introduced into nutrient broth and onto a blood nutrient agar plate. Two tubes of L-form broth and two plates of L-form agar are similarly inoculated. The inoculum on the agar plates is carefully streaked out with a sterile cotton-tipped applicator. All cultures are incubated aerobically at 37°C. Samples of the sediment are placed on two microscope slides and air-dried. One slide is used for Gram staining and the other is fixed in cold absolute methanol and stained with Giemsa. Both slides are examined under oil immersion for typical L-forms (Fig. 2-2).

The nutrient broth and blood nutrient agar cultures of the hypertonic sediment are employed to ensure that classic bacterial forms are not present in the filtrate. If growth occurs in these cultures, all the cultures from that specimen are discarded. The L-form culture plates are examined every 48 hours with a microscope for typical L-form (Fig. 2-3) or classic bacterial colonies. The plates are kept for four weeks before they are reported as negative. The culture tubes are examined daily for turbidity, an indication of L-form reversion to classic parent forms. In the event that the broths do not become turbid, they are subcultured at weekly intervals in a medium that would support L-form growth. In the event that reversion does occur, the classic parent colony can be handled in the routine manner for an antibiogram profile and microbial speciation.

Clinical Biochemistry of Renal Disease

The primary functions of the kidney are the regulation of water, acid-base and electrolyte balance, the maintenance of osmotic pressure of body fluids, and the removal of metabolic waste products and certain toxic substances. The biochemistry of renal disease, specifically related to the measurements of metabolic waste products, will be discussed here. Automated methods of analysis are in widespread use. However, since these are not always available, a brief discussion of standard methods of analysis is included in the appendix to this chapter (p. 236). Techniques for the determination of urea clearance are also mentioned, since the clearance test still remains one of the simplest and most rapid methods for the clinical assessment of renal function.

UREA

Urea is the chief end product of the metabolism of proteins and amino acids. Under normal conditions it comprises about half the total urine solids and is therefore the most abundant urinary constituent except water. Urea has a molecular weight of 60, a molecular size of 3 Å, is 47 percent nitrogen, and is the same size as a molecule of water. Thus it can pass through almost all biologic membranes to produce identical concentrations in various body components, calculated on a water content basis, provided fluctuations in concentration on one side of the membrane do not occur too rapidly.

The liver is believed to be the only organ capable of making urea. Studies have been made of urea formation in liver slices which were respiring in an oxygenated medium containing ammonium salts. From these studies a series of reactions which comprise the ornithine cycle were formulated. Ammonium and bicarbonate ions are activated to form carbamyl phosphate, which is incorporated into a molecule of ornithine and citrulline. Citrulline combines with aspartic acid to form arginosuccinic acid, which is cleaved into arginine and fumaric acid. Finally, arginine is hydrolyzed to urea and ornithine. During these enzymatic processes, carbon dioxide from the catabolism of carbohydrates, fats, and proteins combines with ammonia from the catabolism of amino acids to form urea. Three molecules of adenosine triphosphate are necessary, and five different amino acids enter into the reaction (acyl glutamic acid, ornithine, citrulline, aspartic acid, and arginine).

Normally urea constitutes approximately 40 to 50 percent of the non-protein nitrogen in the blood. The level of blood urea nitrogen (nitrogen is approximately 50 percent of the urea molecule) is related directly to protein intake and inversely to glomerular filtration rate. Increased protein catabolism (e.g., trauma, fever, and certain drugs such as corticosteroids and tetracycline) also leads to blood urea nitrogen increase, as does proteolysis of blood in large hematomas or in hemorrhage in the gastrointestinal tract. Urea clearance and excretion vary directly with urine flow. The effects of all these factors on blood urea nitrogen are exaggerated as glomerular filtration rate decreases.

Methods for the determination of urea may be based on reaction with diacetyl monoxime or similar compounds or on urease action.

Urea at temperatures of about 125°C and above is hydrolyzed to NH_3 and CO_2. Because of the inconvenience of autoclaving, this technique is not very popular, although from time to time it is resurrected. In a newer method urea is precipitated as diaxanthylurea by addition of an alcoholic solution of xanthydrol, and the precipitate is weighed. This is the only truly specific method, but it is too laborious for normal clinical practice. When it is converted to a photometric procedure, a six-hour waiting period is required, and some interference from thiourea and allatoin occurs.

The enzyme urease specifically hydrolyzes urea to carbamic acid, which then decomposes directly to CO_2 and NH_3. Although the quantity of urea originally present can be determined by gasometric measurement of the carbon dioxide formed, most of the urease techniques measure the ammonia. The ammonia may be titrated following its isolation by aeration or isothermic distillation (Conway technique). Recovery of ammonia by aeration is extremely difficult and unreliable. Nesslerization applied directly to a protein-free filtrate obviates this difficulty and shortens the procedure. A reaction between ammonia and phenol in the presence of hypochlorite yields a blue color due to dissociated indophenol. This reaction is ten times more sensitive for ammonia than nesslerization.

Urea in concentrations greater than 800 mg per 100 ml in in-vitro studies inhibits glucose utilization. The possibility cannot be excluded that high levels of urea may cause shifts in biosynthetic processes and thus cause the accumulation of other toxins which cause the uremic syndrome. It seems reasonable to conclude at this time that the contribution of urea itself to the biochemical abnormalities of chronic renal failure is modest if not negligible. However, blood urea nitrogen levels as a measure of the progress of renal failure are still useful.

CREATININE

Creatinine is the end product of muscle metabolism and is the anhydride of creatine. Creatinine is excreted from plasma by glomerular filtration and also, in man, by tubular secretion. Therefore creatinine clearance exceeds glomerular clearance. In contrast to urea clearance, creatinine clearance is not flow dependent. The concentration of serum creatinine is less dependent on protein catabolism than urea concentration but is dependent on muscle catabolism.

Current methods for measuring creatinine include noncreatinine chromogens, leading to error when creatinine clearance is used to approximate glomerular filtration rate, since the noncreatinine chromogens are not filtered.

URIC ACID

Uric acid is a metabolite of nucleic acids. The bone marrow may be a major site of formation, and possibly the liver or muscles also, but this is not yet certain. Uric acid is present in the bloodstream and is excreted mainly in urine, to a lesser extent in digestive fluid, and in small amounts in sweat and saliva. It is probably not destroyed in human tissues, but that portion of it entering the intestine may be destroyed by bacterial action. Variations in uric acid levels are affected by the rates of formation and excretion.

Production of uric acid is influenced by factors that affect metabolism of protein, carbohydrate, and fat, as well as by those that affect degradation of exogenous and endogenous nucleic acids and nucleotides. The body contains a uric acid pool of about 1.2 gm, of which more than 50 percent is turned over daily and an additional amount destroyed by bacterial action. Increased values may be observed in the presence of nitrogen retention. Uricosuric drugs, such as salicylates, corticosteroids, and mercurial diuretics, administered in small doses may decrease uric acid excretion.

AMMONIA

Under ordinary dietary conditions, a normal subject excretes 30 to 50 mEq of ammonia daily. One mechanism for the elimination of hydrogen ions and the conservation of cation is the production of ammonia. Urinary ammonia is formed in the tubule cells, especially in the distal portion of the tubule, the major site of acidification. Most of the ammonia is derived from amide and amino nitrogen groups of glutamine (by the action of glutaminase). Dissolved NH_3 diffuses into the lumen of the tubule, combining with H^+ ions in the acidified fluid to form NH_4^+ ions. This facilitates removal of H^+ ions and thus permits conservation of Na^+. Ammonia excretion is increased in metabolic acidosis and negligible in alkalosis.

Ammonia production is impaired in renal insufficiency and is a major cause of acidosis.

AMINO ACIDS

Renal conservation of the free amino acids of the plasma is quite efficient; under normal conditions, less than 5 percent of the amount entering the tubules in the glomerular filtrate escapes reabsorption into the bloodstream. When the exogenous supply is increased, only a fraction is excreted in the urine, the bulk of the excess being metabolized mainly to urea in the liver. Since renal clearance of the amino acids varies widely under normal conditions, there is no uniform correlation between the amounts of particular amino acids in the urine and their concentrations in the blood.

Renal forms of aminoaciduria are identified on the basis of normal plasma amino acid concentrations and increased renal clearance of the amino acid involved, which occurs because of decreased tubular reabsorption. Aminoaciduria may exist either as an isolated phenomenon or in association with other reabsorptive defects. It may represent a congenital abnormality of tubular function or may occur as a result of or in association with acquired disease. Several clinically distinct entities of this type have been described.

Methods have been developed for determination of alpha amino acid nitrogen in blood and urine. One method is based on the color produced with sodium beta-naphthoquinone-4-sulfonate. The gasometric ninhydrin method remains the reference method for the determination of alpha amino acid nitrogen in biologic fluids but is too tedious for routine analyses. Automatic analysers are available for the measurement of individual amino acids.

GUANIDINES

Methylguanidine and guanidino succinic acid are at present the most commonly studied compounds suspected of being uremic toxins. Guanidino succinic acid (GSA) limits internal platelet transformation in response to exogenous adenosine diphosphate, possibly accounting for the hemostatic abnormalities found in renal failure. In addition GSA may play a role in uremic neuropathy, since it inhibits transketolase, an enzyme vital for the formation of myelin.

Methylguanidine may be responsible for the gastrointestinal, neurological, and other symptoms seen in uremia. Dogs intoxicated with methylguanidine have been reported as having these symptoms. Further studies are required, especially regarding the levels found in uremic patients, to substantiate these findings.

Methods for measuring methylguanidine and GSA are not yet suited for routine clinical use.

OTHER COMPOUNDS

Phenols and indoles accumulate in uremia but seem to play no role in production of uremic symptoms.

DETERMINATION OF UREA BY UREASE AND THE BERTHELOT REACTION

Reagents

BUFFERED UREASE SOLUTION. 150 mg urease (activity ca. 1000 units/ gm) and 1 gm ethylenediaminetetraacetic acid (EDTA) per 100 ml aqueous solution, adjusted to a pH of 6.5. Any medium-grade urease (such as Urease, type II, ca. 800–1000 Sumner units/gm, marketed by Sigma Chemical) is satisfactory. The urease solution should be kept refrigerated, under which condition it is stable for one month. Stability is much greater in the frozen or lyophilized state.

PHENOL COLOR REAGENT. 50 gm AR grade phenol and 0.25 gm AR grade sodium nitroprusside per liter. Stable at least two months if kept cool and in amber bottle protected from light.

ALKALI-HYPOCHLORITE REAGENT. 25 gm AR grade sodium hydroxide and 2.1 gm sodium hypochlorite per liter. Commercial bleach (Clorox), which contains 5.25 gm NaOCl per 100 ml, can be used: combine 25 gm sodium hydroxide and 40 ml Clorox, dilute to 1 liter. Stable at least two months if kept cool and in amber bottle protected from light.

UREA STANDARD. Place 0.429 gm urea in a 1-liter volumetric flask and make to volume with distilled water. Add a few drops of chloroform as a preservative. Store in refrigerator. 1 ml contains 0.2 mg urea N (nitrogen).

Procedure for Serum or Plasma

1. Set up the following test tubes (or cuvets):
   Blank   0.2 ml buffered urease solution.
   Standard   0.2 ml buffered urease solution and 20 μl urea standard.
   Unknown   0.2 ml buffered urease solution and 20 μl serum or plasma.
                The 20 μl aliquots of standard and unknown are added by micropipets, Sahli hemoglobin pipets being satisfactory if their accuracy has been checked.
2. Incubate tubes in a water bath at 37°C for 15 minutes or at 25°C for 30 minutes (minimum times).
3. Add 1 ml phenol color reagent to each tube, mix, then add 1 ml alkali-hypochlorite reagent, and mix promptly again. It is mandatory that the phenol reagent be added and mixed first.
4. Incubate tubes at 50°–60°C for 3 minutes, at 37°C for 20 minutes, or at 25°C for 40 minutes.
5. Add water equally to all tubes to bring absorbance readings into desirable absorbance range (preferably 0.2–0.8). For Beckman DU spectrophotometer with 1-cm cuvets add 8 ml water. For Klett photometer with #54 filter add 3 ml water.
6. Read absorbances of blank (Ab), standard (As), and unknown (Ax) against water at 630 mμ or with a filter with normal wavelength in this region. If Ax is greater than 0.8, dilute the blank and unknown further with water equally, read absorbances again, and make proper corrections in calculation.

CALCULATION

$$\text{mg urea N}/100 \text{ ml} = \frac{\text{Ax} - \text{Ab}}{\text{As} - \text{Ab}} \times 20$$

Procedure for Urine

In blood the preformed NH_4^+ content is negligible compared with that formed from urea by urease action. For urine, however, this is not the case; normally, the preformed NH_4^+ is about 5 percent of the total present after conversion of the urea to ammonia. Hence, unless an independent analysis for preformed ammonia is made and subtracted from the final result, the value obtained represents urea nitrogen + preformed ammonia nitrogen.

Since the average output of urea nitrogen is of the order of 10 gm per day, the concentration in urine is about 50 times that in blood. The test, therefore, uses 20 μl of a 1:50 dilution of urine instead of 20 μl of serum or plasma. The standard in this instance is equivalent to 1000 mg urea N per 100 ml urine. Preformed ammonia may be determined in the urine simply by omitting the incubation with urease and substituting water for the urease solution.

DETERMINATION OF UREA NITROGEN BY UREASE AND NESSLERIZATION

Reagents

FOLIN-WU PROTEIN PRECIPITATING REAGENTS.

KOCH'S GLYCEROL-UREASE EXTRACT (or any active urease preparation). Koch's extract can be either prepared or bought commercially. Stable at least one year at refrigerator temperature.

PHOSPHATE BUFFER. pH about 6.5. Dissolve 6 gm KH_2PO_4 and 2 gm Na_2HPO_4 in 1 liter distilled water. Store in refrigerator.

SODIUM CITRATE. 15%.

NESSLER'S REAGENT.

UREA STANDARD. Place 0.429 gm urea in a 1-liter volumetric flask and make to volume with distilled water. Add a few drops of chloroform as a preservative. Store in refrigerator. One milliliter contains 0.2 mg urea nitrogen.

Macro Procedure for Blood, Serum, or Plasma

1. Set up in test tubes:
   Blank   0.5 ml water.
   Standard   0.5 ml urea standard.
   Unknown   0.5 ml serum (preferable) or whole blood (do not use ammonium oxalate as anticoagulant).
2. To each tube add 1 ml phosphate buffer and five drops urease solution, mix, and incubate for 30 minutes at 55°C, 1 hour at 37°C, or 90 minutes at room temperature. Whole blood should not be incubated much longer, but for serum and urine there is no time limit.
3. Add 8.5 ml water to blank and to standard, and mix. If the unknown is blood, add to it 6.5 ml water and 1 ml 0.67N sulfuric acid, and mix; then add 1 ml 10% sodium tungstate, mix, and filter through What-

man #1 filter paper. If the unknown is serum, add to it 7.5 ml water and 0.5 ml acid, mix, then add 0.5 ml tungstate, mix, and filter.

4. Transfer 1 ml blank, standard, and unknown separately to large test tubes (15–20 mm diameter). Add 3.8 ml water and 0.2 ml 15% sodium citrate to each. Mix.

5. Add 1 ml Nessler's reagent, while mixing, as rapidly as feasible.

6. Within one minute after adding Nessler's reagent, read all tubes against water at 420 mμ. Obviously, if a series of determinations is being run, the samples must be nesslerized one or two at a time. If a filter photometer is used, see that the filter has a nominal wavelength of 420 mμ, and read standard and unknown against the reagent blank. If absorbance is too high, develop color again with a smaller aliquot of the protein-free filtrate.

CALCULATION.   For spectrophotometer at 420 mμ:

$$\text{mg urea N/100 ml} = \frac{\text{Ax} - \text{Ab}}{\text{As} - \text{Ab}} \times 20$$

To convert urea N to urea:

$$\text{urea} = 2.14 \times \text{urea N}$$

Procedure for Urine

Use 0.5 ml of a 1:50 dilution of the urine and treat as for serum, using half quantities of precipitating reagents (as for serum) to precipitate any protein that is present. If the solution is clear after addition of protein precipitants, filtration is not necessary.

CALCULATION.   For spectrophotometer at 420 mμ:

$$\text{mg urea N/100 ml} = \frac{\text{Ax} - \text{Ab}}{\text{As} - \text{Ab}} \times 1000$$

If the absorbance of the unknown is less than one-half or greater than four times that of the standard, the color development should be repeated with an appropriate aliquot of the urease-treated sample and the required correction made in the calculation.

DETERMINATION OF UREA NITROGEN BY DIACETYLMONOXIME

Reagents

ACID MIXTURE.   Add, slowly and with constant swirling, 75 ml 85% phosphoric acid to 100 ml water. Add slowly, with swirling, 25 ml concentrated sulfuric acid.

DIACETYLMONOXIME.   5% in 95% ethanol. Keeps indefinitely when refrigerated.

ACID DIACETYL.   Add 1 ml 5% diacetyl to 25 ml acid mixture. Make fresh daily.

TUNGSTIC ACID REAGENT. Mix equal volumes of 0.15N sulfuric acid (4.15 ml concentrated sulfuric acid to 1 liter water) and 2.2% sodium tungstate dihydrate.

STOCK UREA. To make 1 mg/ml, dissolve 100 mg urea in water and dilute to 100 ml in a volumetric flask.

WORKING STANDARDS. First, to make 0.01 mg/ml, dilute 1 ml stock to 100 ml. Second, to make 0.02 mg/ml, dilute 1 ml stock to 50 ml (standards a and b).

Procedure

1. Add 0.1 ml blood to 3.9 ml tungstic acid reagent. Use water instead of blood for the blank and standard for the controls.
2. Shake well, let stand for 2 minutes, and centrifuge.
3. To 2 ml supernatant fluid, add 2 ml acid diacetyl and mix thoroughly.
4. Heat in a boiling water bath for 10 minutes. Keep away from light.
5. Cool and read the sample and controls against the blank at 480 mμ.

   CALCULATION (using standards a and b)

$$(a)\ \frac{ODu}{ODs} \times 40 = \text{mg urea}/100 \text{ ml}$$

$$(b)\ \frac{ODu}{ODs} \times 80 = \text{mg urea}/100 \text{ ml}$$

To convert mg percent urea to mg percent urea nitrogen, multiply by 0.467.

DETERMINATION OF CREATININE

Reagents

PICRIC ACID. 0.040M. 9.16 gm anhydrous or 10.17 gm reagent grade picric acid (containing 10–12% added water), made up to 1 liter with distilled water. Solution can be aided by heat. Recrystallization is not necessary. Exact standardization of the acid is not required. If creatinine is not to be determined, a saturated solution of picric acid can be used. Solutions are stable at room temperature but should be protected from sunlight.

SODIUM HYDROXIDE. 0.75N 30 gm/liter solution.

SATURATED AQUEOUS OXALIC ACID.

LLOYD'S REAGENT. Approximately 100 mg aliquots of the powder are used in each adsorption. After one such sample has been weighed out, the amounts thereafter may be approximated on the tip of a spatula. An alternative is to use 1 ml of an aqueous 10% suspension. It has been claimed that not all brands of Lloyd's reagent will adsorb creatinine.

STOCK CREATININE STANDARD. 1.5 mg/ml in 0.1N hydrogen chloride. Stable indefinitely in refrigerator.

Procedures without Lloyd's Reagent

Serum Creatinine

1. To 2 ml of serum add 3 ml water, 1 ml 10% sodium tungstate, and 2 ml 0.67N sulfuric acid. Mix and centrifuge.
2. Set up in test tubes:
   Reagent blank   3 ml water.
   Standard   1 ml working standard and 2 ml water.
   Unknown   3 ml protein-free centrifugate.
3. To each tube add 1 ml picric acid and 1 ml 0.75N sodium hydroxide, and mix.
4. At exactly 20 minutes read against reagent blank at 520 mμ.
   CALCULATION

$$\text{mg creatinine}/100 \text{ ml serum} = \frac{Ax}{As} \times 2$$

Urine Creatinine

1. For unknown use 3 ml of a 1:100 dilution of urine. If there is proteinuria, remove protein by making a 1:10 Folin-Wu protein-free filtrate in the manner ordinarily employed for blood. Make a further 1:10 dilution of this filtrate to yield the desired 1:100 dilution of the original urine.
2. For standard use 2 ml working standard and 1 ml water.

Procedures with Lloyd's Reagent

Serum Creatinine

1. To 2 ml serum add 3 ml water, 1 ml 10% sodium tungstate, and 2 ml 0.67 sulfuric acid. Mix and centrifuge.
2. Set up in test tubes:
   Reagent blank   5 ml water.
   Standard   1 ml working standard and 4 ml sulfuric acid.
   Unknown   3 ml protein-free centrifugate and 2 ml sulfuric acid.
3. Add 0.5 ml saturated aqueous oxalic acid to each tube.
4. Add approximately 100 mg Lloyd's reagent to each tube or, alternatively use 1 ml 10% aqueous suspension of Lloyd's reagent.
5. Close tubes with rubber stoppers and shake them intermittently for 10 minutes.
6. Centrifuge, decant, and drain.
7. Add to each tube 3 ml water, 1 ml picric acid, and 1 ml 0.75N sodium hydroxide.
8. Close tubes with rubber stoppers and shake them intermittently for 10 minutes. Centrifuge.

9. Read supernates at 520 mμ against reagent blank at any time after 20
   minutes after step 7.

   CALCULATION

$$\text{mg creatinine}/100 \text{ ml serum} = \frac{Ax}{As} \times 2$$

Urine Creatinine

Same as for serum, except:
1. For unknown, use 3 ml of a 1:100 dilution and 2 ml water. In case
   of proteinuria, remove protein as outlined in step 1 of Urine Creatinine,
   Procedures without Lloyd's Reagent.
2. For standard, use 2 ml working standard and 3 ml water.

   CALCULATION

$$\text{mg creatinine}/\text{ml urine} = \frac{Ax}{As}$$

Urea or Creatinine Clearance Tests

On the morning of the test the patient should not have any breakfast.
Starting at 7:30 A.M. he should drink one glass of water every half hour until
the test is completed. At 9:00 A.M. he should empty his bladder completely,
and the urine should be discarded. At 9:30 A.M. 5 cc of clotted blood should
be drawn and kept. At 10:00 A.M. the patient should empty his bladder
completely, and all urine should be kept. Catheterization is necessary if
there is any doubt about the patient's capacity to empty his bladder completely. If desired, a second collection period may follow, with another
blood sample. If the patient is a child, his height, weight, and sex should
be recorded.

   CALCULATION

1. If the volume of urine excreted is more than 2 ml/min, calculate the
   maximal clearance (Cm) by the following formula:

$$Cm = UV/P$$

   where U = urea concentration of urine

   P = urea concentration of plasma

   V = volume of urine excreted per minute

   The range of normal is 75–90 ml/min, and the percentage of the normal
   equals 1.33 × UV/P.
2. If the rate of excretion is less than 2 ml/min, the standard clearance
   (Cs) is calculated according to the following formula (not recommended):

$$Cs = U\sqrt{\overline{V}}/P$$

   In the normal subject, the rate of creatinine clearance exceeds that of
inulin by approximately 10 to 15 percent.

DETERMINATION OF AMMONIA

To obtain a basal level, patients should be fasting for at least 6 hours prior to the test.

Special Apparatus

DIFFUSION BOTTLES. Vaccine bottles, ca. 50–65 ml capacity, dimensions ca. 2.5 by 1.5 in.

RUBBER STOPPERS. One set of solid stoppers to fit the diffusion bottles. A second set of one-holed stoppers that fit the receiving rods.

RECEIVING RODS. 6- by 80-mm glass rods with 0.5 in. of one end ground so that when dipped in acid it retains an acid film over its surface. The rods are set in the one-holed rubber stoppers in such a way that the ground end of the rod extends about halfway into the stoppered bottle.

STAINLESS STEEL RODS. Approximately 8 mm in diameter and 40 mm long. Three are required per bottle. (Glass rods do not work; they are not sufficiently heavy).

ROTATOR. A wheel rotating about 50 rpm, with the axis horizontal, to which spring clamps are attached to hold the diffusion bottles about 8 cm from the axis, with the flat bottom of the bottles against the wheel.

Reagents

ALKALINE BUFFER MIXTURE. Two parts potassium carbonate, 1.5 parts water, and 1 part anhydrous potassium bicarbonate. Mix thoroughly, but do not powder. Store in a closed container over aqueous saturated K_2CO_3.

SULFURIC ACID. 1N. Add 1 ml concentrated sulfuric acid to 35 ml distilled water.

PHENOL COLOR REAGENT. See Reagents under Determination of Urea by Urease and the Berthelot Reaction.

ALKALI-HYPOCHLORITE REAGENT. See Reagents under Determination of Urea by Urease and the Berthelot Reaction.

WORKING AMMONIA STANDARD. 3 μg nitrogen per milliliter. Dilute 3 ml stock ammonia standard (0.1 mg ammonia nitrogen per milliliter).

Procedure for Blood

1. Set up a series of diffusion bottles (two blanks, two standards, and two for each unknown) each containing 3 gm alkaline buffer mixture and three dry stainless steel rods. Stopper, using the solid stoppers, and lay them on their sides in preparation for use.
2. When ready to use the bottles, set them up in the following order:

    Blank   Add 2 ml distilled water to bottle and immediately stopper. Lay aside.

    Standard   Add 2 ml working standard (6 μg NH_3N) to bottle and immediately stopper. Lay aside.

    Unknown   Add 2 ml blood (collected with anticoagulant) to bottle and immediately stopper. Mix on rotator for 1 minute.

3. Working with one bottle at a time, wet the ground portion of a receiving rod in 1N sulfuric acid, remove the solid stopper from the bottle while it is lying on its side, and quickly insert the receiving rod with one-holed stopper, taking care not to touch the neck of the bottle with the rod.
4. Place all bottles on rotator and rotate at 50 rpm for 40 minutes.
5. Remove all bottles from rotator and lay them down gently on their sides. Remove the receiving rods carefully, one at a time, taking great care that the rods not touch the necks of the bottles. Wash the acid off each receiving rod, into a test tube, with 1 ml phenol color reagent. Next, wash off each rod, into the test tube, with 1 ml alkali-hypochlorite reagent and 1 ml distilled water successively.
6. Incubate the tubes in a water bath at 50°–60°C for 3 minutes, at 37°C for 20 minutes, or at 25°C for 40 minutes.
7. Add water equally to all tubes to bring absorbance readings into desirable absorbance range (preferably 0.2–0.8). For Beckman DU with 1-cm cuvets add 7.0 ml water; for Klett photometer using #54 filter add 2 ml water.
8. Read absorbances of blank (Ab), standard (As), and unknown (Ax) against water at 630 mμ or with a filter with nominal wavelength in this region. If Ax is 0.8, dilute the blank and the unknown with water equally, read absorbances again, and make proper corrections in calculation.

CALCULATION

$$\mu\text{g ammonia N/ml blood} = \frac{Ax - Ab}{As - Ab} \times 3$$

Procedure for Urine

The ammonia content of urine can be determined by applying the color reaction directly.
1. Set up the following in tubes:

Blank   1 ml phenol reagent.

Standard   1 ml phenol reagent and 20 μl standard (70.7 mg AR grade $(NH_4)_2SO_4$/100 ml; 20 μl = 3 μg NH_4^+ N).

Unknown   1 ml phenol reagent and 20 μl 1:5 dilution of urine. The 20 μl aliquots of standard and unknown should be added from micropipets, Sahli hemoglobin pipets being satisfactory if their accuracy has been checked.

2. Add 1 ml of alkali-hypochlorite reagent to each tube, and mix.
3. Proceed as in steps 6, 7, and 8 under Procedure for Blood.

CALCULATION

$$\text{mg ammonia N/100 ml urine} = \frac{Ax - Ab}{As - Ab} \times 75$$

Normal Values

The normal range for venous whole blood has been reported to be 0.75–1.96 μg ammonia nitrogen per milliliter, for plasma 0.56–1.22 μg/ml, and for erythrocytes 0.96–3.31 μg/ml. There is evidence that the whole blood ammonia level of newborn infants averages somewhat higher than adult levels. The normal 24-hour output of ammonia nitrogen in urine has been reported to be 0.14–1.47 gm for adults and 0.56 to 2.93 gm for infants.

DETERMINATION OF AMINO ACID BY AMINO ACID NITROGEN–FOLIN-WU PRECIPITATING REAGENT METHOD

Reagents

STOCK AMINO ACID SOLUTIONS. Prepare two stock solutions. First, dissolve 268 mg glycine (pure) and 1 gm sodium benzoate in enough 0.07N hydrochloric acid to make 500 ml. Second, dissolve 526 mg glutamic acid and 1 gm sodium benzoate in enough 0.07N hydrochloric acid to make 500 ml.

STANDARD AMINO ACID SOLUTION (0.03 mg nitrogen per milliliter). Place 15 ml glycine stock solution and 15 ml glutamic acid stock solution in a 100-ml volumetric flask. Add to the mark 0.07N hydrochloric acid containing 2 gm sodium benzoate in 1000 ml acid. This standard is used for the analysis of filtrates prepared from unlaked blood.

STANDARD AMINO ACID SOLUTION (0.05 mg nitrogen per milliliter). Place 25 ml glycine stock solution and 25 ml glutamic acid solution in a 100-ml volumetric flask and add to the mark 0.07N hydrochloric acid containing 2 gm sodium benzoate in 1000 ml acid.

BORAX SOLUTION. Dissolve 1.5 gm borax in about 50 ml distilled water in a 100-ml volumetric flask. Dilute to the 100 ml mark with distilled water.

SODIUM B-NAPHTHOQUINONESULFONIC ACID. Freshly prepared 0.5% solution. Transfer 100 mg quinone to a small flask. Add 20 ml distilled water and shake. Complete solution takes place rapidly.

BLEACHING SOLUTIONS. Two solutions are necessary for the bleaching of the excess B-naphthoquinonesulfonic acid reagent. (1) A 0.1M solution of sodium thiosulfate, and (2) an acid formaldehyde solution prepared by mixing 75 ml 1.5N hydrochloric acid and 25 ml glacial acetic acid with 100 ml 0.15M formaldehyde. The 0.15M formaldehyde may be made by diluting 11.3 ml 40% formaldehyde to 1 liter.

SULFATE-TUNGSTATE SOLUTION. Dissolve 15 gm anhydrous sodium sulfate and 1.5 gm sodium tungstate in enough distilled water to make 1125 ml.

Procedure

1. Pipet 10 ml protein-free blood filtrate and Folin reagent to a large (1- by 8-in.) test tube labeled U for unknown.
2. Pipet 1 ml standard solution (1 ml = 0.05 mg) to a similar-sized test tube labeled S for standard.

3. Add 2 ml 1.5% borax solution to tube U.
4. Add 2 ml freshly prepared 0.5% B-naphthoquinonesulfonic acid to each.
5. Mix thoroughly.
6. Set both the U and the S tube in a dark closet for from 18 to 24 hours.
7. Add 2 ml acid formaldehyde solution and 2 ml 0.1M sodium thiosulfate solution to each.
8. Dilute each to 25 ml with distilled water.
9. Mix thoroughly and allow to stand four or five minutes to allow for complete bleaching of excess quinone reagent.
10. Read in a colorimeter.

CALCULATION

$$\frac{\text{Reading of unknown}}{\text{Reading of standard}} \times 5 = \text{mg amino acid}$$

Normal: 2.3–3.74 mg in 100 ml blood.

Ophthalmic Diagnosis of Renal Disease

Ocular examination is an essential component of the evaluation of patients with renal disease. Positive findings, however, are not absolute indications, as there are no ocular pathologic changes specific for kidney disease. For example, calcific deposits in the cornea and conjunctiva may result from secondary changes in calcium and phosphate metabolism concomitant with renal failure. Similarly, pathologic changes in the optic nerve and retina result from vascular alterations due to systemic hypertension. Eye changes, therefore, result not from renal pathology per se but from secondary changes induced in systemic blood pressure or in mineral metabolism. Consequently, no ocular sign may be considered pathognomonic, although it should be taken as a warning.

CONJUNCTIVAL METASTATIC CALCIFICATION

A striking finding is that of conjunctival metastatic calcification in uremic patients with low or normal serum calcium. Calcium phosphate microcrystals are found in the superficial conjunctival layers in a majority of patients with advanced acute or chronic renal disease (Fig. 4-1). The deposits are at times associated with ocular irritation and are the cause of the "red eyes of renal failure." In the majority of instances, however, the eyes are white and the patient entirely asymptomatic.

The occurrence of conjunctival metastatic calcification in hypercalcemia of diverse etiology is relatively rare as compared to its incidence in advanced renal failure with low or normal serum calcium. It would seem that the requirement for this phenomenon is a serum calcium and phosphate product in excess of 70. In most instances the elevated plasma inorganic phosphate level is chiefly responsible for the increased value of the calcium and phosphate product.

In all but the most evident cases biomicroscopy is essential to detect the microcrystals which are invariably located in the palpebral fissure. Crystals lie immediately beneath the conjunctival epithelium, which is elevated over them. Small crystals are white, but large crystals tend to be flat and colorless. The deposits are superficial to the episcleral vessels and do not move with blinking.

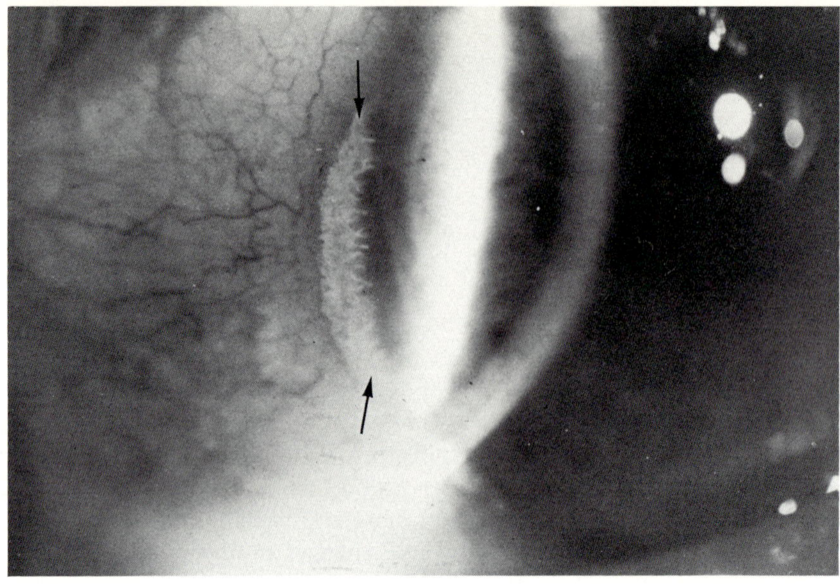

Fig. 4-1. Slit lamp photograph of limbal calcific deposits in a 26-year-old uremic male patient. (Serum calcium, 9.0; serum phosphorus, 9.4; serum calcium-phosphorus product, 84.6.)

Similar conjunctival calcific deposits have been noted in renal disease with hypercalcemia. In such cases calcium deposition in the superficial corneal layers may occur in a horizontal linear distribution to produce band keratopathy. This finding, when marked, is grossly visible and may significantly impair visual acuity. Commonly, band keratopathy results from ocular disease such as uveitis rather than from systemic alterations in mineral metabolism. Therapy by local debridement in conjunction with chelating agents is frequently effective.

HEPATOLENTICULAR DEGENERATION

Corneal pigmentation may antecede central nervous system manifestations in hepatolenticular degeneration and may therefore be an important diagnostic sign. Other ocular findings may include sunflower cataract, internal and/or external ophthalmoplegias, and the Kayser-Fleischer ring. This last varies in color from ruby red to green or, sometimes, yellowish-brown. Starting close to the corneal limbus, it usually extends onto clear cornea for several millimeters. The extent of the ring is apparently unrelated to the severity or stage of disease. Corneal changes do not interfere with vision and, thus, require no therapy. They tend to disappear when agents such as penicillamine are given systemically.

HEREDITARY CHRONIC NEPHRITIS

In hereditary chronic nephritis reduced visual acuity may occur from one of several ocular causes. These may include bilateral progressive anterior lenticonus and/or subcapsular cataracts, or retinopathy and/or maculopathy. Hyaline deposits in the optic nerve heads are also seen but usually do not result in alterations in visual acuity.

HYPERCALCEMIA

Band keratopathy may be seen in hypercalcemia resulting from any etiology. Unlike the corneal and conjunctival calcific deposits noted with low or normal serum calcium, it may significantly impair visual acuity. Band keratopathy has been noted in the aminoacidurias, such as Fanconi's syndrome, as well as in hypophosphatasia. Visual acuity may be restored by mechanical debridement or the use of topical chelating agents or both. These procedures may, however, require repetition upon reaccumulation of the corneal calcific material.

HYPERTENSIVE RETINOPATHY

The response of retinal blood vessels to elevated intravascular pressure is determined by their premorbid state. For example, sclerotic and narrowed arterioles do not respond in the same manner as healthy arterioles which are unprotected, so to speak, by fibrotic changes. The clinical appearance of the fundi of patients with high blood pressure is, therefore, modified by the presence or absence of preexisting retinal vascular disease.

With elevation of blood pressure, pathologic alterations occur in the retinal vasculature to produce clinically visible retinopathic changes similar to those seen in essential hypertension. There is hypertonic narrowing of retinal arterioles, hyperplasia of the vessel walls with caliber variation, and arteriovenous crossing changes due to hyperplasia of arteriolar walls. There may also be retinal hemorrhages, exudates, venous occlusions, and, in long-standing hypertension, diffuse arteriolar sclerosis and narrowing.

Although retinopathy may result from either acute or chronic renal disease, the latter is much more commonly associated with the development of what has been erroneously termed "renal retinopathy" (arteriolar narrowing and sclerosis, intraretinal hemorrhage, and exudate formation).

Renal disease in the absence of systemic hypertension does not cause retinopathy. Therefore "renal retinopathy" is not a specific clinical entity and appears only when there is associated hypertension.

Intraretinal hemorrhages are commonly seen in all types of hypertensive retinopathy. It is important to note that the shapes of these hemorrhages, as well as of exudates, are determined by the retinal architecture. The innermost layer* of the retina is formed by the long axons of the ganglion

* The layers of the retina are numbered from the back of the eyeball inward. Layer 1 is epithelial; 2, rods and cones; 3, bipolar cells; 4, ganglion cells. Looking into the eye from the front, the "deeper" layers are *behind* the ganglion cell layer. "Innermost" layers are 3 and 4, reading from the back of the eye in.

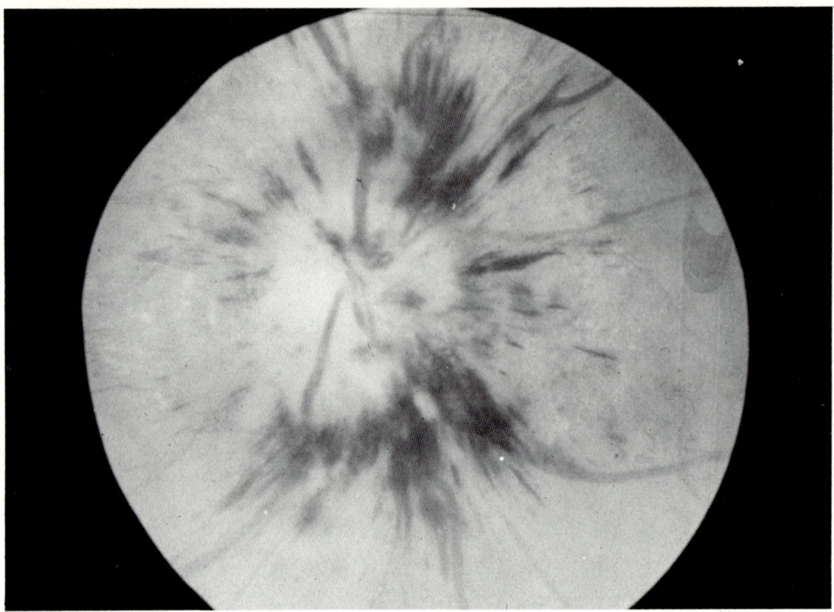

Fig. 4-2. Papilledema which developed during the malignant phase of hypertension associated with chronic renal failure. The disc margins are blurred, the cup obliterated, and numerous superficial flame-shaped retinal hemorrhages and venous engorgement are seen.

cells running parallel to the deeper layers of the retina. Consequently, hemorrhages or exudates arising in this layer will have a feathered or paintbrush-type border and, if not dense, will appear to be bright red and striated. Bleeding in the innermost retinal layers, then, gives rise to so-called flame-shaped hemorrhages (Fig. 4-2), while exudate formation in this same layer produces the clinical appearance of a cotton-wool spot (Fig. 4-3).

Round hemorrhages are also seen in the retina and result from the same pathologic process as flame-shaped hemorrhages, but lie in the deeper layers of the retina. The configuration of their borders is determined in part by the arrangement of Müller's fibers, which are vertically oriented to the plane of the retina. Deeper retinal hemorrhages, therefore, have a dot or blot appearance. Regardless of whether they are located in the deep or in the superficial layers of the retina, retinal hemorrhages anterior to the equatorial plane of the eye have a round or blotchy configuration because of the reduced number of ganglion cells and axons in the periphery.

Although massive hemorrhages are not a typical component of renal hypertensive retinopathy, they can and do occur either as a result of vascular necrosis, or more commonly, as bleeding secondary to venous oc-

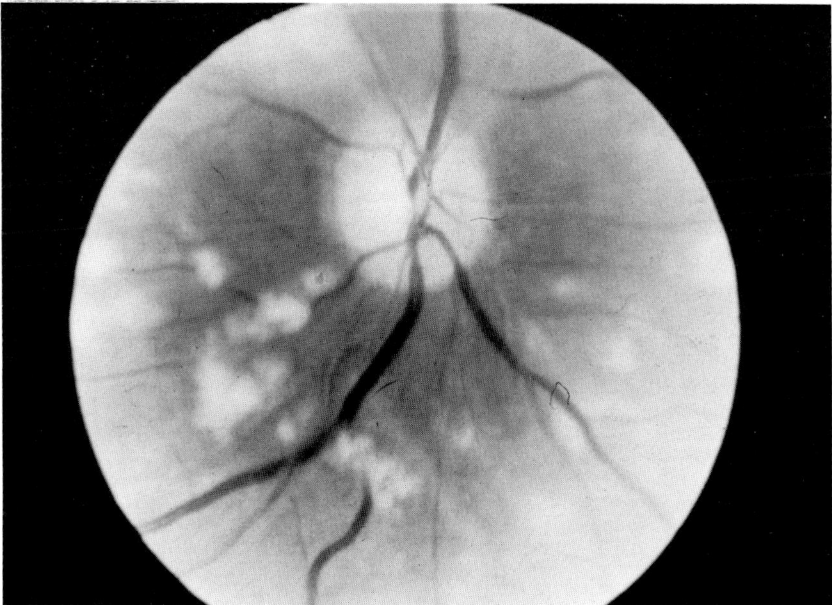

Fig. 4-3. Classic cotton-wool exudates which have formed in the innermost layer of the retina. The superficial location of these exudates is clearly demonstrated in areas where exudates have obscured retinal veins.

clusion resulting from compression by arteriolar walls at arteriovenous crossings.

The evolution and disappearance of superficial cotton-wool exudates has been well documented. Superficial retinal hemorrhages may have a less variable course and may persist without noticeable change for long periods. Those seen in association with cotton-wool spots, however, frequently seem to disappear at the same rate as the exudate.

COTTON-WOOL SPOTS

There is now general agreement that the cotton-wool spot or superficial exudate is the clinical manifestation of a focal ischemic lesion of the inner layers of the retina. Experimental data indicate that less than 24 hours of ischemia are required for the formation of this lesion. The human lesion begins as a small, pearly gray area, generally ill defined, which increases in size over a two- to three-day period. It looks white and fluffy and develops frayed edges due to its location in the inner retinal layers. Most such lesions are less than 1 disc diameter in size. Hemorrhage located in the nerve fiber layer is frequently seen at the circumference of the cotton-wool spot.

Soft exudates may overlie arteries and veins or cause them to become deflected. They are generally fully developed at the end of three or four days and begin to decrease in size within a month, disappearing completely within two to eight weeks. Fluorescein angiographic studies performed in the early stages of development of these lesions often reveal leakage of dye from small arterioles and a state of poor capillary perfusion in the area within which the cotton-wool spots form. In hypertensive patients without diabetes, circumferential microaneurysms may also be seen in the vicinity of the lesions. The important characteristics that distinguish between cotton-wool spots and hard exudates are color, location, configuration of edges, and length of life cycle.

The cotton-wool spot, then, represents a retinal vascular lesion resulting from obliteration of the capillary flow and altered permeability of small vessels and consists primarily of altered, edematous neurons. The lesion is in no way pathognomonic and may be seen in diabetes without systemic hypertension, following retinal emboli, and in any other condition resulting in focal retinal ischemia.

HARD EXUDATES

The presence of hard exudates indicates chronicity of the hypertensive state. They are not unlike the exudates seen in diabetic retinopathy and probably are formed from serous accumulation of fluid leaking from deeper retinal capillary beds. Their configuration is determined by the retinal architecture, so that they are either punctate or, when they coalesce, plaque-like with sharply crenated borders. When present in the macula, hard exudates form a star-like figure radiating out from the central foveal pit due to the arrangement of Henle's fiber layer (Fig. 4-4). The development of a circinate ring around the macula, although frequently seen in hypertensive states, is not specific for this disease. This ring is seen in any condition in which the perimacular vasculature undergoes functional or pathologic alterations leading to proteinaceous leakage. Absorption of these exudates is extremely variable, but in general they persist for months to years.

PAPILLEDEMA

Malignant hypertension, especially in young patients with healthy vessels, may produce additional ocular changes characterized primarily by the development of papilledema. Concomitantly, there is often widespread edema involving the retina at the posterior pole, superficial hemorrhages and cotton-wool exudates, and massive choroidal transudation producing bullous elevation of the retina.

In the early stages it is difficult to distinguish, by the appearance of the disc alone, between papilledema due to an intracranial lesion and papilledema secondary to malignant hypertension. Elevation of the disc is first seen nasally in all cases, because the axons of the ganglion cells are more densely packed in this region and hence a greater quantity of myelin is present there. When myelin begins to imbibe fluid as a consequence of

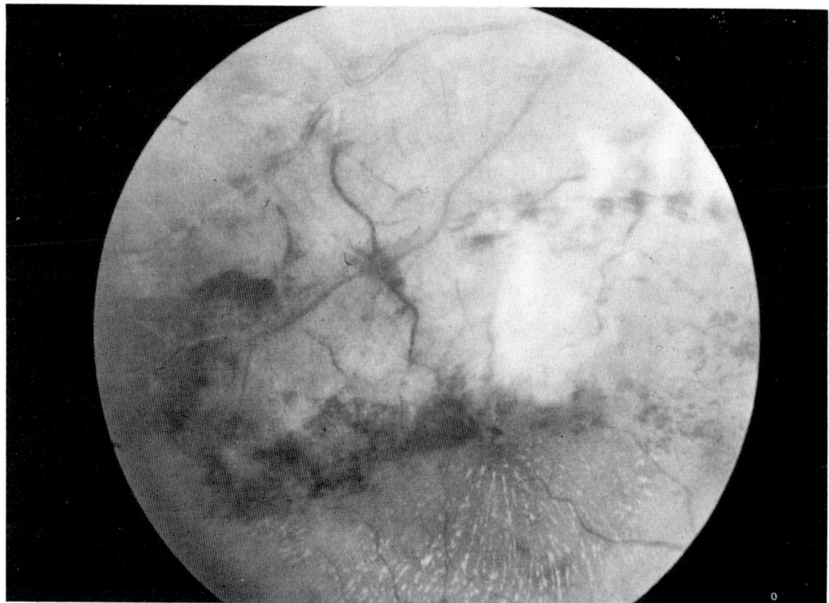

Fig. 4-4.   Superficial hemorrhages and exudates are seen superior to the macula. There are also deep retinal hemorrhages nasal and temporal to the macula and deep exudates in Henle's fiber layer which radiate out from the central foveal area, clearly defining the unique architecture of the inferior half of the macula.

the rise in venous pressure, this area of greatest myelin density initially is visibly swollen. However, the fully developed picture of hypertensive papilledema is characterized not only by imbibition of fluid by the myelin but also by diffuse intraretinal edema which surrounds, and may offset, the disc. Since the macular region frequently is edematous as well, central visual acuity is often reduced.

With increased intracranial pressure, elevation of the nerve head is higher and more mushroom-like in appearance than with hypertensive papilledema, because intraretinal edema formation around the disc is minimal. Although superficial hemorrhages and exudates are seen in both instances, they are generally more extensive in patients with systemic hypertension. Of course, the finding of either attenuated, or even sclerosed, arterioles in association with papilledema tends to support the diagnosis of hypertensive etiology.

Fluorescein angiography is of no help in differentiating between these two entities, since diffuse leakage of dye from the disc occurs with both conditions. This diagnostic technique is most helpful, however, in ruling out pseudopapilledema resulting from congenital variations or hyaline deposits within the optic nerve, since dye does not leak in these instances.

Finally, the presence of a secondary bullous retinal detachment in association with papilledema strongly points to a hypertensive etiology.

EXUDATIVE RETINAL DETACHMENT

Exudative (secondary) retinal detachment is common in young patients with severe elevation of blood pressure because of chronic renal disease. Fluid, probably a transudate from the choroidal vasculature, accumulates in the potential space between the pigment epithelial and neuroepithelial layers of the retina, causing anterior displacement of the retina and bullous elevation of the inner retinal layers. The origin of this fluid from the choroidal vasculature can be demonstrated by fluorescein angiography (Fig. 4-5).

Retinal elevation is greatest when the patient is upright, because the fluid rapidly shifts and accumulates inferiorly to produce bullous detachment of the inferior portion of the retina. Changes in head position alter the location of fluid, causing bullous elevations in the dependent regions and reattachment of the retina in opposite areas. These gravitational shifts

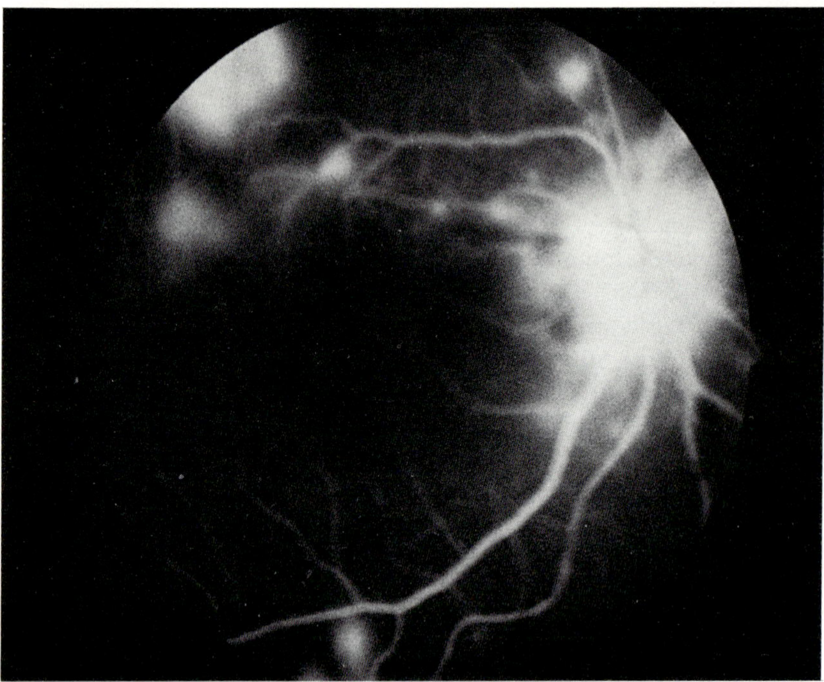

Fig. 4-5. Fluorescein angiogram, mid arteriovenous phase, demonstrating early leakage of dye from the optic nerve as well as accumulation above and below the macula, presumably from damaged choroidal vessels. Retinal vessels are out of focus due to the presence of associated, secondary, shallow retinal detachment.

in fluid readily distinguish a secondary retinal detachment from a primary detachment due to a retinal tear; in the latter case there is no dependent fluid accumulation.

Exudative bullous retinal detachments occur in those hypertensive states associated with chronic renal disease and in eclampsia. Reversal of the detachment takes place with normalization of the blood pressure. The ultimate visual prognosis is related to the duration of the detachment as well as to the presence of intraretinal hemorrhage and exudate formation, which can result in scarring. Following reattachment, widespread retinal pigmentary disturbances can be seen, but visual function, especially associated with eclamptic detachments, is surprisingly unimpaired.

5 Radiologic Techniques Used in the Diagnosis of Renal Disorders

Radiologic examinations of a patient with suspected renal disease almost invariably begin with a plain or scout film of the abdomen or KUB (kidneys, ureters, and bladder) followed by intravenous pyelography. A variety of specialized radiologic procedures may then be used to obtain more detailed information about kidney function, to reveal the presence of cysts, to locate obstructions or abnormalities in the urinary tract (a procedure which may be combined with cystoscopy), or to indicate the presence of renal vascular disease or carcinoma.

The illustrations in this section are arranged according to the type of procedure. In some cases normal anatomic variations are included as well as a representative sample of anatomic anomalies or pathologic conditions. Unless otherwise noted, the projections are in the anteroposterior plane.

Plain Film

A plain film can reveal calcifications in the kidney or urinary tract; it may also yield information about kidney size and indicate the presence of hydronephrosis, cysts, tumors, or displacements of the kidney caused by abnormalities in surrounding tissue.

Intravenous Pyelography (Excretory Urography)

Intravenous pyelography is used to indicate kidney size, shape, and position. It provides gross information about function, especially in the case of past or present infection. An IVP can also reveal congenital anomalies, such as a double collecting system or crossed ectopia, and pathologic conditions, such as medullary sponge kidney or cystic calcifications.

Rapid Sequence Urography

In rapid sequence urography the rate of dye concentration and its time of appearance in the pelves and ureters is measured and can be compared for the two kidneys. It is used especially when there is a difference in kidney size. A delay in the visualization of dye in one or both kidneys indicates the presence of unilateral or bilateral renal artery stenosis. Greater concentration of dye in a kidney affected by renal artery stenosis distinguishes this condition from unilateral chronic pyelonephritis.

Nephrotomography

Nephrotomography is used to obtain vertical sections through the kidney in order to pinpoint certain abnormalities.

Retrograde Studies

Retrograde studies are used to obtain detailed information about obstructions or abnormalities in the renal pelves or upper ureters.

Cystography

Cystography is used to detect abnormalities in the lower urinary tract, particularly bladder neck obstructions and reflux.

Renal Angiography

Renal arteriograms are used in the diagnosis of renal tumors and in the detection of renal artery stenosis. If an intravenous pyelogram indicates a small kidney, the arteriogram may determine whether the diminished size is congenital or caused either by infection or by vascular disease. Renal venograms can demonstrate renal vein thrombosis or the invasion of the vein by carcinoma.

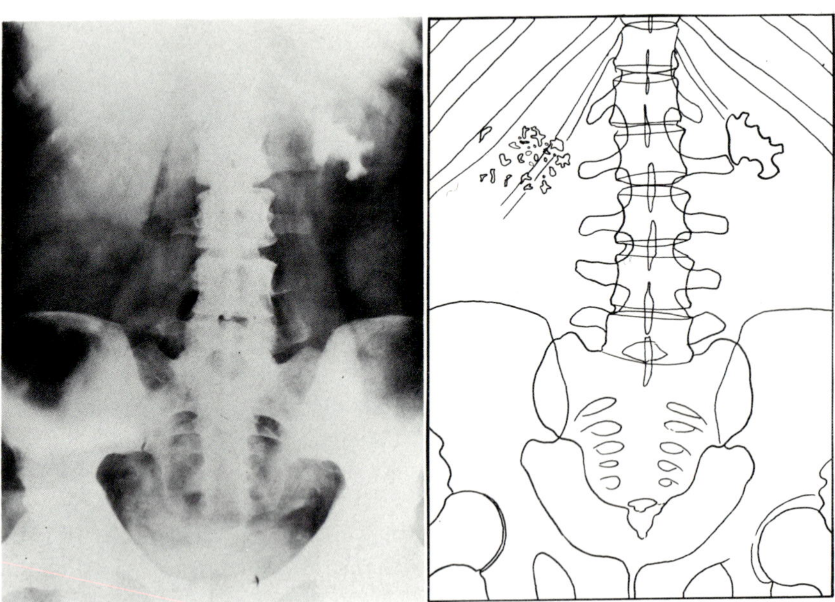

Fig. 5-1. Plain film of abdomen showing nephrolithiasis—staghorn calculi of left renal pelvis and multiple calculi of right collecting system.

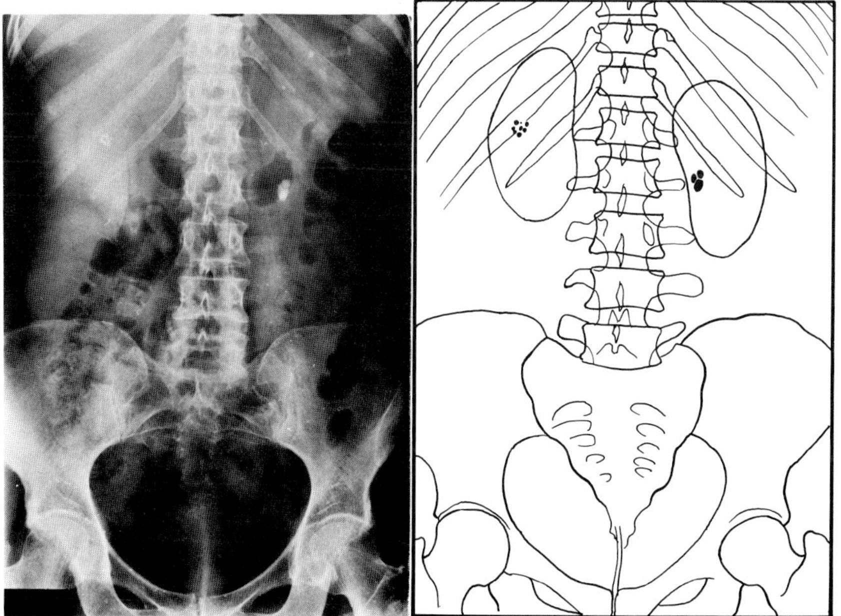

Fig. 5-2. Plain film of kidneys, ureters, and bladder, showing bilateral renal calculi.

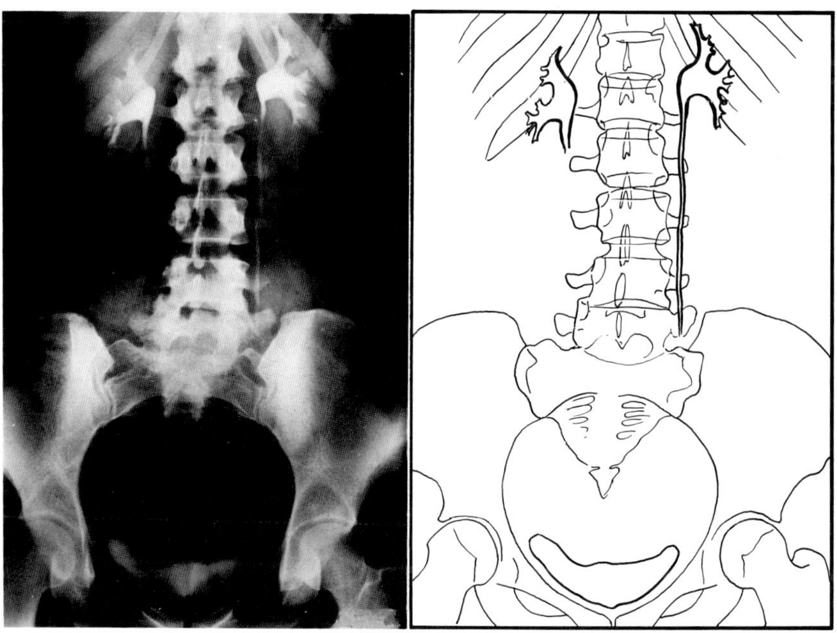

Fig. 5-3. Intravenous pyelogram of 24-year-old female, showing normal structures.

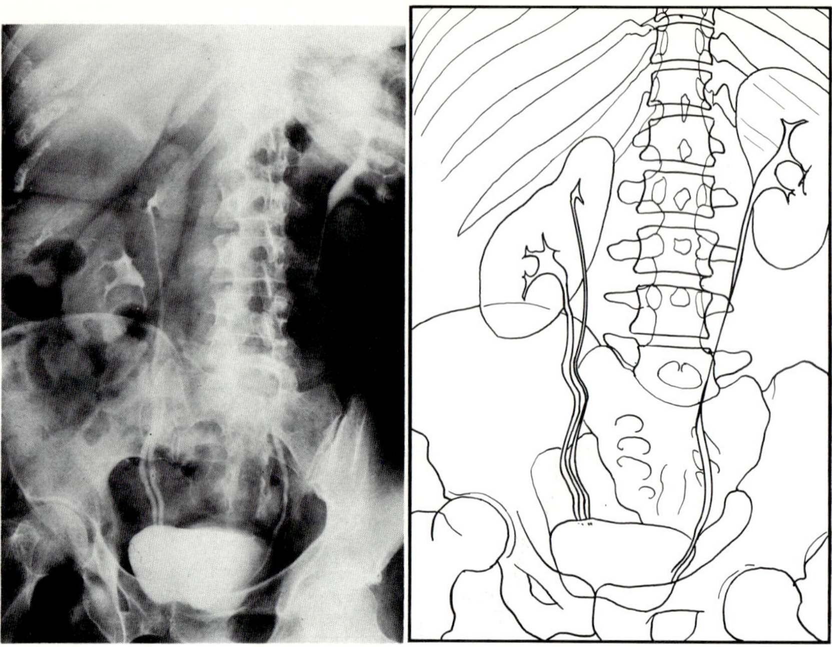

Fig. 5-4.   Intravenous pyelogram showing double collecting system and ureter on the right.

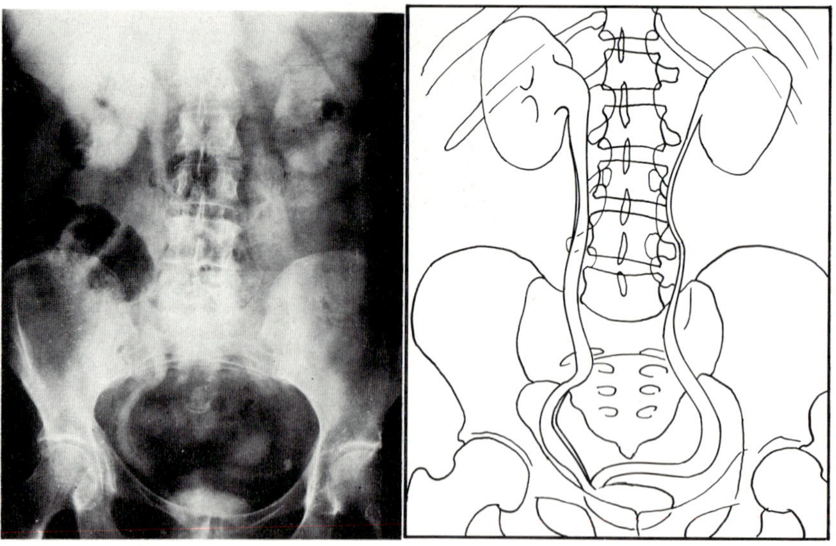

Fig. 5-5.   Intravenous pyelogram showing double collecting system on the right with single ureteral orifice. The ureters join in the wall of the bladder.

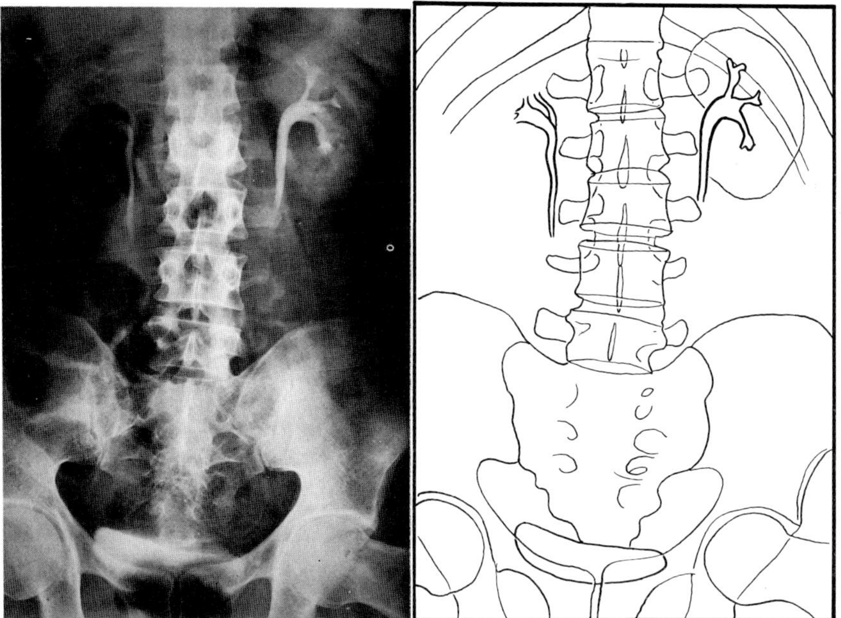

Fig. 5-6. Intravenous pyelogram showing normal collecting system on the left. There is a double collecting system on the right which clears less contrast medium; this indicates the presence of a vascular lesion.

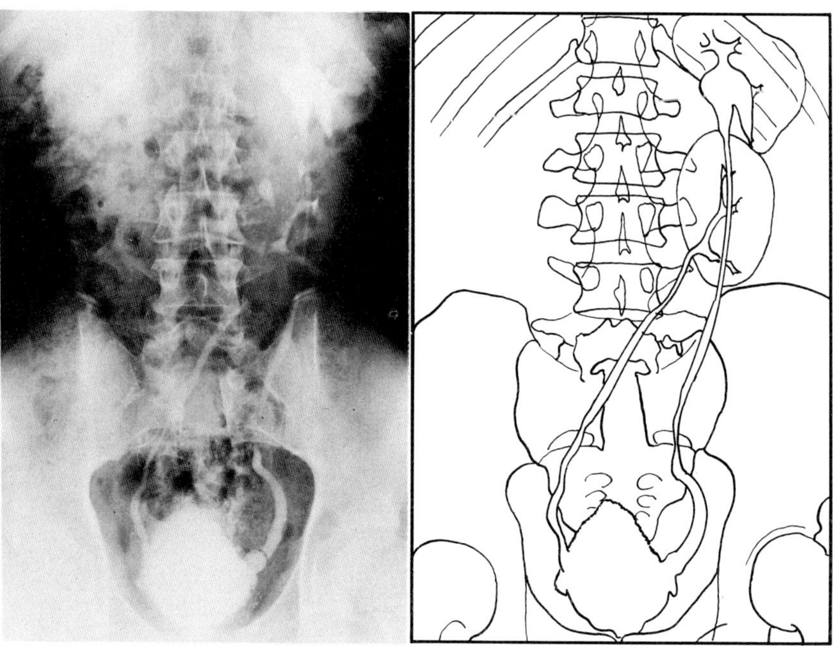

Fig. 5-7. Intravenous pyelogram showing crossed ectopia, neurogenic bladder, and spina bifida.

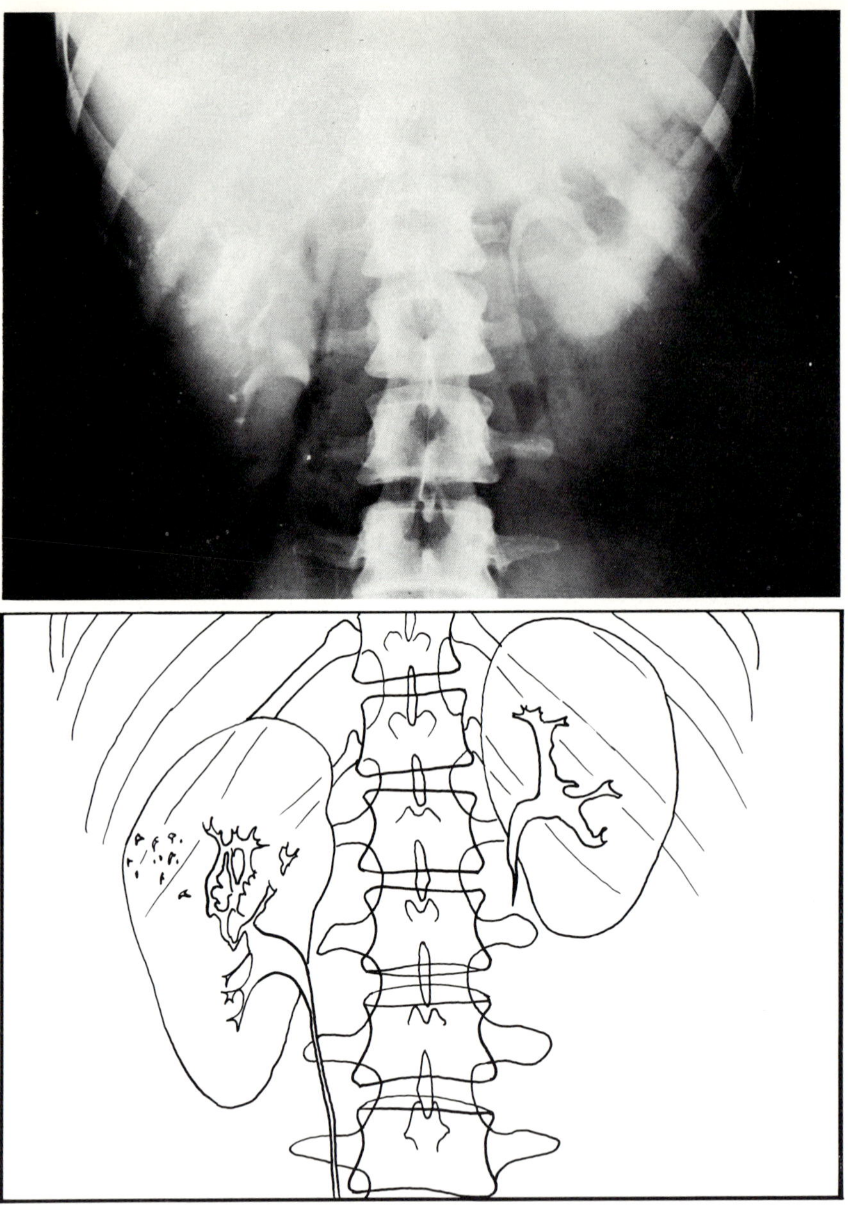

Fig. 5-8. Intravenous pyelogram of patient with medullary sponge kidney and cystic calcifications.

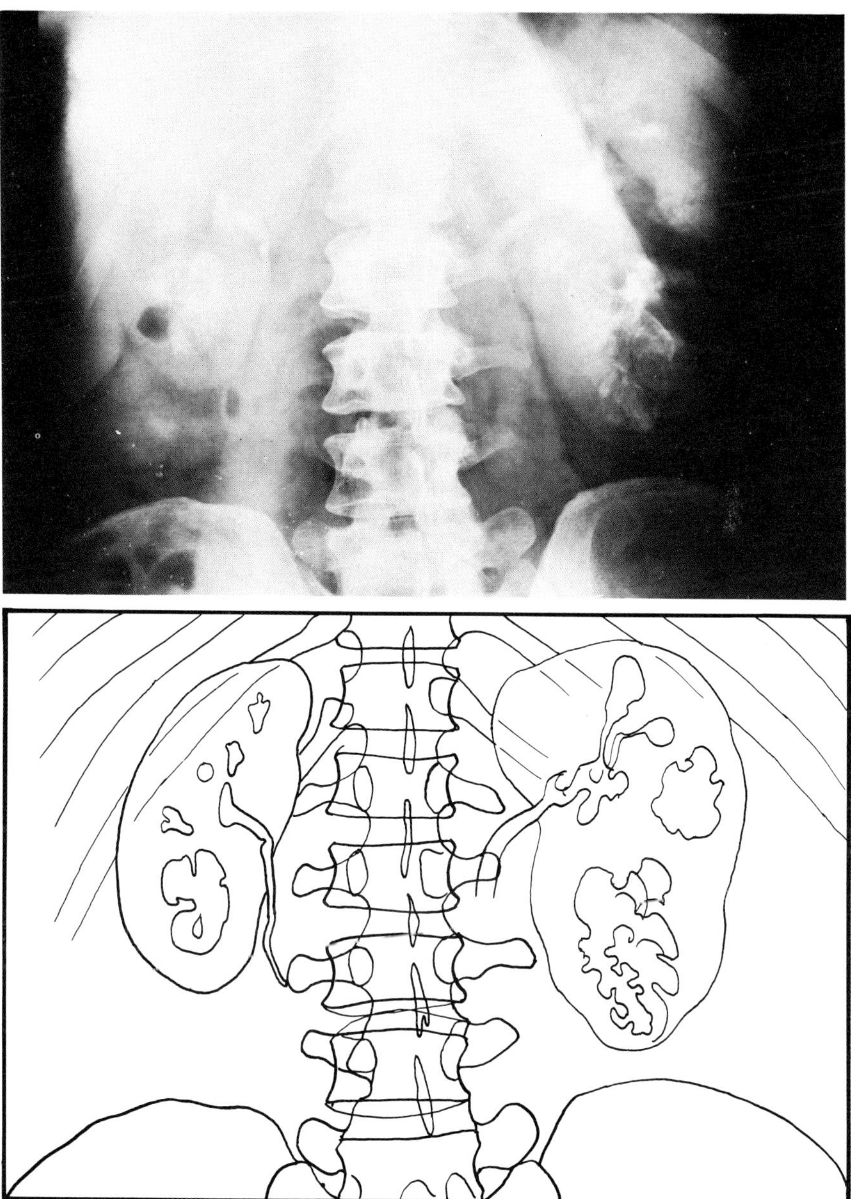

Fig. 5-9. Intravenous pyelogram of patient with severe medullary sponge kidney. Note the rapid filling of the cysts, particularly in the left kidney.

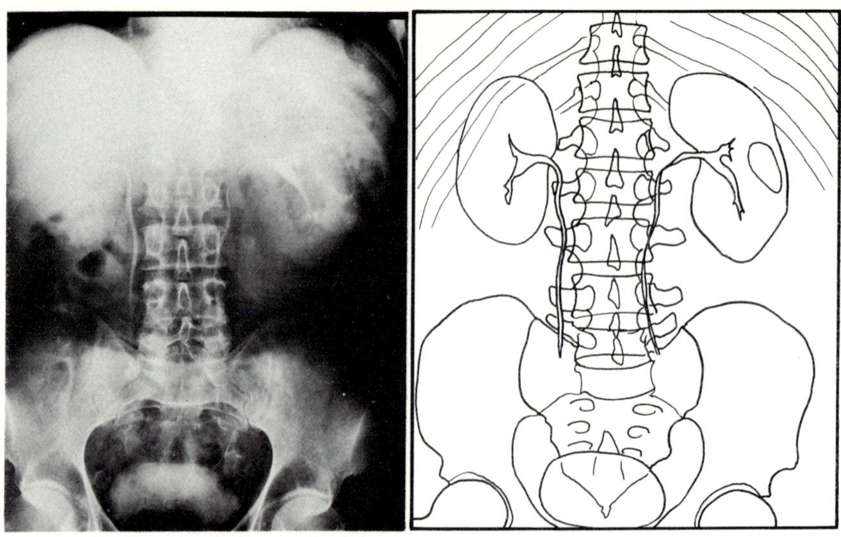

Fig. 5-10. Intravenous pyelogram showing benign renal cyst in the left kidney.

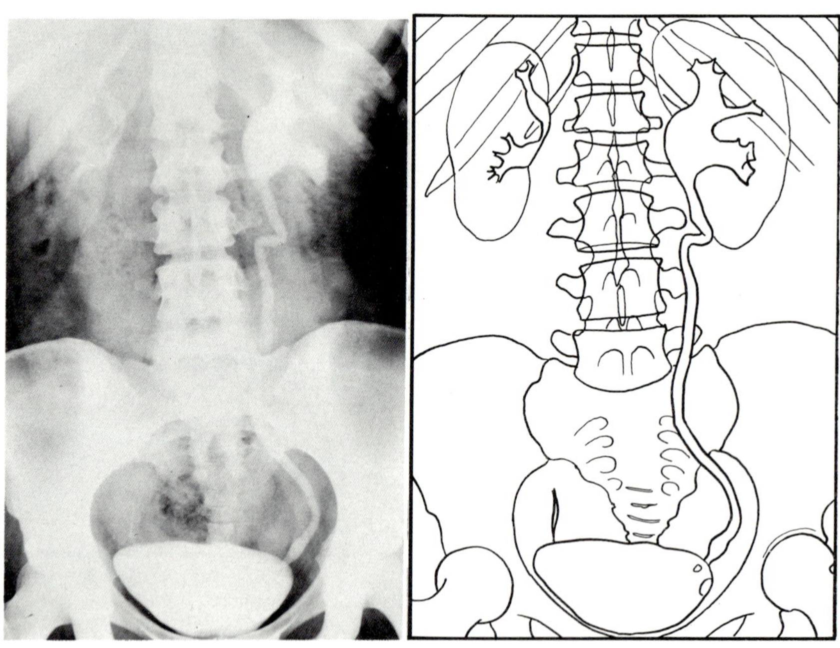

Fig. 5-11. Intravenous pyelogram revealing left vesicoureteral stone and resultant dilated ureters and pelvis. A phlebolith is also visible underlying the bladder shadow.

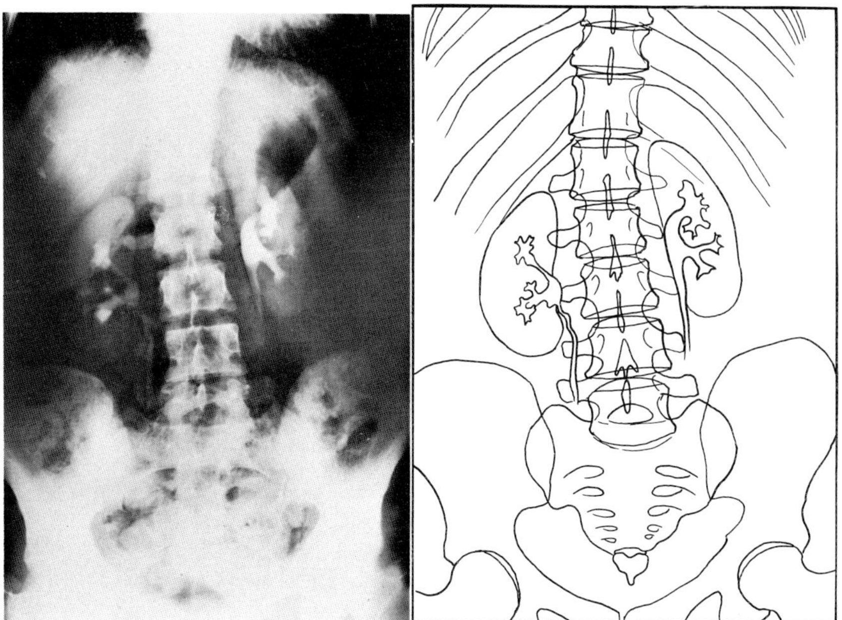

Fig. 5-12. Intravenous pyelogram showing clubbing of the calyces without shrinkage, which suggests pyelonephritis.

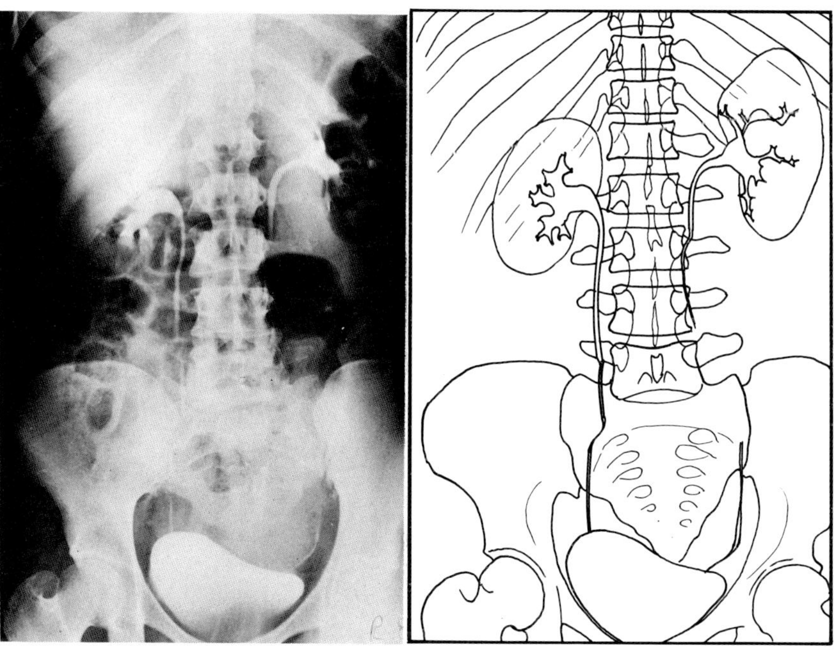

Fig. 5-13. Intravenous pyelogram in a patient with diabetes mellitus and greater than 10^5 bacteria (enterococci) per milliliter of urine. Papillary necrosis is present.

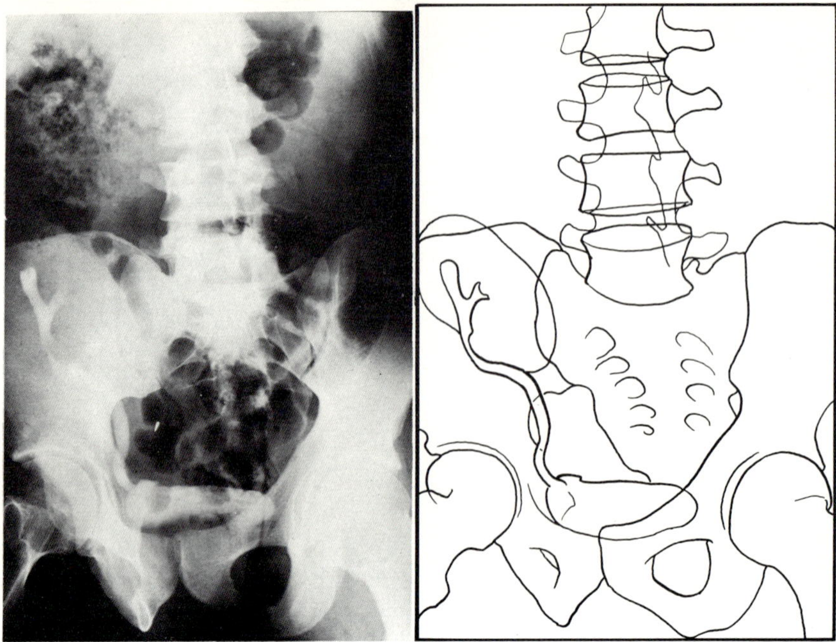

Fig. 5-14. Intravenous pyelogram showing transplanted kidney in the right iliac fossa.

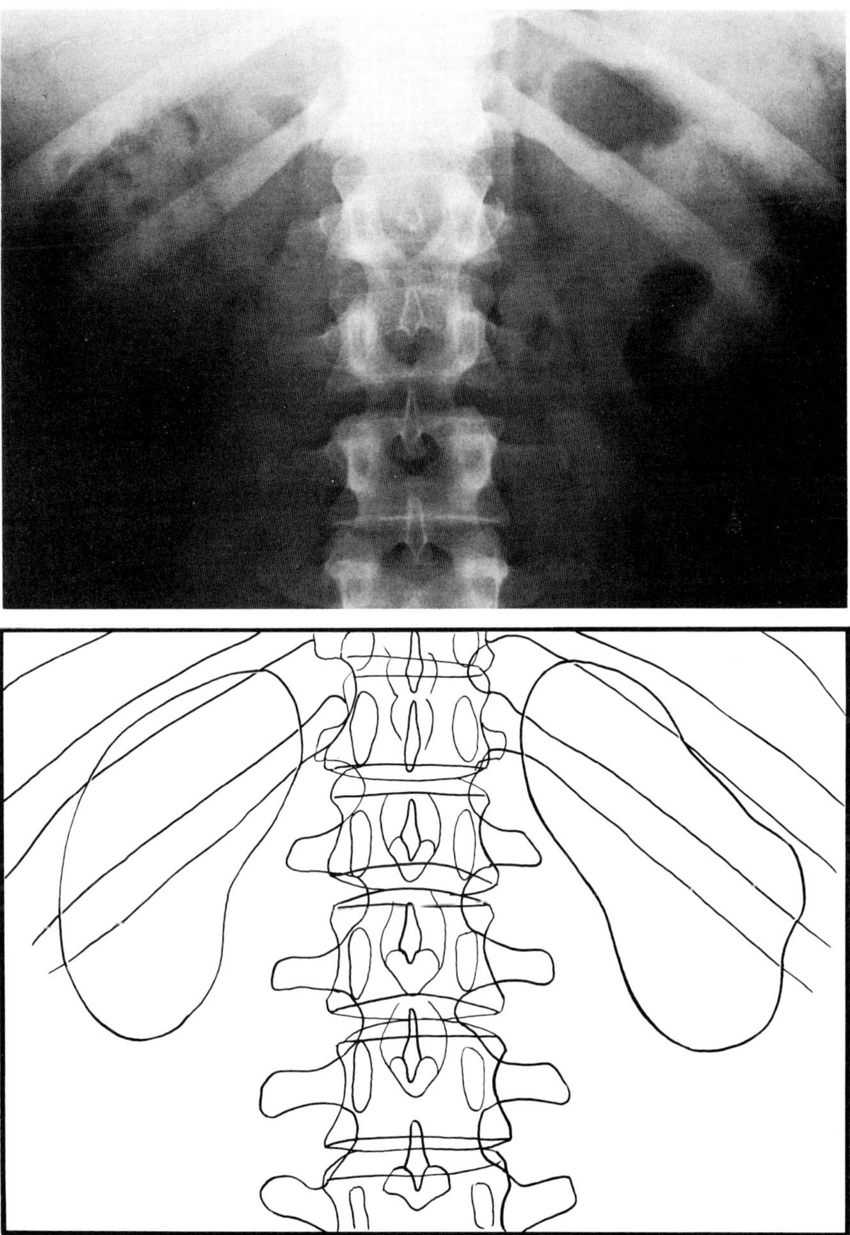

Fig. 5-15. Rapid sequence urography. **A.** Plain film showing kidneys of normal size without calculi.

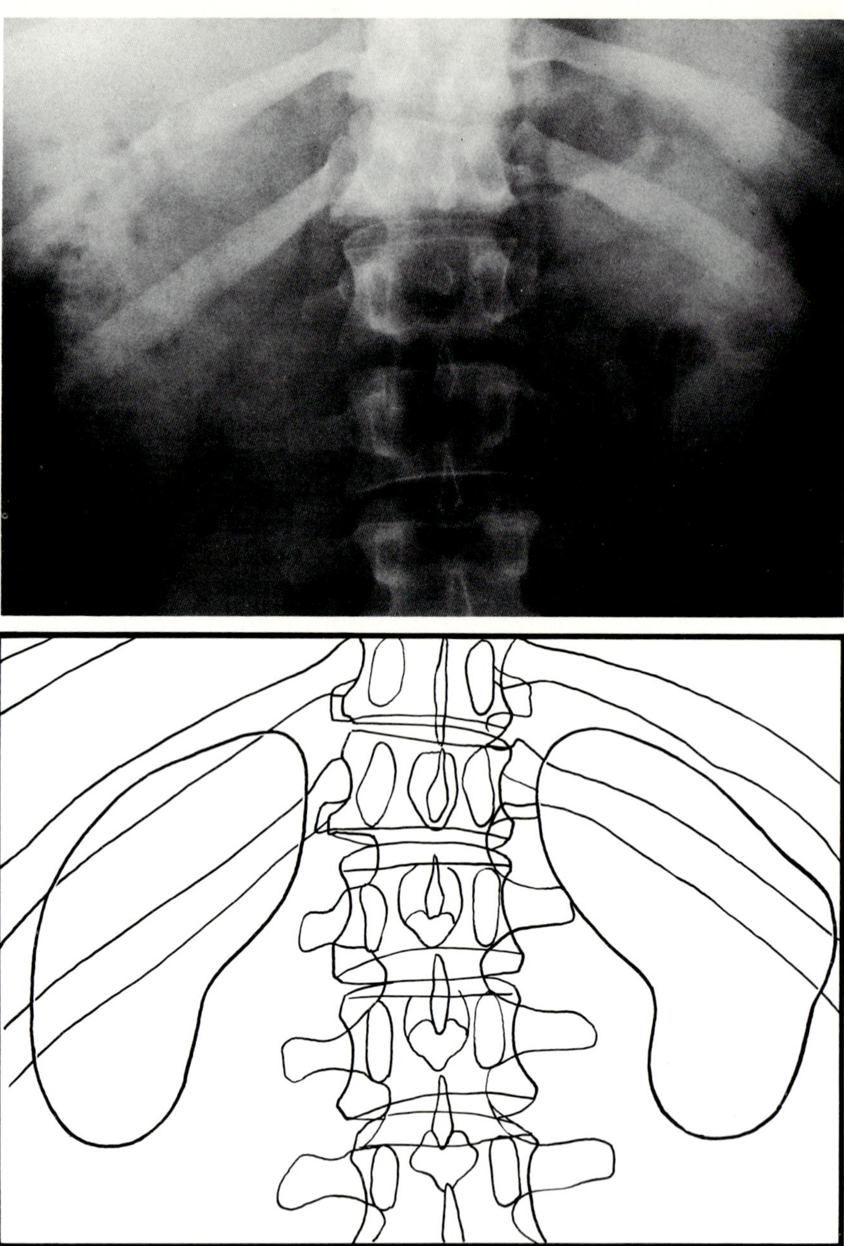

Fig. 5-15B. One minute after injection of radiopaque contrast medium. Normal nephrogram.

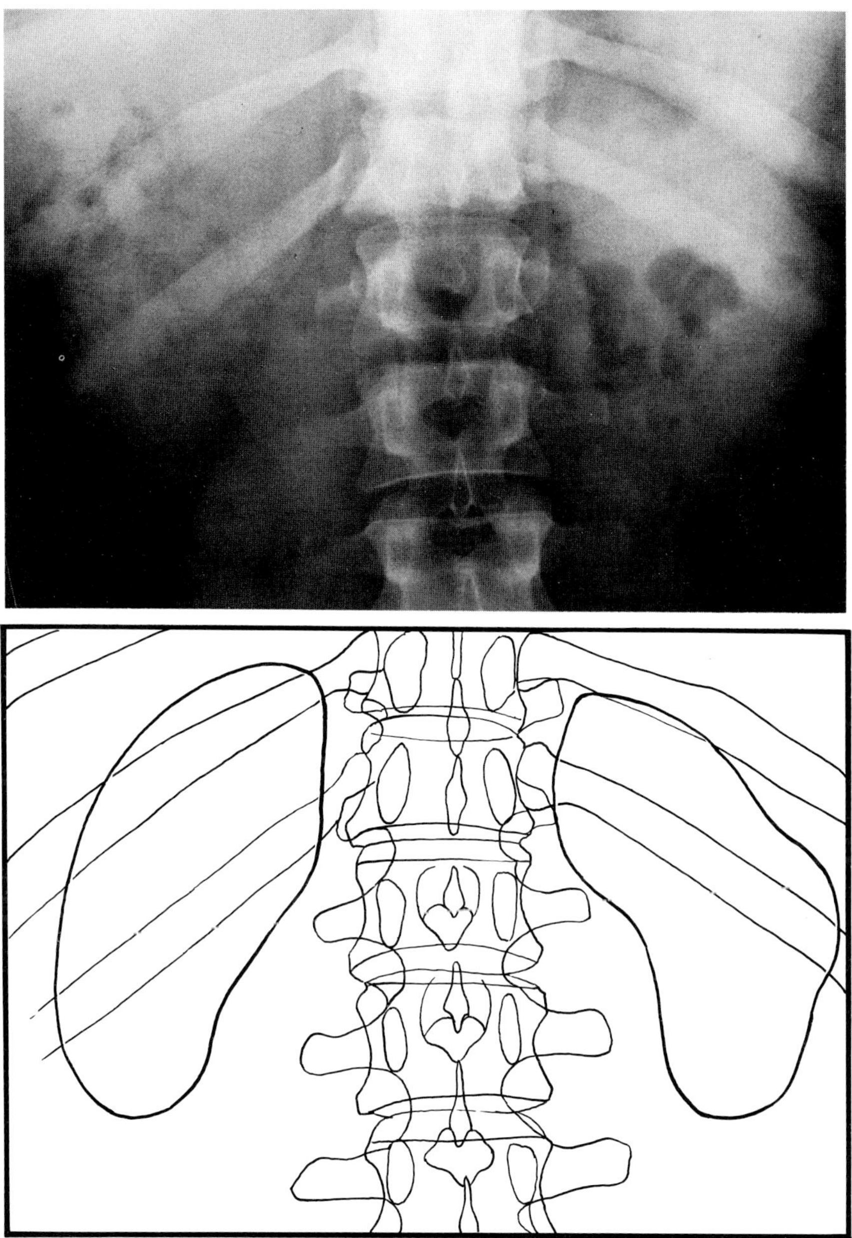

Fig. 5-15C. Three minutes after injection. Symmetric nephrogram with kidneys of equal size.

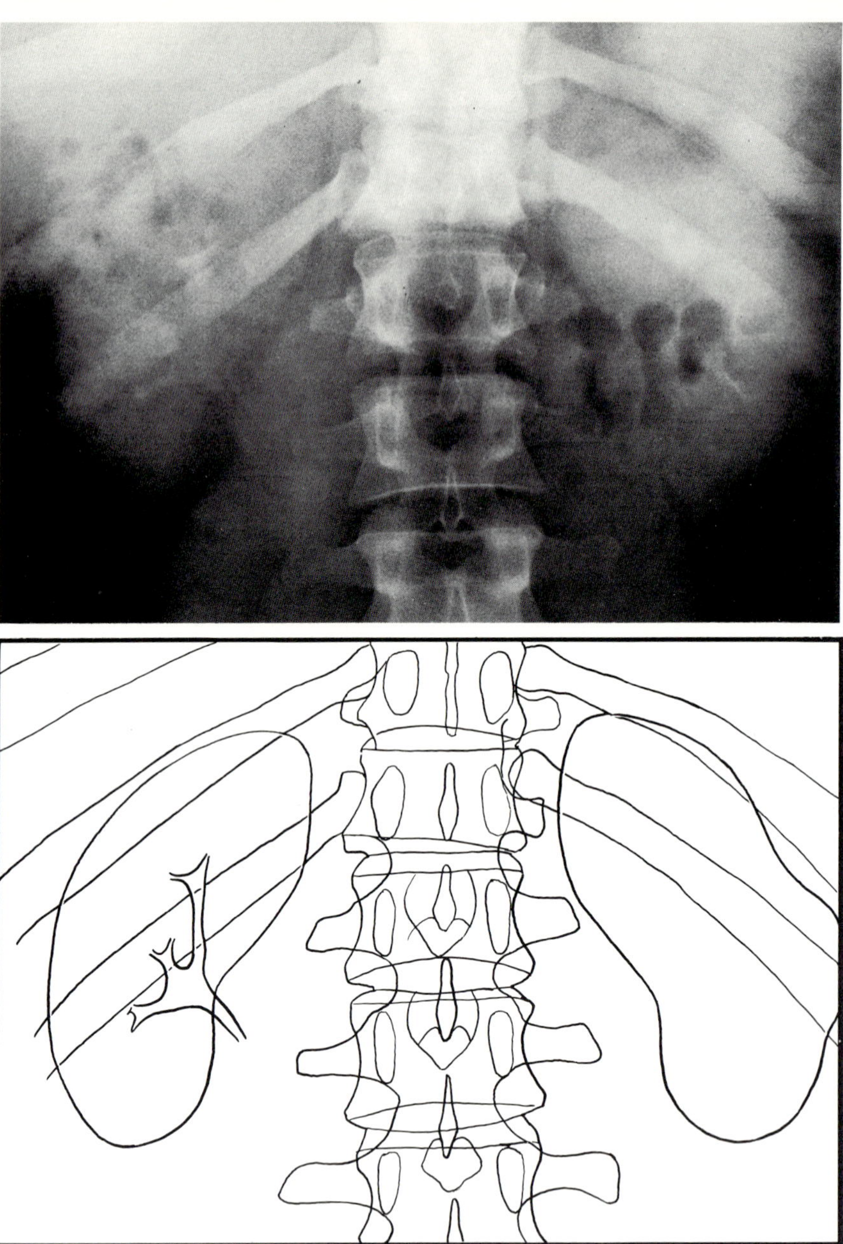

Fig. 5-15D.   Four minutes after injection. Contrast medium is seen in both kidneys.

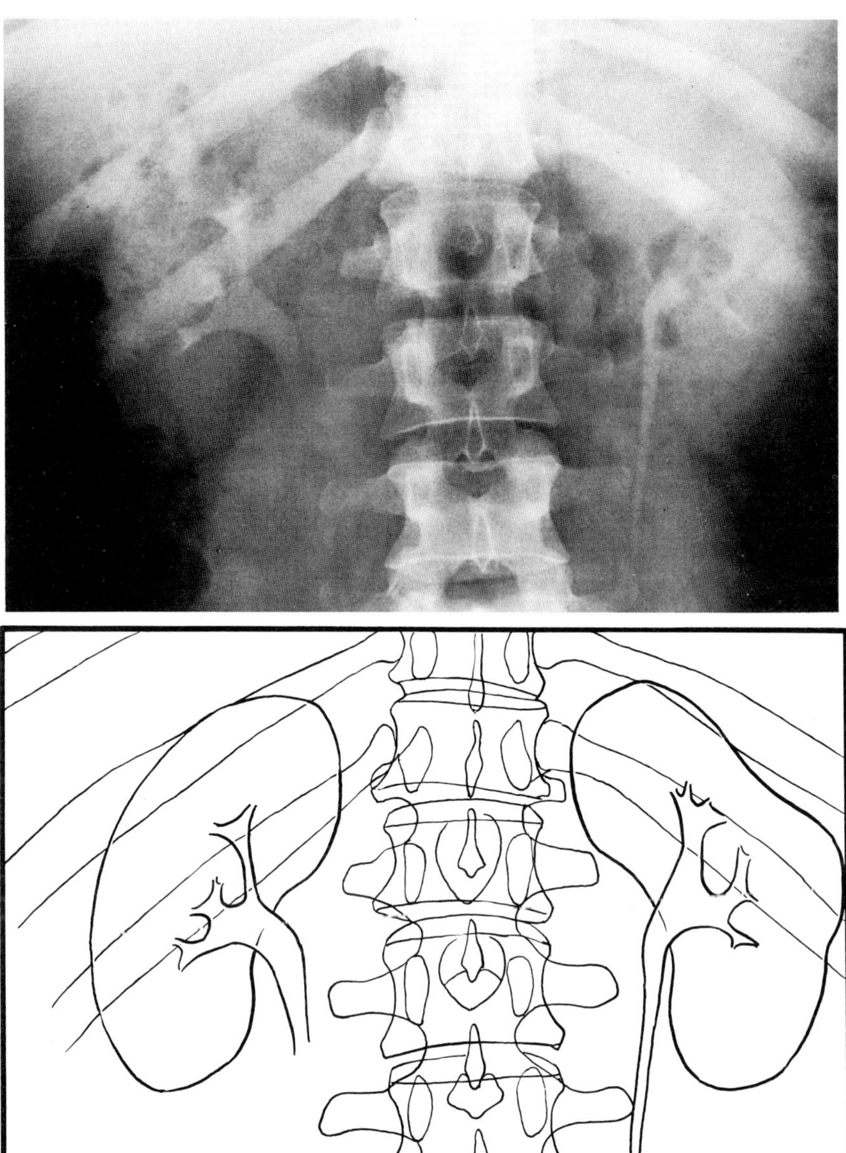

Fig. 5-15E.   Five minutes after injection. Symmetric calyceal system; i.e., each kidney is clearing the same amount of contrast medium.

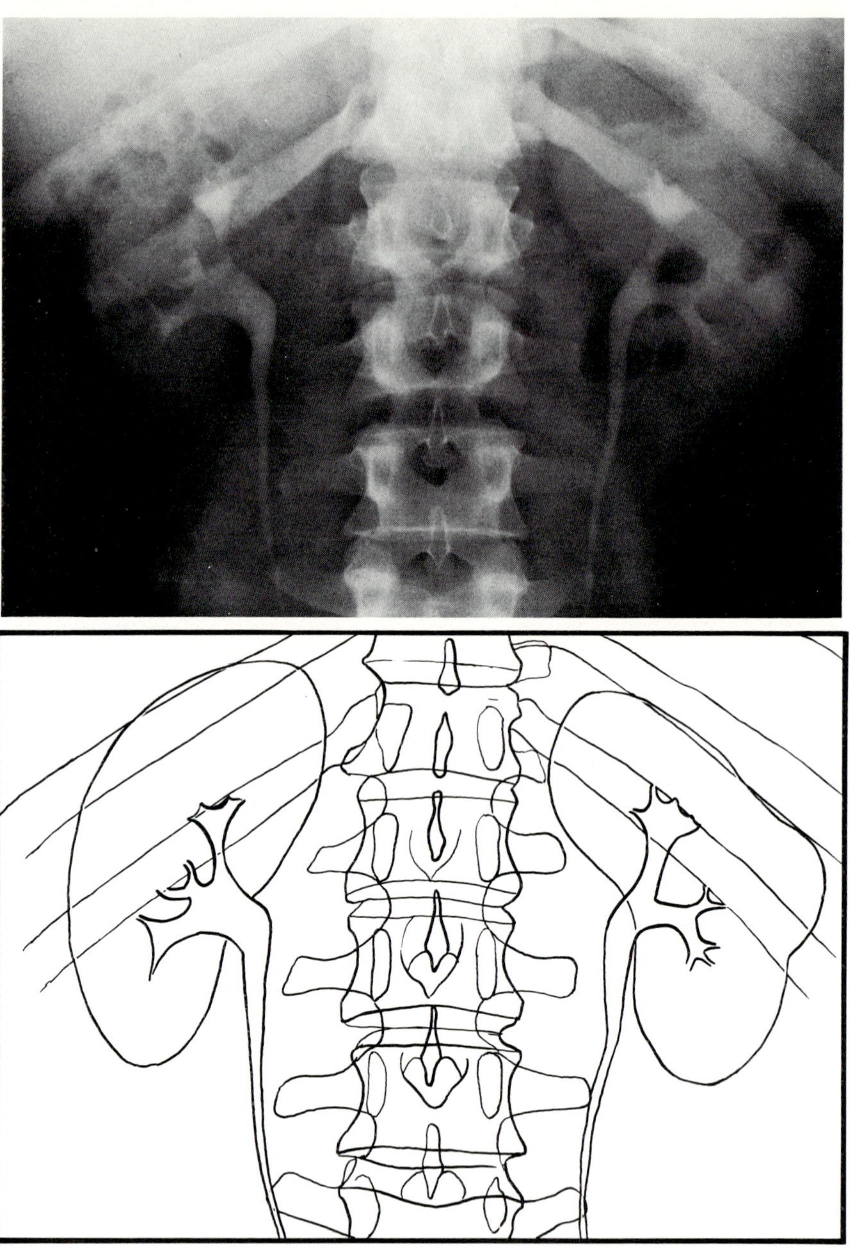

Fig. 5-15F.   Ten minutes after injection. Collecting systems are normal.

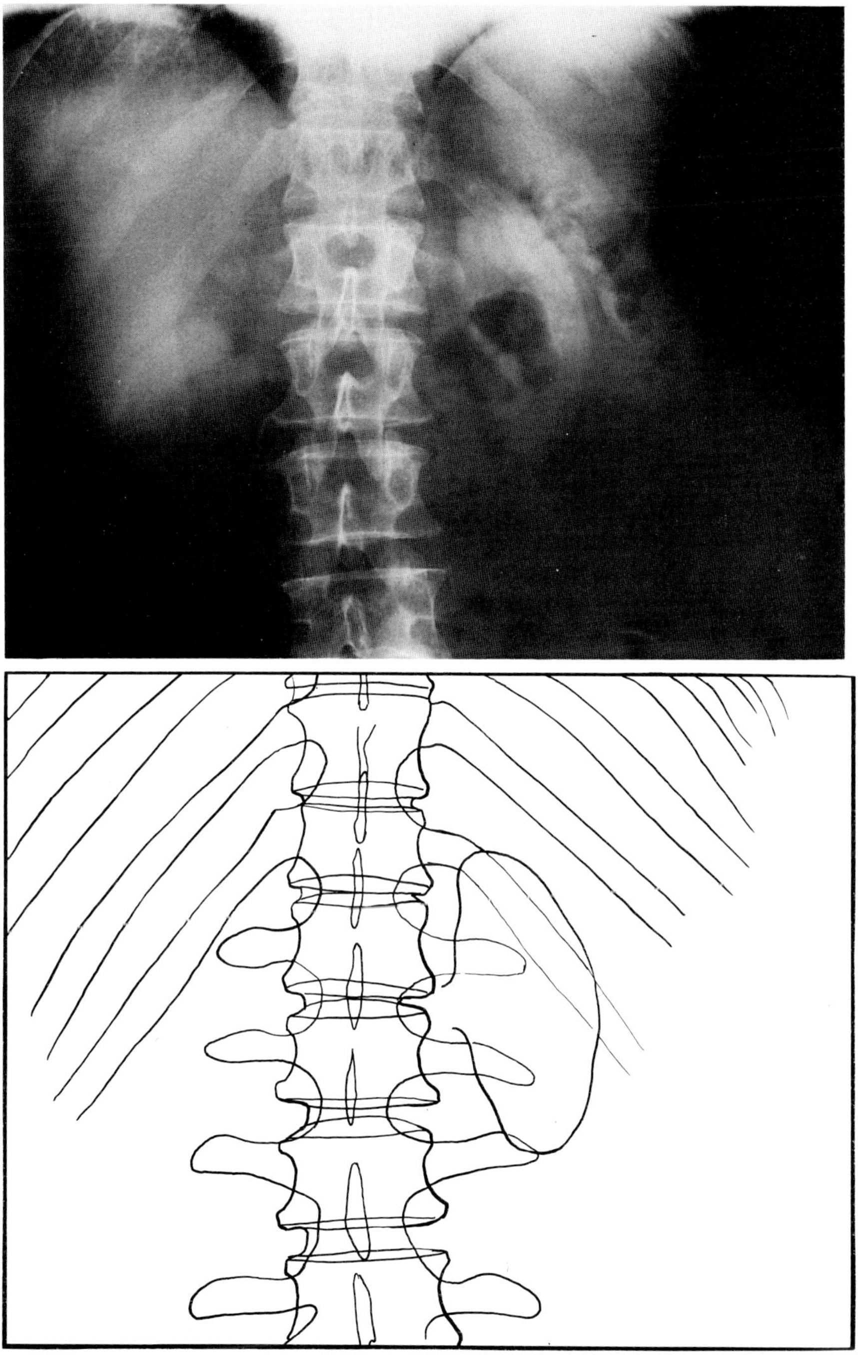

Fig. 5-16. Rapid sequence urography one minute after injection of contrast medium. Delayed nephrogram on right side indicates arterial vascular disease.

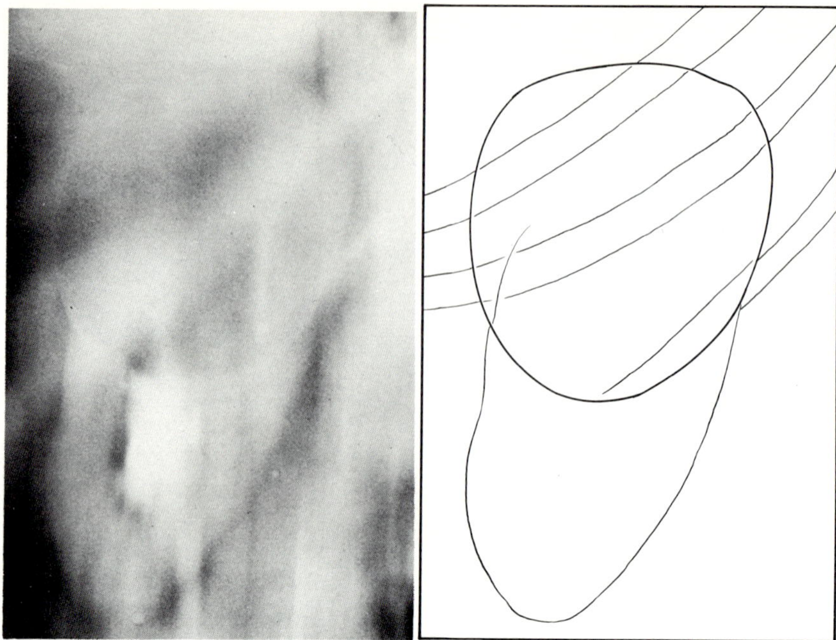

Fig. 5-17. Nephrotomogram. A large mass, sharply outlined and lucent at the center, occupies the upper pole of the right kidney. The wall of the mass is paper thin, indicating a benign cyst.

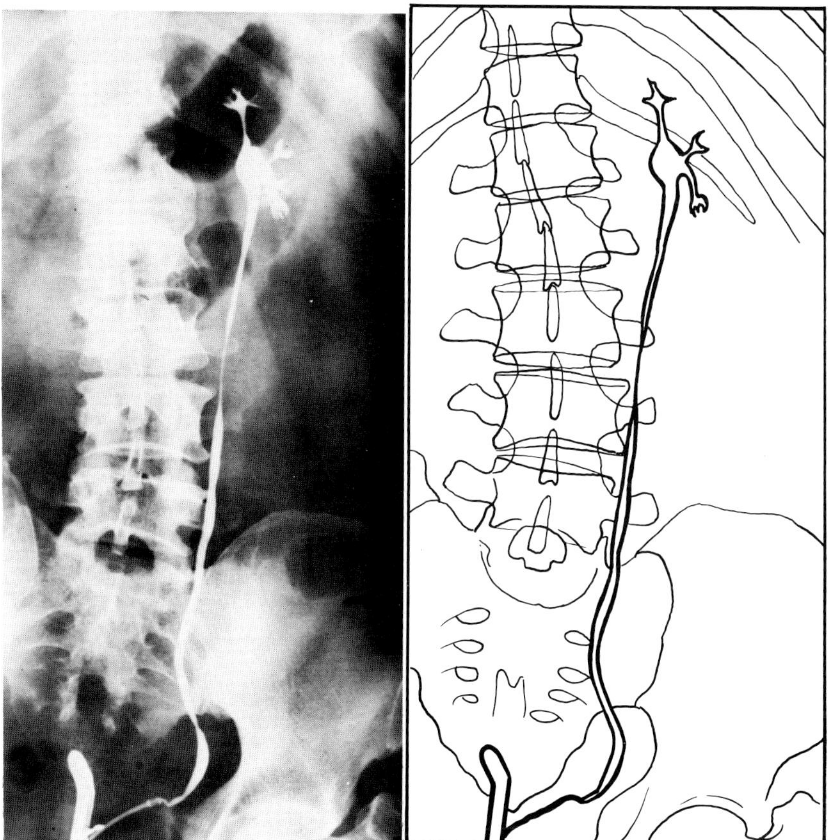

Fig. 5-18. Normal retrograde pyelogram. A cannula is introduced through the urethra and into the distal portion of the left ureter. The contrast material is injected with moderate pressure and outlines the entire collecting system. The renal outline is not seen here.

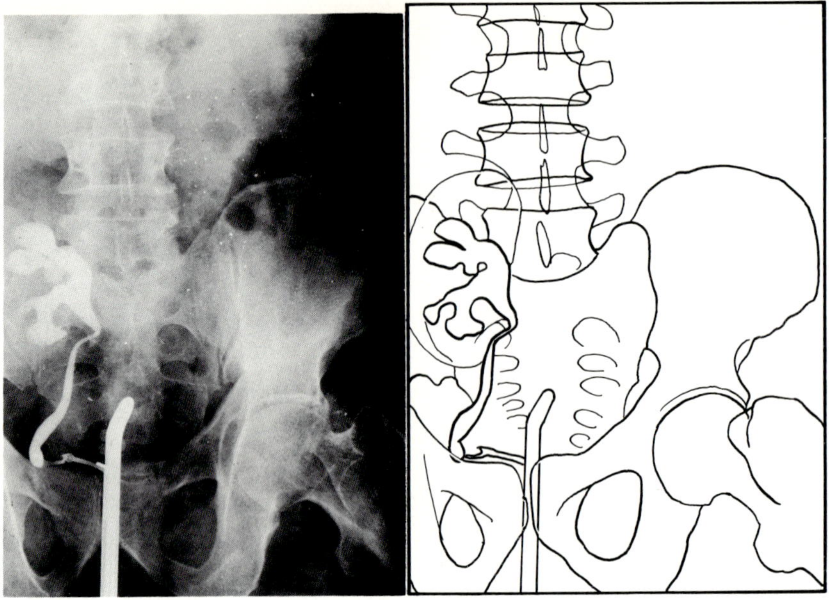

Fig. 5-19.   Retrograde pyelogram showing a right pelvic kidney with vesico-ureteral reflux.

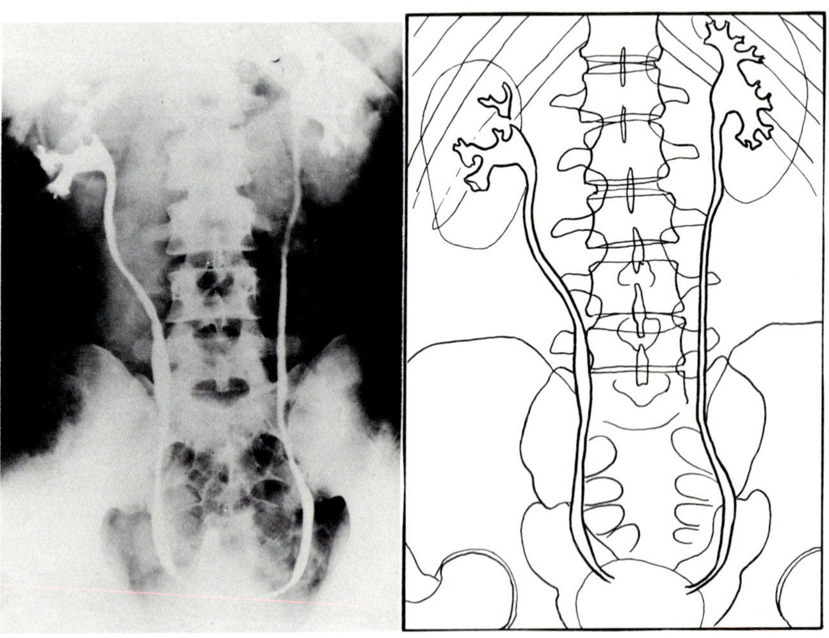

Fig. 5-20.   Retrograde pyelogram showing tuberculosis in right kidney.

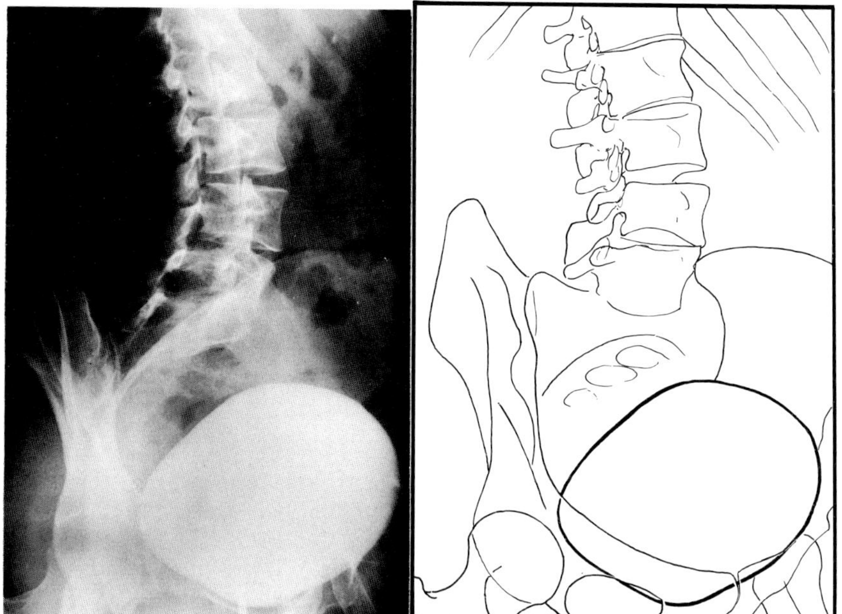

Fig. 5-21. Normal cystogram in a 24-year-old female.

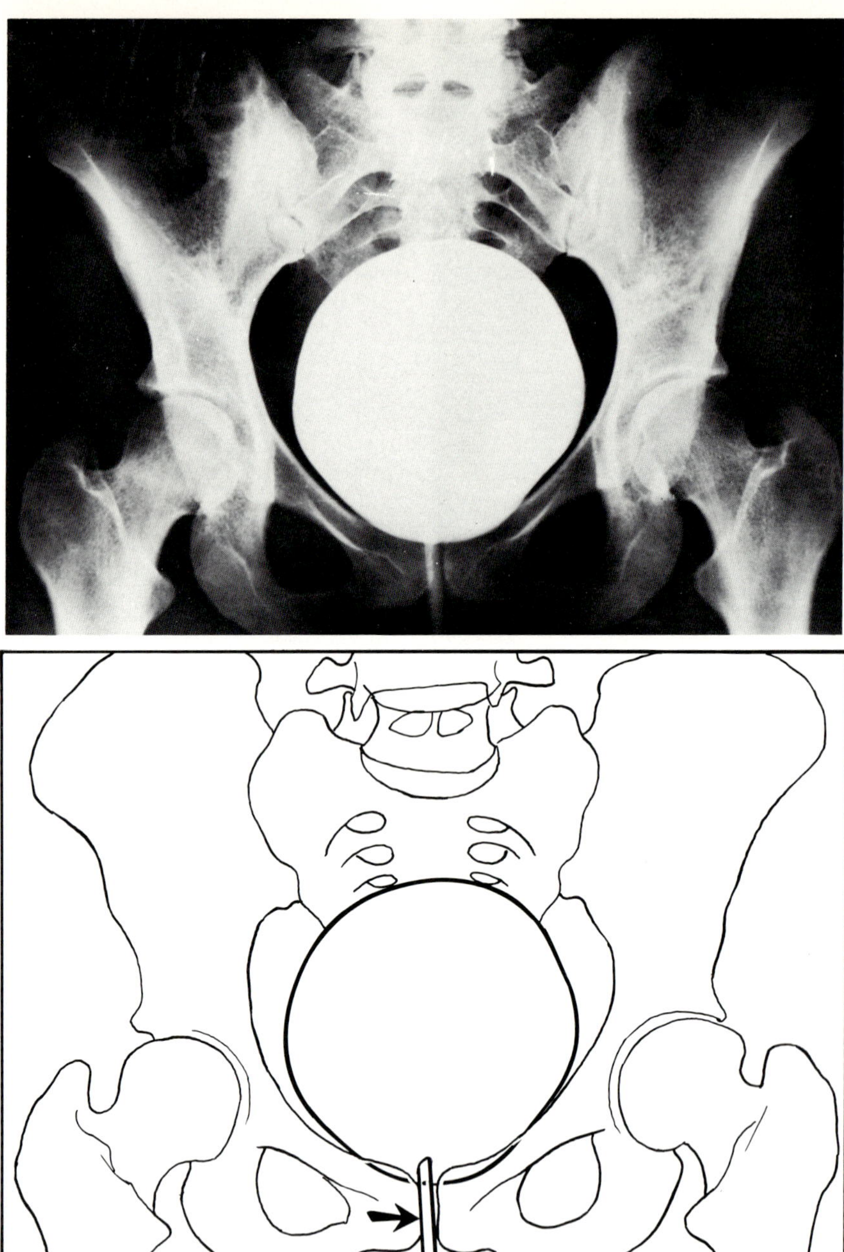

Fig. 5-22. Cystogram. Contrast material has been introduced in retrograde fashion through a catheter (*arrow*). Bladder outline is normal.

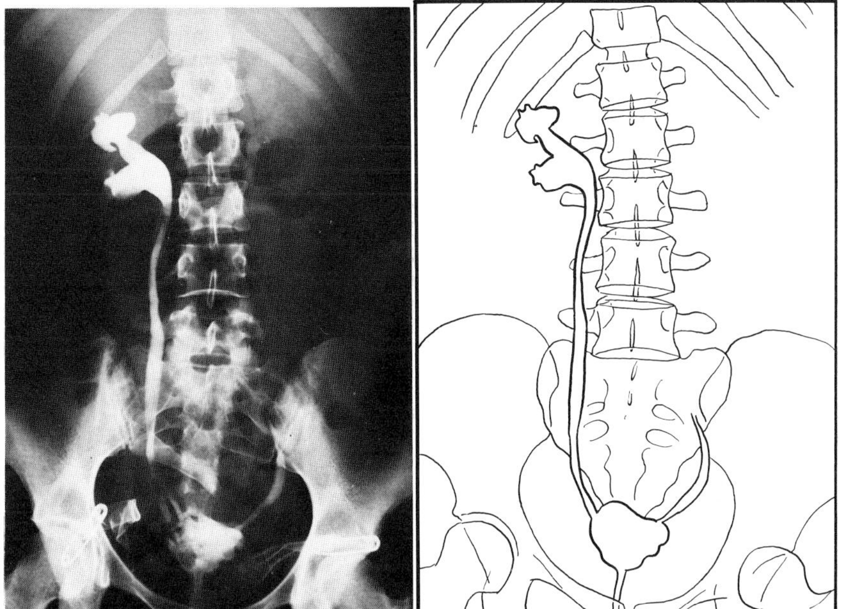

Fig. 5-23. Cystogram showing bilateral vesicoureteral reflux which is more marked on the right.

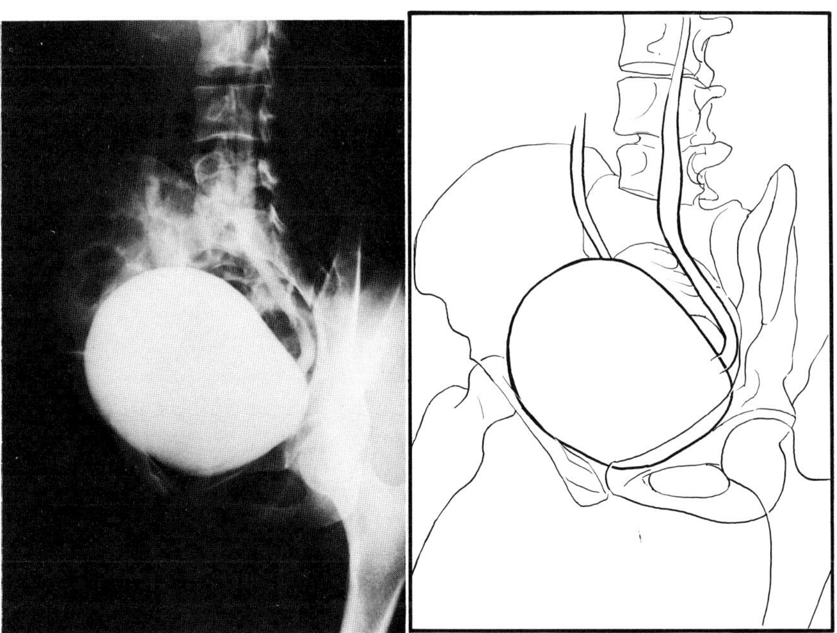

Fig. 5-24. Cystogram showing bilateral ureteral reflux in a 5-year-old female.

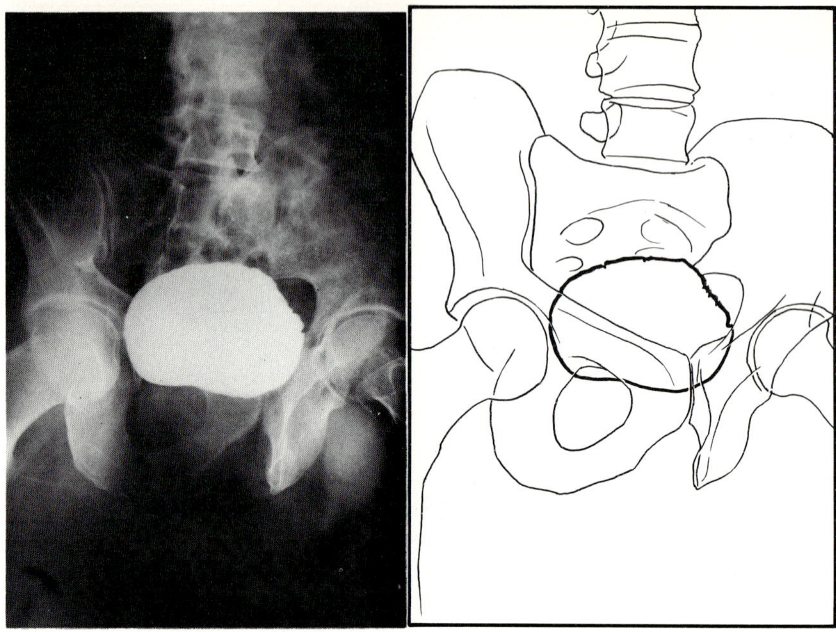

Fig. 5-25. Cystogram showing trabeculation of bladder dome.

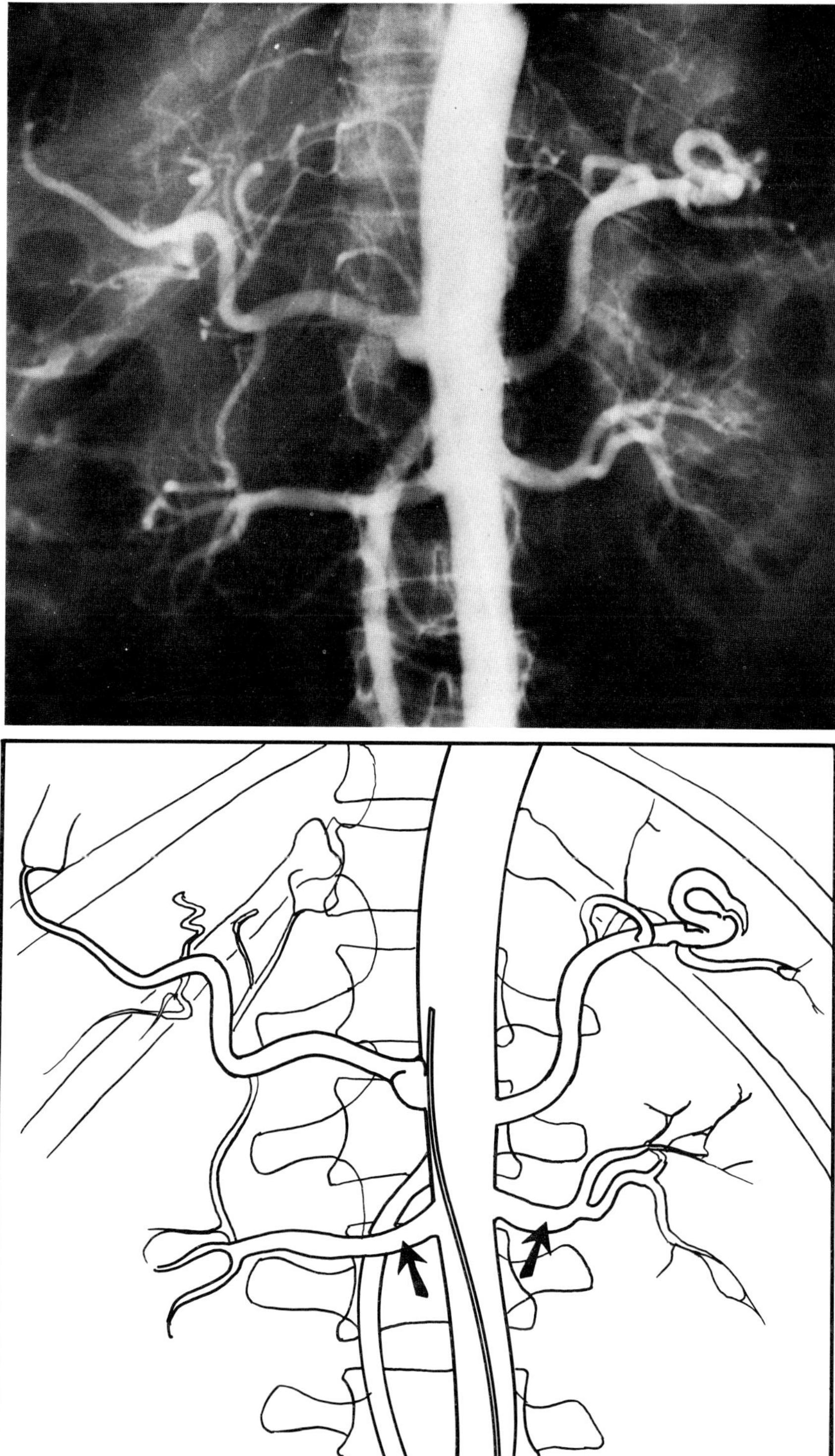

Fig. 5-26. Normal aortogram. The catheter was introduced from the femoral artery and placed above the origin of the celiac axis. The origin of the major vessels arising from the aorta shows up clearly. Both renal arteries are normal (*arrows*).

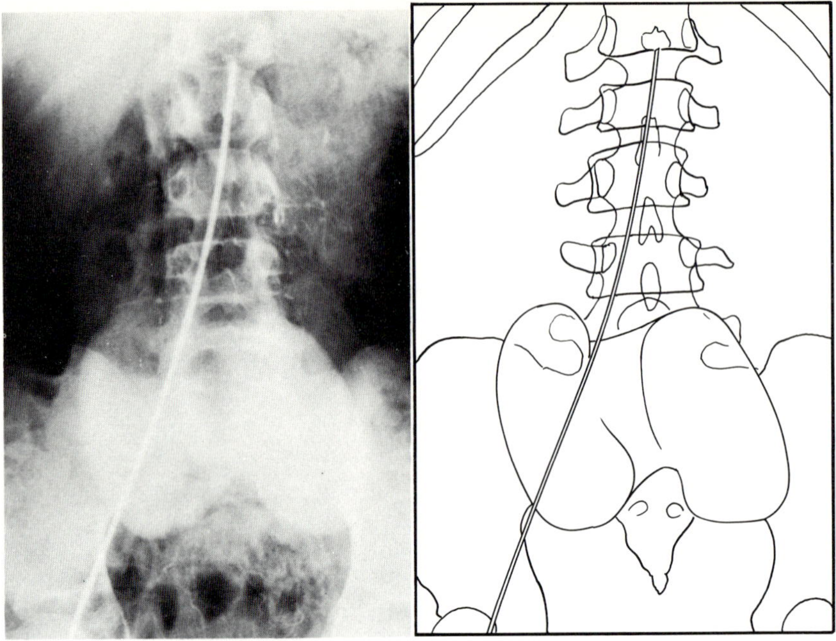

Fig. 5-27. Aortogram revealing a fused pelvic kidney.

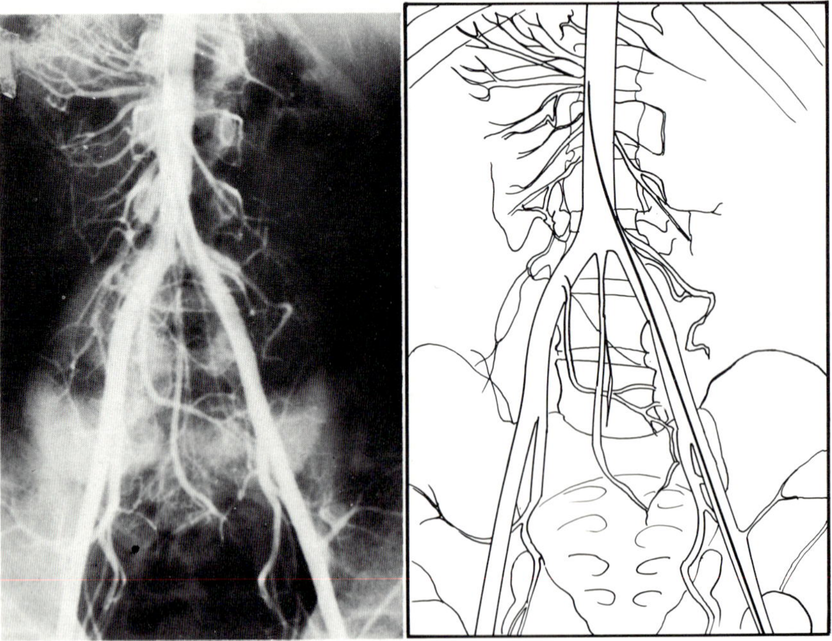

Fig. 5-28. Normal arteriogram. The catheter was introduced through the left femoral artery and extends up the aorta to level just below the kidneys.

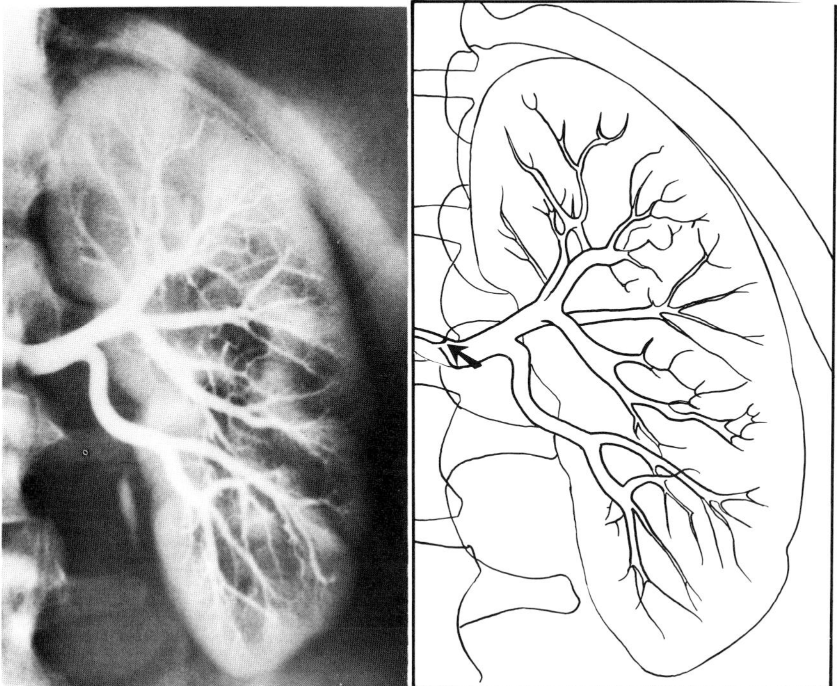

Fig. 5-29. Arterial phase of a normal selective left renal arteriogram. The tip of the catheter has been introduced well inside the renal artery (*arrow*).

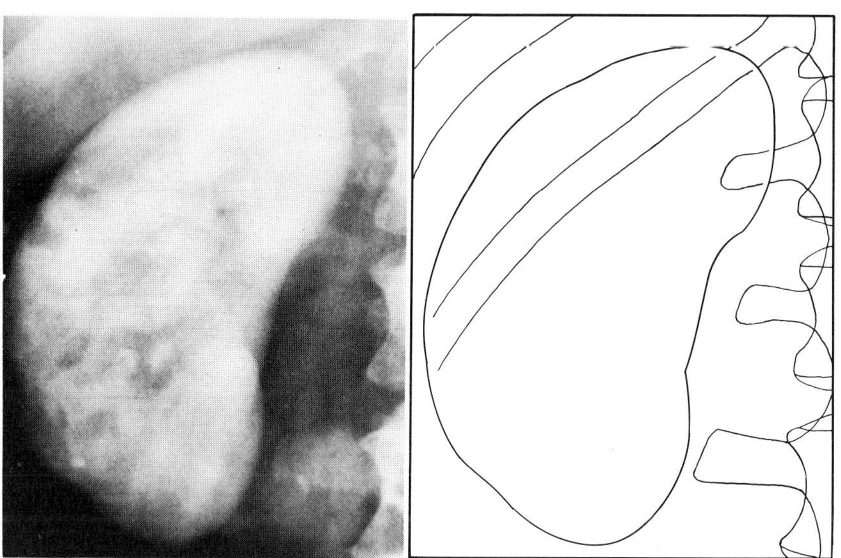

Fig. 5-30. Nephrogram effect obtained during a selective right renal arteriogram. This kidney is normal and demonstrates normal cortical thickness with no defects.

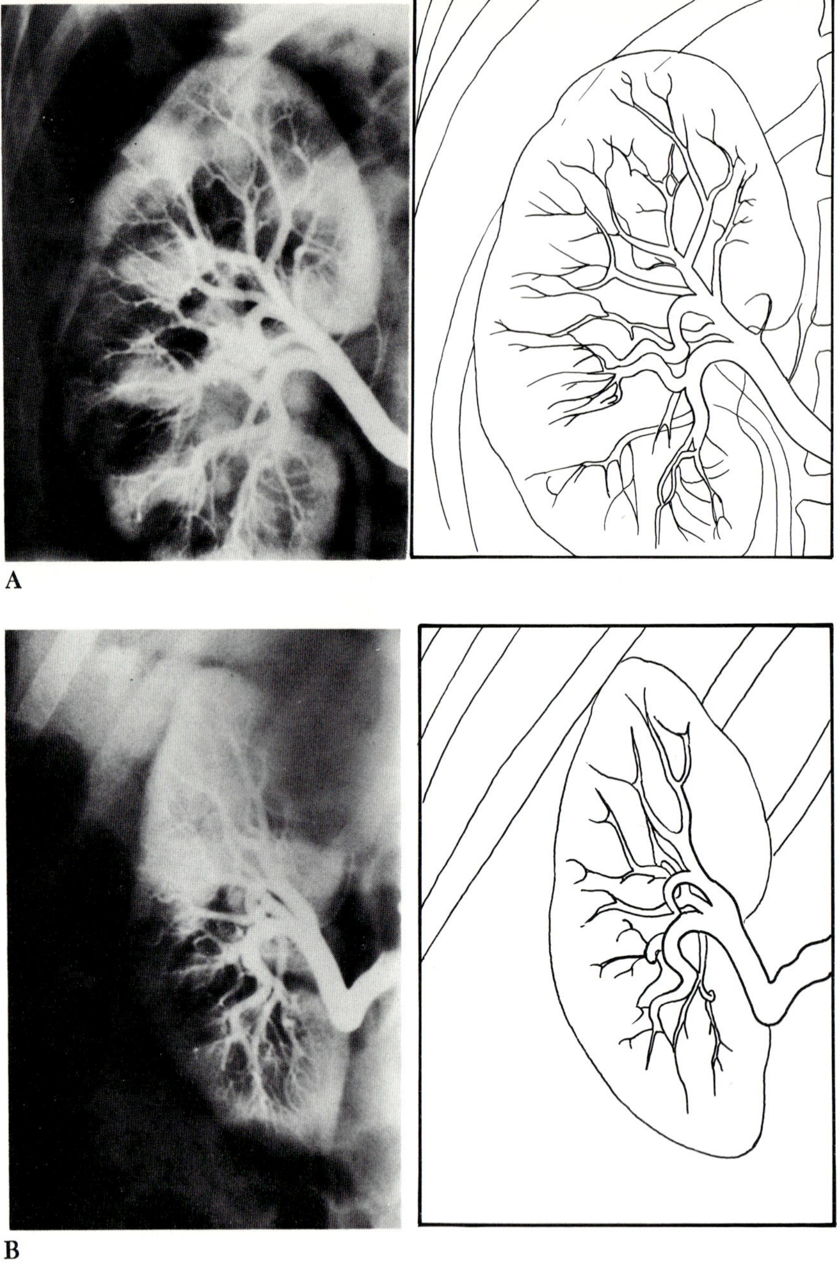

A

B

Fig. 5-31. Selective renal arteriogram of the right kidney. **A.** The arterial phase is normal.

Fig. 5-31B. Oblique projection reveals a mass occupying the posterior aspect of the upper pole. The arteriogram shows that no "tumor" vessels are present.

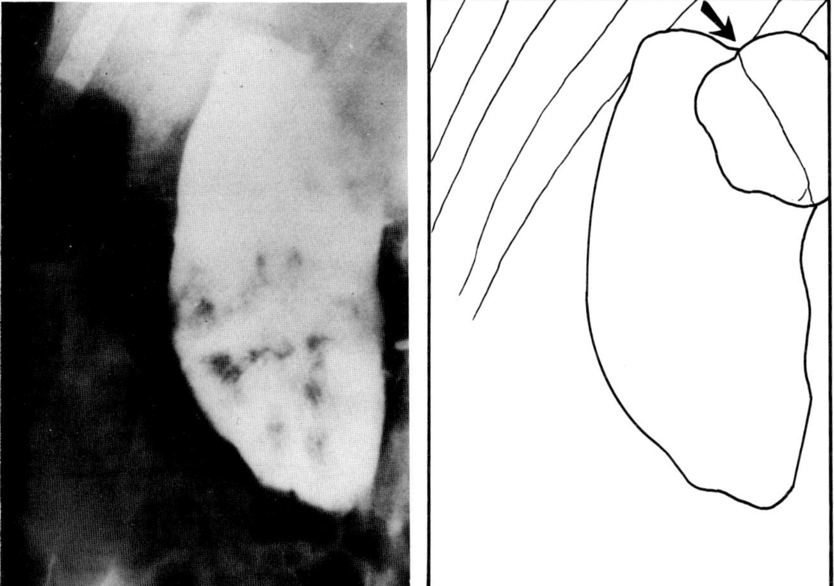

Fig. 5-31C. Nephrogram phase reveals the presence of "lips" (*arrow*) usually associated with a benign cyst. The lip represents the junction of the normal kidney and the cyst wall.

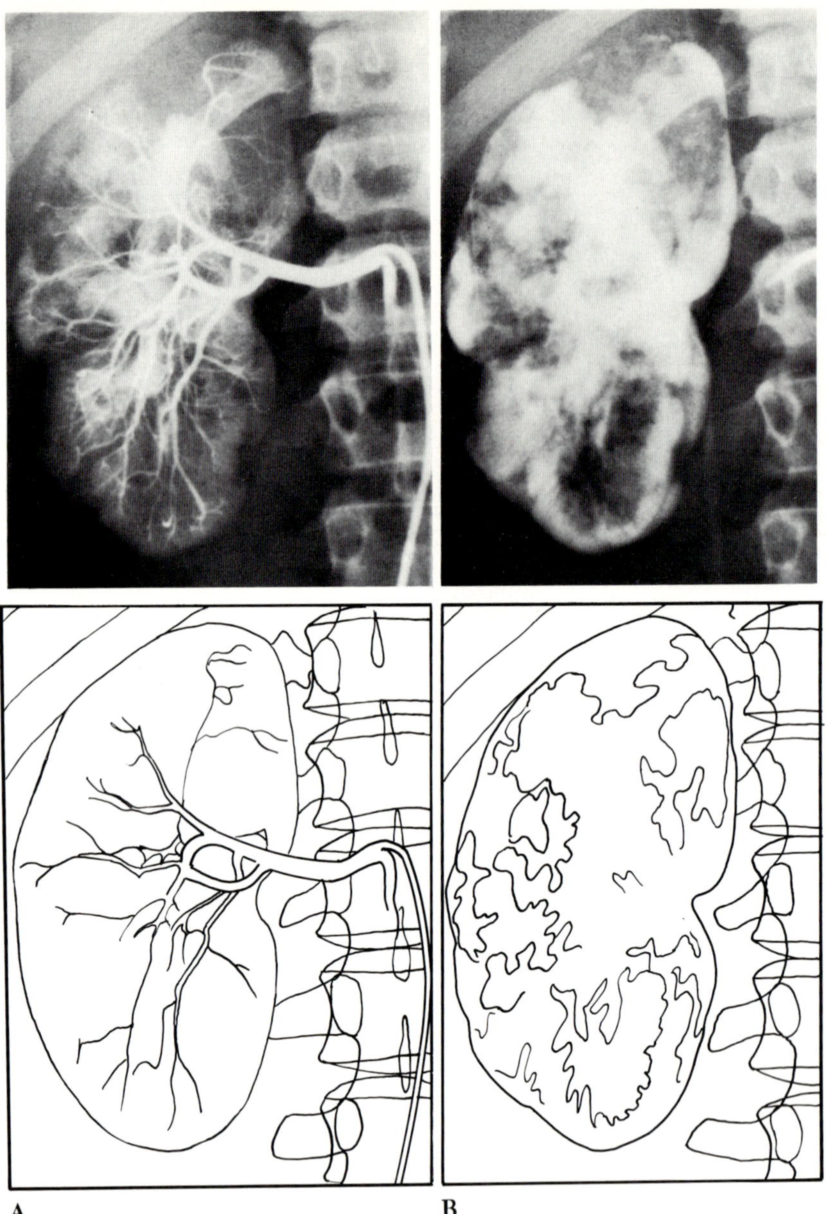

A   B

Fig. 5-32. Selective right renal arteriogram. **A.** Arterial phase reveals very slender arteries, indicating poor perfusion of a kidney which in addition demonstrates many filling defects.

Fig. 5-32B. Nephrogram effect reveals the presence of multiple cysts. This patient has polycystic kidney disease.

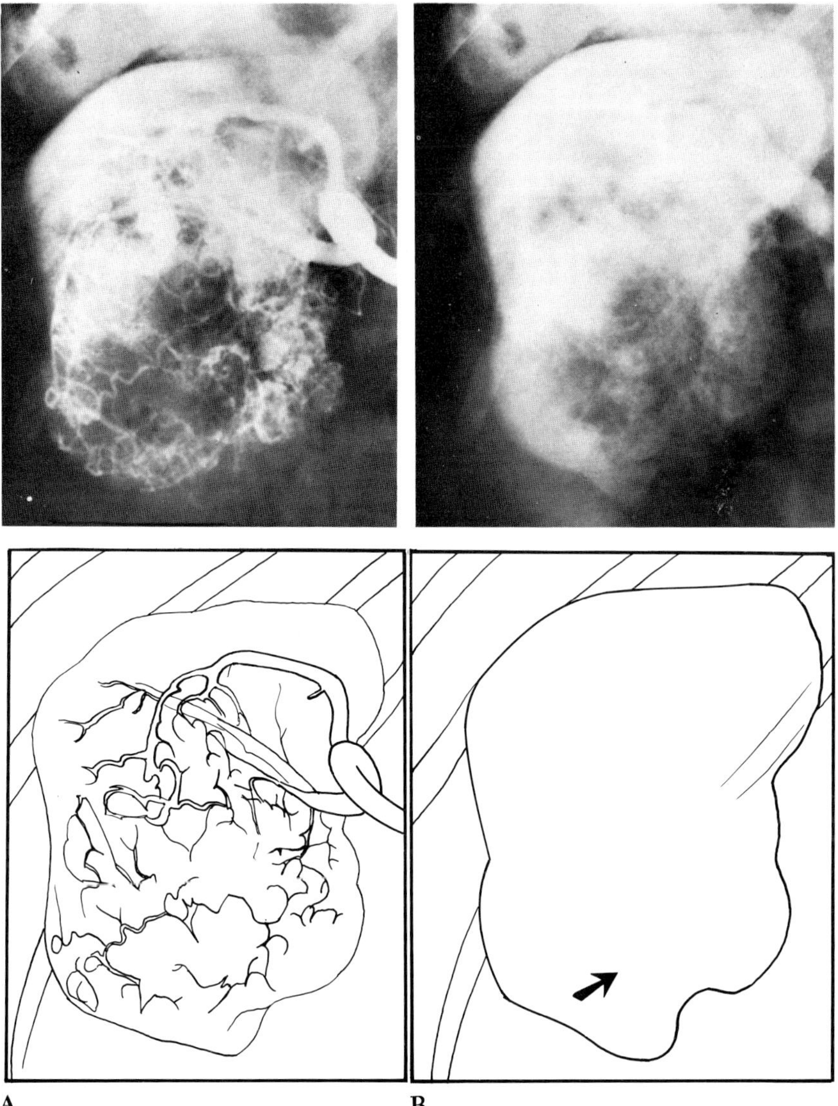

A   B

Fig. 5-33. Selective renal arteriogram. **A.** Arterial phase demonstrates a large tumor occupying the lower pole of the right kidney. The vessels are disarranged and are typical "tumor" vessels.

Fig. 5-33B. Nephrogram phase reveals a lucency within the tumor, indicating necrosis. The main renal vein arising from this kidney (*arrow*) seems to be uninvolved.

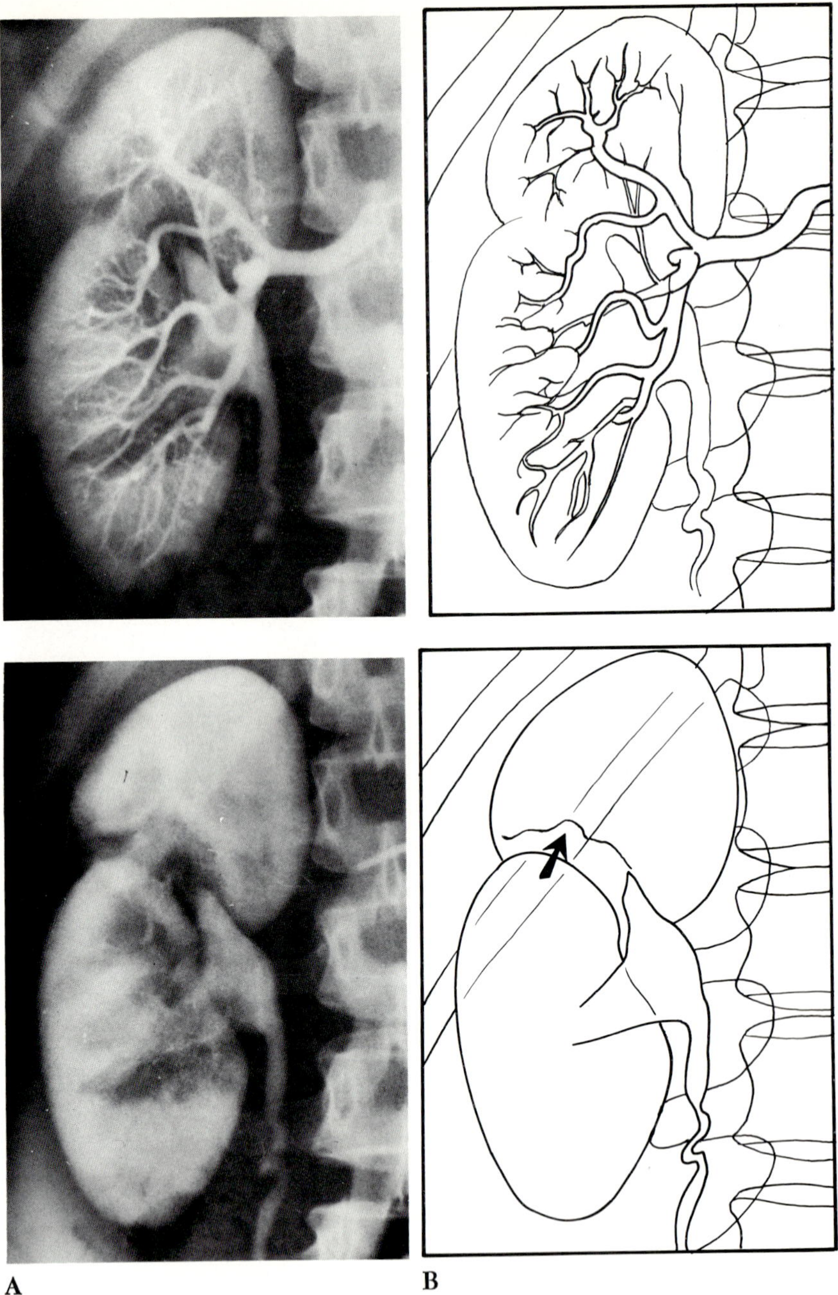

Fig. 5-34. Selective right renal arteriogram. A. Arterial phase reveals a disruption of the continuity of the kidney. There is no extravasation of contrast, and the vessels appear to be normal.

Fig. 5-34B. Nephrogram effect reveals a fracture through the kidney partially separating the upper pole (*arrow*).

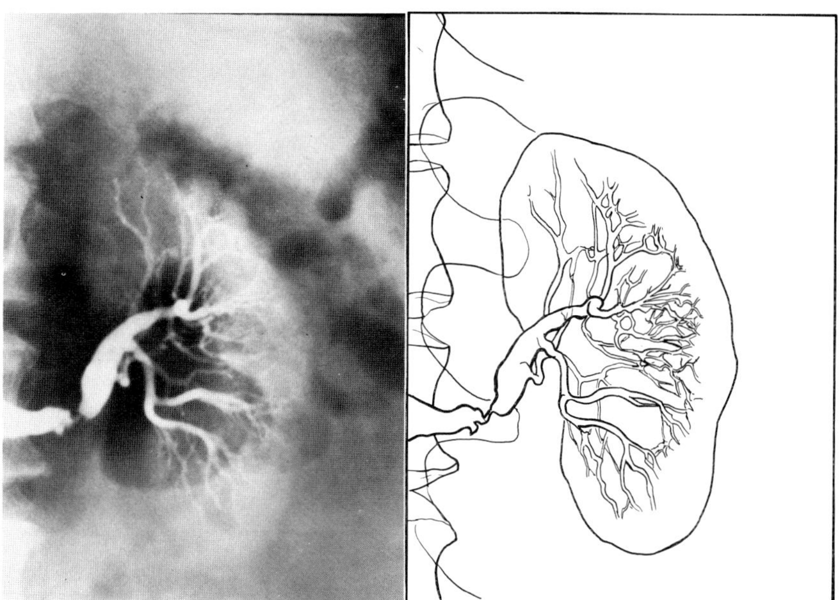

Fig. 5-35. Selective injection of the left renal artery, showing an area of stenosis with poststenotic dilatation.

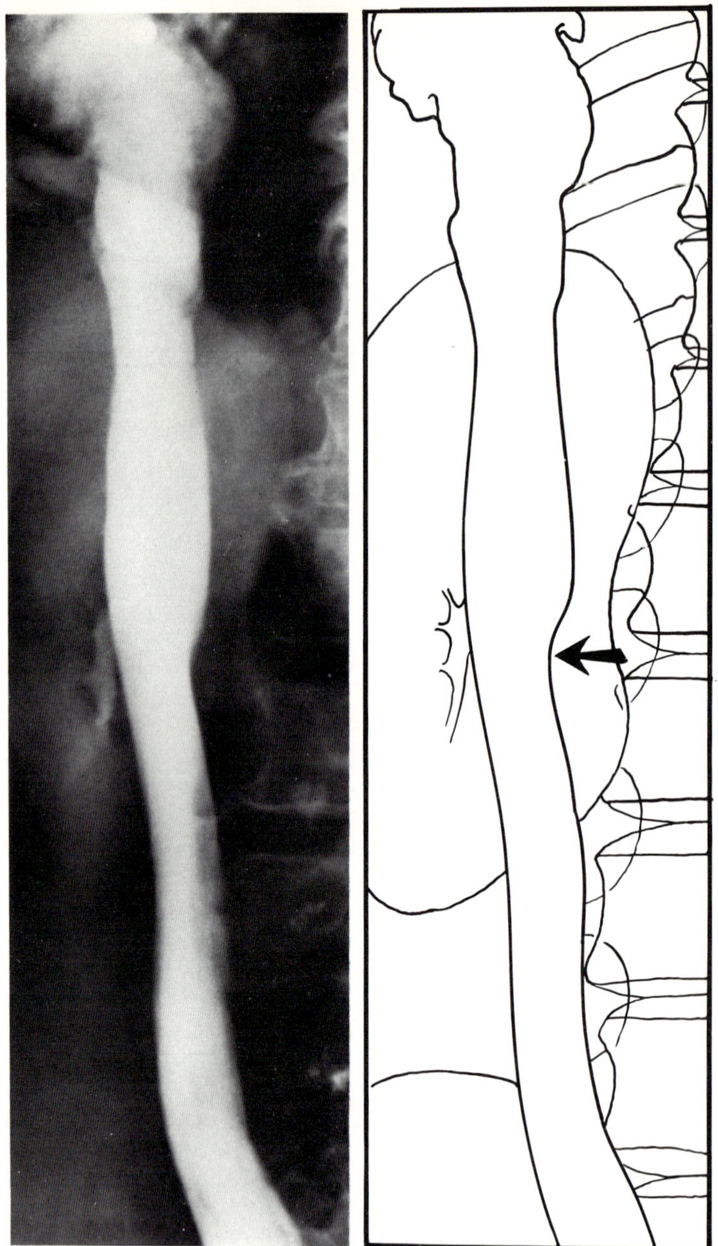

Fig. 5-36. Oblique projection of an inferior venacavogram. The posterior impression (*arrow*) is produced by the right renal artery, which passes behind the inferior vena cava. This is a normal finding.

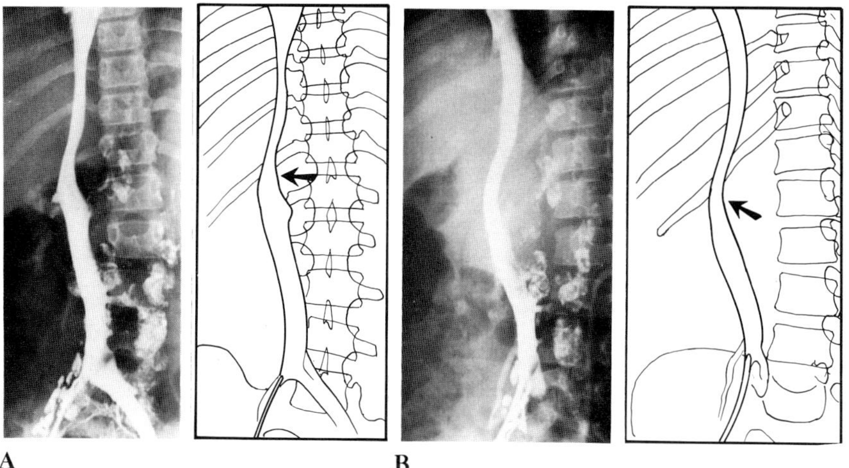

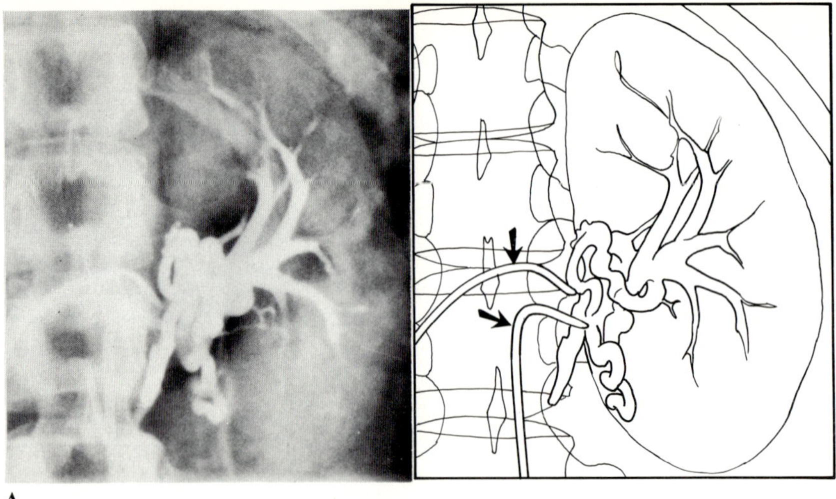

A

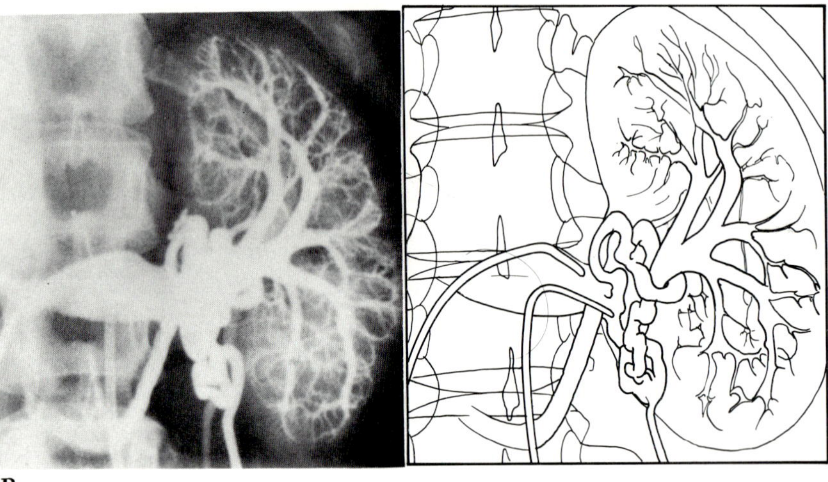

B

Fig. 5-38. Normal selective renal venogram. **A.** Note the presence of two catheters, one in the renal artery (*arrow*) and the other in the renal vein (*arrow*). The successful opacification of the entire venous system is due to simultaneous injection of epinephrine into the renal artery and renal vein, which prevents venous washout and in turn yields an excellent phlebogram.

Fig. 5-38B. The effect of the epinephrine is transient, since the contrast is already clearing after a few seconds.

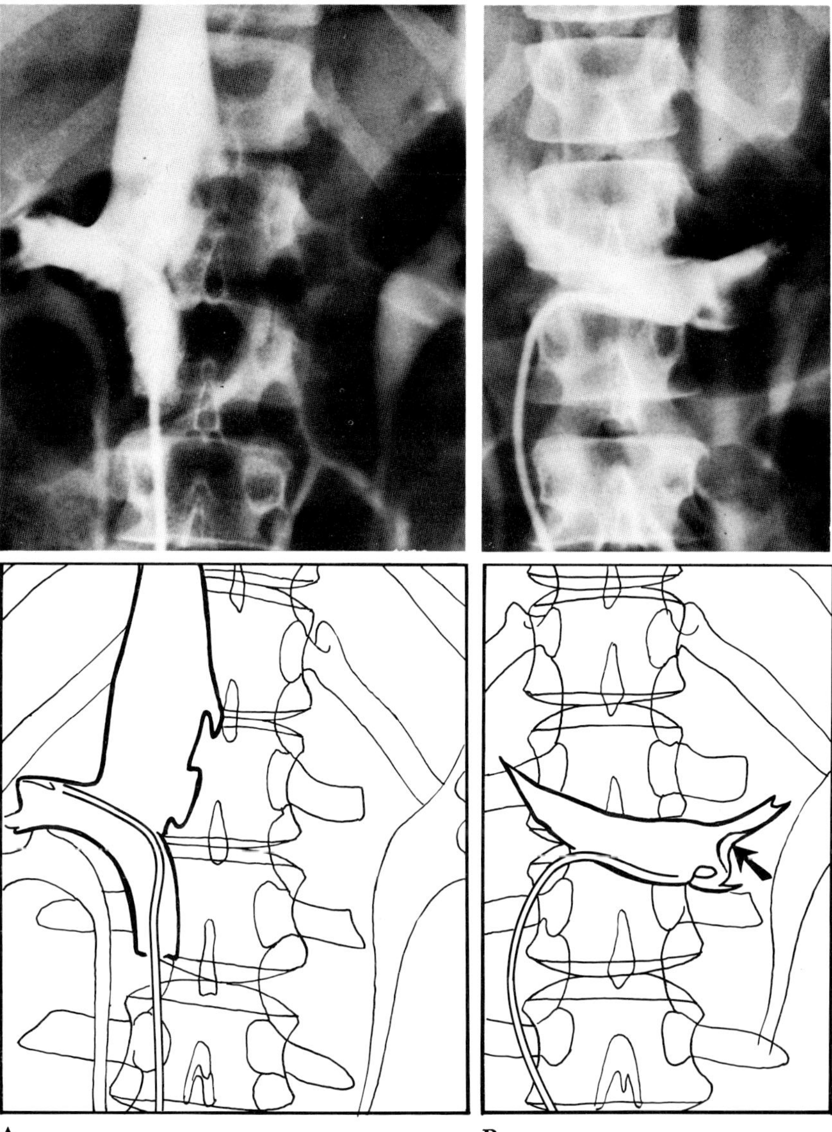

Fig. 5-39A.   A catheter has been placed selectively into the right renal vein. No occlusion is noted.

Fig. 5-39B.   The catheter has been placed into the left renal vein and a filling defect representing a large blood clot can easily be seen (*arrow*).

Nephron Dissection

The technique of microdissection allows isolation of the complete nephron, precise identification of each segment, and localization of the site of any pathologic lesions. Before microdissection can be undertaken, however, care must be taken to ensure that the tissue selected is cut in such a way that the continuity of the nephron can be maintained. Once the tissue is macerated, separation of each nephron becomes an easy matter. Two techniques are available: acid maceration and collagenase maceration.

SELECTION OF MATERIAL

Formalin-fixed or fresh tissue according to the technique to be employed is selected from coronally dissected kidney. A wedge-shaped piece of tissue is cut so that it includes the cortex and medulla in continuity from the capsule to the tip of the pyramid. The slices should vary in size according to the size of the kidney and the area of kidney selected but should not be more than 2 mm thick.

Tissue from biopsy material also can be used for dissection provided it lies in the right plane and is at least 60 μ thick.

ACID MACERATION

For acid maceration tissue should be fixed in neutral formal saline for at least a week; the longer the tissue is fixed, the longer the time necessary for maceration. Alcohol-fixed material is difficult to dissect, since after maceration the tissue becomes brittle and the nephrons are likely to break.

A number of samples representative of various areas of the kidney should be transferred to a widemouthed glass-stoppered jar containing sufficient hydrochloric acid (sp.gr. 1.150 to 1.160 at 20°C) to more than cover the tissue. To prevent damage to the tissue an acid-resisting plastic spoon rather than a metal needle should be used for this purpose. A portion of slide suitably marked with a diamond should be added to the jar as an identifying label.

To obtain reproducible results it is best to use an incubator maintained at 18°C. For example, the standard maceration time at 18°C can safely be taken to be 48 hours but will vary slightly according to the length of time the tissue has been fixed and the degree of fibrosis present in the material to be examined. In some cases in which maceration needs to be accelerated, as, for example, in the preparation of tissue for autoradiography with an isotope having a short half-life, the container can be placed in a 37°C incubator. Maceration then may be complete in less than 30 minutes, but because rate of maceration is so critical to the process, early disintegration of the tissue may occur, with loss of the specimen.

Experience is usually necessary to decide whether tissue is ready for dissection. As soon as it is ready, the hydrochloric acid should be removed and the tissue washed carefully in four or five changes of distilled water to remove as much as possible of the remaining acid. The tissue should then be allowed to equilibrate in distilled water for a further 24 hours, after which time the nephrons will have lost their rubbery consistency. The material is now ready for transfer to the dissecting dish.

COLLAGENASE MACERATION

The advantage of the collagenase technique is that nuclear staining is preserved as well as certain enzyme and transport functions. Fresh, unfixed renal tissue is prepared as previously described and submitted to 30% ethanol in glacial acetic acid overnight or, preferably, for a few days. It is then treated in running water for a minimum of 4 hours or overnight and is ready for maceration.

Maceration solution consists of 0.25 mg per milliliter of histolyticum collagenase and 0.1 mg per milliliter of chloramphenicol (to prevent bacterial growth during maceration) in 0.067M phosphate buffer at pH 7.2.

The tissue is transferred to a glass stoppered bottle or wide-bore tube and macerated in a bath of this solution at 37°C overnight or for a time which varies with the condition of the tissue. After maceration the tissue is fixed in a fresh solution of 30% ethanol in glacial acetic acid. Before dissection, selected portions of tissue are carefully rinsed in water and, if desired, placed on slides and stained with 0.1% aqueous basic fuchsin in a moist chamber for 1 hour. The stained tissue is then rinsed again and is ready for maceration. Stained macerated tissue can be preserved in 1% formalin solution in water for a week or so before dissection. This form of maceration tends to make dissection more difficult, however, and it is often only possible to obtain portions of tubules from tissue so treated.

MICRODISSECTION TECHNIQUES

The macerated tissue is carefully transferred to a Perspex or glass dissecting dish filled with water. The amount of water should be sufficient to keep the tissue immersed during manipulation. The dish is placed under a binocular stereoscopic microscope with a magnification range of ×5 to ×20. Incident illumination with either a powerful lamp or a lucite rod usually proves to be satisfactory.

The dissection is carried out with ordinary domestic or embroidery sewing needles, gauge 10 or 12, preferably nickel plated to prevent rusting, and suitably mounted; or, for delicate work, it may be performed using Singer's Microdissectors. Although the method of dissection is a matter of experience, it is usually preferable to isolate a portion of the proximal convoluted tubule and to follow the tubule both up and down until the glomerulus and distal convoluted tubules are identified.

If it is desired to follow the renal arterial tree only, maceration should be reduced by about four hours.

MEASUREMENT OF THE NEPHRON

For comparative purposes it is advisable to select tissues for measurement from the same part of the kidney each time. Usually this part has been the left lower lobe between equatorial and polar areas. It is also advisable to select an equal number of representative nephrons from the subcapsular (outer), midcortical (middle), and juxtamedullary (inner) zones, since they vary in size.

After dissection, midline drawings are made, using a Leitz or similar drawing attachment, of the displayed proximal convoluted tubules and glomeruli at $\times 60$ magnification. The tubular length is then measured with a planometer. The diameter of the tubule is measured at twenty points spaced at regular intervals, and the proximal convoluted tubular volume is computed as a cylinder, using the length and the mean of the diameter. The maximum and minimum glomerular diameters are measured with a filar micrometer eyepiece and the glomerular surface areas computed from the mean diameter, assuming the glomerulus to be a sphere.

In order to assess their possible functional anatomic relationship, the index of the glomerulus to the proximal convoluted tubule has been computed, i.e., the glomerular surface area divided by the proximal convoluted tubular volume. This value has been designated as γ, and the mean γ values of any one kidney have been shown as R.

AUTORADIOGRAPHY OF THE ISOLATED NEPHRON

The autoradiograhic technique is used to pinpoint the location of a suitably labeled substance within the nephron. The animal is injected with a labeled substance and killed at a time when the substance is likely to be concentrated maximally within the nephron. For this purpose tritium, ^{125}I, ^{14}C, and ^{35}S have proved most satisfactory. Tritium is particularly good, since its track is short ($2\ \mu$) and ensures the substance is localized in the epithelium rather than in the lumen. The dose is determined by the substance used and the half-life and specific activity of the isotopes, for example, usually 2 mC[1] of H^3 is adequate.

The nephron is dissected by one of the methods previously described, and a series of nephrons is transferred to a coverslip or slide in the dissecting dish. The slide is then removed, drained, and dried at room temperature in a Petri dish to prevent dust contamination. When the slide is dry, it is taken into a darkroom and previously melted photographic emulsion is painted or poured over it. Kodak NTB-3 and 1 Ilford L-4 emulsions have proved to be satisfactory. The slide is allowed to dry on a warm hotplate, then is placed in a light tightbox, sealed, dated, and put in a refrigerator at 0° to 40°C to reduce background. At the appropriate time the box is opened in the dark room and the slide developed in the ordinary way. The box is then resealed to continue further incubation. The developed slide is examined under the low-power microscope ($\times 10$) for evidence of "blackened" areas. Such areas of the nephron are identified, and the developed areas are compared with the background.

Stripping film has not proved satisfactory, since it is technically laborious to handle and difficult to bring into close apposition to the nephron.

PERMANENT RECORD AND PHOTOGRAPHS

In practice it has not been found satisfactory to photograph nephrons or portions of nephrons on the dissecting dish. The selected tissue should be transferred to a slide by means of a fine Pasteur pipet or by immersing in the dissecting dish a coverslip or slide previously smeared with petroleum jelly along each edge, transferring the tissue to this slide by means of dissecting needles, and then removing the slide.

The nephron is mounted wet, covered with a slide or coverslip which forms a wet chamber, and then sealed with Glyceel (George T. Gurr, Limited, London) to provide a permanent record. For formalin-fixed material, staining can be done by placing the appropriate stain on one side of the coverslip and allowing it to diffuse through the liquid medium. The process can be accelerated by drawing the stain through by small portions of filter paper on the other edge of the coverslip.

Photography of the nephron or tubule often proves difficult, since the nephron has many different planes. The most satisfactory method is to photograph it in sections so that each area is in focus; select a lens with as wide a depth of focus as possible and obtain the magnification by extending the bellows. From the resulting photographs a mosaic is prepared, showing the nephron in focus throughout its length. The mosaic can then be rephotographed in its entirety.

Laboratory Aids in Treatable Causes of Hypertension

PHEOCHROMOCYTOMA

Pathology

Pheochromocytomas are tumors that arise from chromaffin cells of adrenal medullary tissue and may be found wherever these cells happen to be located. Accessory adrenal medullary tissue has been found in the urinary bladder, in the sympathetic nerve ganglia and plexuses, and in the organ of Zuckerkandl at the lower end of the aorta. Ninety-eight percent of pheochromocytomas are of intraabdominal origin (80 percent arise in the adrenal glands), and about 1 to 2 percent occur in the intrathoracic paravertebral sympathetic chain. Of those that arise in the adrenal glands, about 10 percent are bilateral. Bilateral tumors have a high incidence of association with thyroid neoplasms, a higher incidence of malignancy than unilateral tumors, and a strong tendency to familial occurrence. Less than 10 percent of all pheochromocytomas are malignant.

Clinical Features

Pheochromocytoma is found in less than 0.5 percent of the hypertensive population. It has no sex predilection and occurs at any age, although its incidence peaks during childhood and again in early adulthood. Ten percent of reported cases are in children, and a similar percentage has been noted in pregnant women. In many instances symptoms of pheochromocytoma have appeared first during pregnancy and have then remitted only to reappear at a later date.

The clinical manifestations of pheochromocytoma are determined by the composition of catecholamines secreted by the tumor. Paroxysmal symptoms such as palpitation, headaches, anxiety, and tremulousness are usually found in patients with tumors which secrete mixtures of norepinephrine and epinephrine and are absent in those whose tumors secrete norepinephrine only. In rare instances the beta-adrenergic vasodilating effects of epinephrine may dominate the whole clinical picture, with hypotension as the major manifestation instead of hypertension.

Common physical findings include hypertension, either persistent or intermittent, and often associated with orthostatic hypotension; excessive sweating; and tachycardia associated with a forceful, thrusting cardiac impulse. In the 5 percent who also have neuroectodermal disorders, the physical examination may reveal neurofibromatosis, café au lait or port wine spots, and conjunctival telangiectasis.

Pathologic Physiology

The physiologic changes seen are the result of the pharmocologic effects of catecholamines. Hypertension is due to increases in total peripheral resistance. Profuse sweating, tachycardia, palpitations, constipation, weight loss, and tremulousness, which are prominent symptoms, have been attributed to the direct effects of catecholamines. Orthostatic hypotension, present in 70 percent of cases, is probably due to functional autonomic blockade with the possibility that catecholamine-induced decreases in plasma and total blood volume play contributory roles.

Diagnosis

Chemical tests

The definitive diagnosis of pheochromocytoma rests with the demonstration of increased urinary excretion of either free catecholamines, vanillylmandelic acid (VMA), or total metanephrines (normetanephrine plus metanephrine). The most widely used diagnostic test is the urinary excretion of VMA, a major end product of both epinephrine and norepinephrine (Fig. 7-1). There is generally no advantage to screening for any

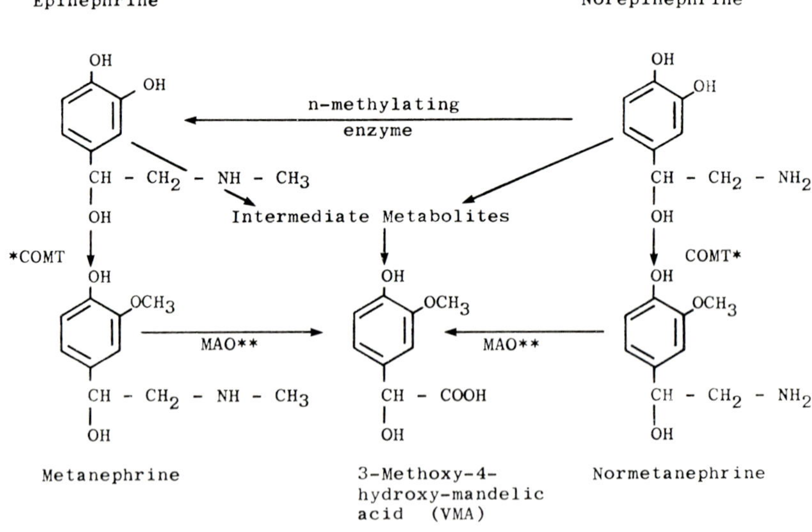

Fig. 7-1.   Metabolic pathways of epinephrine and norepinephrine.

Table 7-1. Normal Values and Substances Interfering with the Determination of Diagnostically Important Catecholamines and Their Metabolites

Catecholamines and Metabolites	Normal Values (24-Hr Excretion)	Increased by	Decreased by
Epinephrine, norepinephrine (Total catecholamines)	20–100 μg	Methyldopa (Aldomet)	Reserpine(?)
Metanephrine, normetanephrine	0.1–0.9 mg	MAO inhibitors, Aldomet	
3-methoxy-4-hydroxymandelic acid (VMA)	2.0–6.0 mg	Raw fruit, coffee, tea, vanilla, nalidixic acid (NegGram)	MAO inhibitors, clofibrate (Atromid-S)

particular end product. However, one should have some understanding of the tests' shortcomings in order to avoid false-positive or false-negative diagnoses (Table 7-1).

CATECHOLAMINES. Catecholamine assays are more difficult than tests for other metabolites because the measurement involves trihydroxyindole fluorometric techniques. Patients receiving alpha-methyldopa (Aldomet) excrete large quantities of d-methyl-catecholamines and metabolites, which results in false elevation of urinary catecholamines.

METANEPHRINES. The 3-methoxy catecholamine metabolites may be measured by either fluorometric or colorimetric assay. The latter, which is based on chemical conversions of the metanephrine to vanillin, is a simple, accurate test which can be performed in any clinical laboratory. Monoamine oxidase (MAO) inhibitors given for hypertension (e.g., pargyline or Eutonyl) or for depression (e.g., isocarboxazid or nialamide) alter the degradation of catecholamines and increase the urinary excretion of metanephrines.

VANILLYLMANDELIC ACID (VMA). VMA assays are more generally available than tests for either the catecholamines or the metanephrines. However, some nonspecific screening tests which are adaptations of phenolic acid color reactions have often resulted in false-positive assays. In patients who ingest quantities of raw fruits, vanilla, coffee, or tea, or who are receiving tetracycline, these crude assays will give high values for urinary VMA approximating those seen in pheochromocytoma. A spectrophotometric assay involving an organic extraction technique followed by conversion to vanillin is the preferred procedure. This assay is not significantly affected by dietary constituents, but the results may be altered by certain drugs. MAO inhibitors will lower VMA excretion by interfering with the degradation of metanephrines. The antibiotic nalidixic acid (NegGram) has been reported to increase VMA values by producing an interfering drug metabolite. Clofibrate (Atromid-S) also decreases VMA values by reducing recovery of the assay.

BLOOD CATECHOLAMINES. Blood catecholamine assay is not used routinely because it is a difficult procedure. Its use is limited to analysis of blood samples at various levels of the vena cava to determine the site of venous drainage from the tumor in a patient who has had an adequate but negative surgical exploration.

Pharmacologic Tests

Pharmacologic tests for the diagnosis of pheochromocytoma are rarely indicated. A provocative test (e.g., a histamine, tyramine, or glucagon test) should be used in only two circumstances: (1) to evaluate the occasional patient who has truly paroxysmal attacks but normal arterial pressure and urinary catecholamines during the quiescent period and (2) to evaluate the hypertensive patient with borderline abnormal excretion of urinary catecholamines and their metabolites.

PRIMARY ALDOSTERONISM

Definitions

The *syndrome of primary aldosteronism* includes all patients with the triad of (1) inappropriate aldosterone secretion rate [ASR], (2) suppressed or normal but unresponsive plasma renin activity [PRA], and (3) provoked or unprovoked hypokalemia. The term *primary aldosteronism,* or *Conn's syndrome,* however, is restricted to a condition resulting from an aldosterone-producing tumor arising from the zona glomerulosa of the adrenal cortex and excludes other conditions with similar or identical clinical and laboratory findings but without demonstrable functioning tumors.

Clinical Features

The peak age distribution is between 30 and 50 years, and women are affected more often than men, in a ratio of 3:1. Arterial hypertension is usually mild, but malignant hypertension has been reported in rare instances. Cardiomegaly and decreases in renal function may be present and result from long-standing hypotension. Nocturia, polyuria, polydipsia, proximal muscle weakness, and paresthesias are common signs and are attributed to potassium deficiency due to prolonged renal potassium wasting. Hypokalemia may also give rise to abnormal glucose tolerance tests, cardiac irregularities, and paralysis, which reverse with repletion of body potassium.

Pathologic Physiology

The secretion of renin with formation of angiotensin II can be stimulated by (1) decreases in renal perfusion pressure, (2) decreases in extracellular fluid volume or by sodium deprivation, and (3) increased activity of the sympathetic nervous system. Angiotensin II acts on the zona glomerulosa of the adrenal cortex to stimulate aldosterone secretion and on vascular smooth muscle to constrict peripheral arterioles. Aldosterone acts on renal tubules to facilitate reabsorpition of sodium in exchange for potassium or hydrogen ions. The extent of this exchange depends on the amount of sodium reaching the distal tubules. The rise in pressure mediated through angiotensin II and the expansion of extracellular fluid volume due to sodium retention act in concert to suppress renin. This results in decreases in both the formation of angiotensin and the secretion of aldosterone.

In primary aldosteronism renin secretion is suppressed because of prolonged extracellular fluid volume expansion, and hypokalemic alkalosis occurs because, in the presence of increased circulating aldosterone, sodium-potassium and sodium-hydrogen exchanges proceed at excessive rates. Suppressed PRA in an ambulatory sodium-depleted patient with aldosteronism is a highly reliable indication of primary excessive aldosterone secretion. In secondary aldosteronism, increased renin secretion is usually the stimulus to aldosterone production. Thus one can readily distinguish primary from secondary aldosteronism by the demonstration of suppressed PRA in the former and increased PRA in the latter.

Diagnosis

Inappropriate secretion of aldosterone can be readily demonstrated by giving high dietary sodium. This test operates on the principle that aldosterone secretion owing to an aldosterone-producing tumor cannot be suppressed normally. The continued excess of circulating aldosterone facilitates sodium-potassium exchange in the renal tubule. Since the extent of this exchange depends on the amount of sodium reaching distal tubules, a high dietary sodium (250 to 300 mEq per day for 7 to 10 days) will exaggerate the exchange and result in renal potassium wasting and decreases in serum potassium concentration. In a normal subject this maneuver would have no adverse effects on potassium balance, since aldosterone secretion would be suppressed to very low values. A positive response to salt-loading (i.e., a fall in serum potassium concentration below 3.5 mEq per liter associated with significant kaliuresis) should be confirmed by estimation of aldosterone production. Aldosterone secretion or excretion determined during salt-loading provides the most informative data. On high dietary sodium, normal subjects have aldosterone excretion rates of less than 5.0 μg per 24 hours; essential hypertensives have slightly higher values at about 7 to 10 μg per 24 hours; and patients with primary aldosteronism have clearly elevated values of 20 μg per 24 hours or higher (see Table 7-2).

Low PRA is not a specific diagnostic aid in finding occult instances of primary aldosteronism. Patients with essential hypertension may exhibit very low PRA levels. But in these patients, whenever levels of PRA are low, those of aldosterone are also low. It appears that, while PRA may help in recognizing primary aldosteronism, the diagnosis depends on the demonstration of oversecretion of aldosterone with its resulting tendency to cause hypokalemic alkalosis.

RENAL ARTERIAL DISEASE

Clinical Features

Renovascular hypertension has no clinical features that are diagnostic. However, a presumptive diagnosis may be made under the following circumstances: (1) hypertension before age 35 or after age 50; (2) acceleration of vascular disease in a patient with essential hypertension, especially following an episode of flank pain; (3) sudden onset of hypertension in a previously normotensive patient; and (4) presence of an upper abdominal bruit, heard best at the epigastrium with radiation to either or both upper quadrants and occasionally in the costovertebral angles.

Diagnosis

Definitive diagnosis of renal arterial disease is made by arteriography, but diagnosis of renovascular hypertension does not necessarily follow. Much attention has been given to the diagnostic and prognostic significance of the finding of disparity of PRA in blood samples taken from two renal veins. Most workers consider a ratio of 1:5 between the involved and non-involved sides as indicating the presence of a renal pressor factor. The dependability of this test is quite good but not absolute. There are a few patients who have not shown disparity but have responded to surgical treatment with normalization of arterial pressure. To increase the accuracy of detection of renovascular hypertension it has been suggested that sampling be done after maneuvers designed to stimulate renin release; these include a low sodium diet with or without the administration of a diuretic and arterial pressure reduction with intravenously administered sodium nitroprusside or hydralazine. There has not been enough experience with any of these maneuvers to prove their value. The best diagnostic test for renovascular hypertension is far from settled.

LABORATORY DETERMINATIONS OF ALDOSTERONE AND PLASMA RENIN ACTIVITY AND THEIR CLINICAL SIGNIFICANCE

Numerous factors affect the secretion of aldosterone and renin. Particular attention must be paid to the state of sodium and potassium balance. Sodium depletion increases aldosterone and renin secretion, while sodium repletion decreases both. Hypokalemia decreases aldosterone production, while it increases renin secretion. On the other hand, hyperkalemia increases aldosterone production, while it tends to suppress renin secretion. Estrogen is well known for its tendency to elevate both aldosterone and renin secretion. Therefore studies to determine integrity of the renin-aldosterone system should be avoided in women during the luteal phase of the menstrual cycle and in those who are on oral contraceptive therapy.

Diuretics and antihypertensive agents (e.g., Apresoline, ganglionic blocking drugs, and adrenergic blocking agents) should be stopped at least a month prior to evaluation of the renin-aldosterone system.

From a clinical point of view the measurement of aldosterone has of necessity been confined to the urine. Since the pH 1 or acid-labile metabolite is converted into free aldosterone, this metabolite has been favored for analysis. Until recently the technique most commonly used was the double-isotope derivative method introduced by Kliman and Peterson; this is time-consuming, expensive, and tedious. The recent success in obtaining specific antibodies to aldosterone has led to the development of radioimmunoassay techniques which are simpler, faster, and less expensive while attaining a high degree of sensitivity and specificity. Several such methods for the measurement of plasma aldosterone have been published, and Seeley and her associates have applied this newer technique to the measurement of urinary excretion rate of the acid-labile conjugate of aldosterone. Their method, which used antibodies induced in sheep by the injection of aldosterone-21-hemisuccinate bovine serum albumin, requires no chromatographic steps; it is rapid and simple, and the values compare favorably with those obtained by double-isotope dilution. The technique employed in one laboratory utilizes antibodies produced against aldosterone-λ-lactone-3-carboxymethyl-oxime coupled to bovine serum albumin. Aldosterone-λ-lactone constitutes the ligand. The method consists essentially of the following steps: (1) extraction with dichloromethane after hydrolysis at pH 1, (2) alkali and water washings of the dichloromethane extracts, (3) periodate oxidation, (4) liquid-partition and (5) radioimmunoassay procedure. Periodate oxidation converts free aldosterone to a λ-lactone derivative, while all other closely related steroids are converted to etianic acids which are readily removed by sodium bicarbonate wash (step 4). This results in purer and highly stable samples. This method has been applied in a variety of clinical situations, in which it has proved highly specific and reliable, and it appears far simpler and more convenient than other existing procedures. The normal values during different levels of dietary sodium are shown in Table 7-2.

Current methods for the measurement of PRA also employ a radioimmunoassay technique as described by Haber and coworkers. Several modifications of this technique have been reported. The commercial availability

Table 7-2. Normal Values of Aldosterone Excretion (μg per 24 hr)

Dietary Na	Mean	SE	SD	Range
Unrestricted	6.5	1.0	3.7	2.1–16.2
Low (4th day)	58.4	11.5	34.5	22–122
High (3rd day)	3.9	0.7	1.9	1.0–7.0

of an antiserum to angiotensin I and ^{125}I-labeled peptide has allowed PRA determinations to be carried out in centers without the facilities for the preparation of these reagents. In this approach angiotensin I generated during timed incubation of plasma at 37°C is measured as a reflection of endogenous renin. No exogenous renin substrate is added, and zero order kinetics are assumed for the enzyme-substrate system. Inhibitors of converting enzyme (e.g., EDTA, DFP) are added prior to incubation to prevent conversion of generated angiotensin I to angiotensin II. The plasma incubation and the radioimmunoassay procedures are depicted in Figures 7-2 and 7-3, respectively.

In general, the values for PRA by radioimmunoassay are two to three times higher than those obtained by bioassay. This difference is probably the result of (1) incubating plasma at pH 7.4 and (2) the presence of nonspecific immunoreactive substances in raw plasma. Indeed, Page and Haber have characterized in human plasma certain proteins that react with the antibodies against angiotensin I. Our laboratory has circumvented this problem by prior processing of blood by the method of Pickens et al. and incubation of plasma at pH 5.5. This has resulted in values not significantly different from those obtained by bioassay. The normal values for PRA using this modification are shown in Table 7-3.

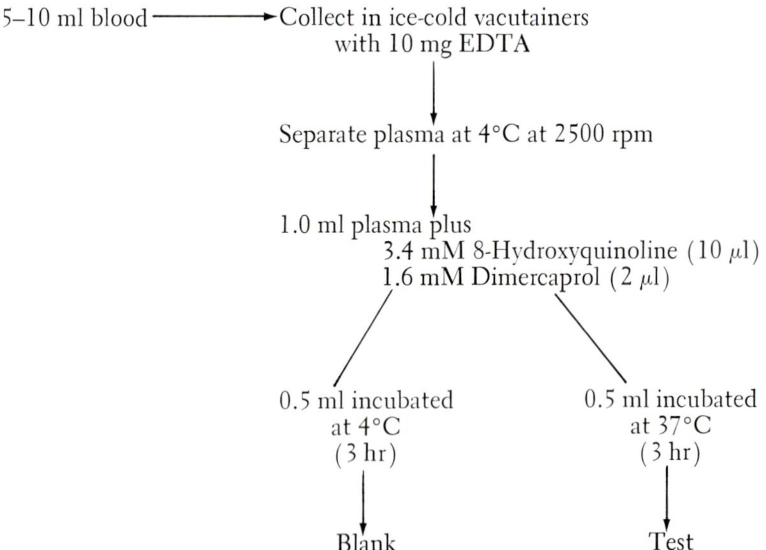

Fig. 7-2. Incubation of plasma.

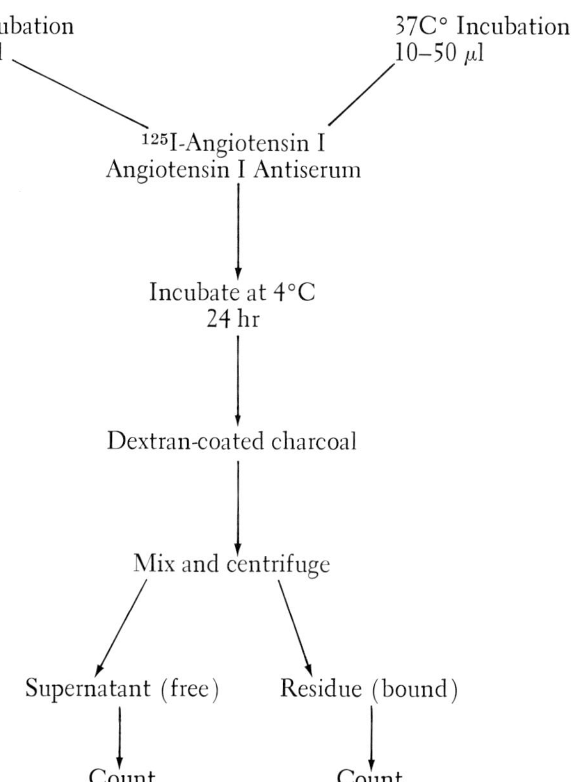

Angiotensin I standards, 0, 100, 200, 300, 400, 500 pg/min in duplicate. Charcoal blank—supernatant left following treatment of ^{125}I-Angiotensin I and Tris buffer with dextran-coated charcoal.

Computation: % Bound $= \dfrac{\text{Activity in supernatant tube (cpm)} \times 100}{\text{Activity in supernatant tube (cpm)} + \text{activity in charcoal tube (cpm)}}$

Fig. 7-3. Radioimmunoassay procedure.

Table 7-3. Normal Values of Plasma Renin Activity (ng/ml/4 hr) in Fasting Patients after 30 to 45 Minutes of Supine Rest

Dietary Na	Mean	SE	SD	Range
Unrestricted	1.2	0.28	0.84	0.4–2.7
Low (4th day)	8.96	1.76	5.28	3.3–15.2
High (3rd day)	1.22	0.32	0.96	0.23–3.5

8 The Metabolic Ward and the Metabolic Laboratory

THE METABOLIC WARD

Few metabolic units have all the features that are desirable for research, diagnosis, and therapy. These necessary features fall into four categories.

First, patients need living conditions as in a hotel. Private bedrooms, adequate storage space, a common dining room, a pleasant TV lounge, and access to a library make for contented subjects.

Second, the collection, processing, and storage of specimens of food, excreta, blood, other fluids, and tissue should be carried out in an adequate space set aside for that function and no other.

Third, specialized research interests are not always compatible with usual hospital routines; they should be kept separate. This principle applies particularly to dietary control, which should be entrusted to a special diet kitchen, not the general hospital kitchen, and to biochemical and other routine laboratory procedures which provide data that are part of the patient's general record. For instance the routine laboratory might be trusted with urea and glucose but usually not with fractionation of individual amino acids or proteins. Although it is tempting to save money by using the routine laboratory as a prime source of research data, there is always a risk of loss of time and accuracy. The allotment of space for research is rarely generous enough.

Fourth, all areas should be planned for flexibility so as to avoid expensive remodeling to accommodate new procedures or new lines of diagnosis, therapy, or research.

The commonest errors of omission or commission in planning and building metabolic wards are poor lighting and dingy decor; inadequate environmental controls for both summer and winter; insufficient outlets for water, air, gas, vacuum, and electricity; inadequate storage space for the needs of patients, laboratories, and kitchens; lack of private or even separate office space for physicians, nurses, and other professional personnel; inappropriate or no recreational facilities; and poor dining facilities.

The Metabolic Importance of the Patient's Environment, Activity, and Level of Nutrition

A patient's immediate past history may have a profound effect on his renal function. For example, his environmental physiology, work physiology, nutritional physiology, and therapeutics may all be responsible for significant alterations.

Exposure to cold may cause diuresis by inhibiting the production of antidiuretic hormone. Exposure to heat may cause oliguria by increasing the circulating antidiuretic hormone. As the rate of sweating increases, there is a compensatory decrease in renal water loss.

Physical activity has much to do with renal function, and different grades of exercise may cause opposite changes. Even altering posture may have effects, as in orthostatic proteinuria. Compared with standing, walking at a pace of around five km per hour generally causes an increase in the rate of urine flow, jogging at 8 km per hour has no effect, and running at 11 km per hour causes oliguria. Prolonged strenuous exercise, as in cross-country running or contact sports, may cause proteinuria, cylindruria, and microscopic hematuria. This syndrome has been termed *athletic pseudonephritis* and is benign and quickly reversible. Hard physical work also induces oliguria. Probably a diminished renal plasma flow leads to this oliguria, as the U/P ratio for creatinine is usually not altered.

The immediate nutritional history is of importance in renal function with respect to acid-base balance and water balance. Habitual acid-ash diets produce a metabolic acidosis from the phosphoric and sulfuric acid precursors oxidized to those acids from protein and amino acids. Habitual alkaline-ash diets lead to an alkalosis by producing mineral bases, especially potassium hydroxide, when organic salts are oxidized. The potential osmotic intake can be calculated as the sum of ingested anions and cations and the urea, ammonia, phosphate, and sulfate equivalents of ingested protein. The water-osmotic balance may then be affected by primary deficiency or excess of water, primary deficiency or excess of osmols, and their mutual interplay. For instance, a primary deficiency of osmols, as in a low-sodium diet, will lead to an obligatory water deficit.

The patient's history with respect to medication, either self-prescribed or physician-prescribed, may be significant. Laxatives lead to loss of base and water. Alkalizers cause alkalosis. Diuretics can induce changes in acid-base or water-osmotic balance. Vomiting is still a common cause of alkalosis, even though self-induced emesis is now rare.

Collection and Processing of Specimens

The collection, processing, and storage of specimens should be carried on away from the patients' quarters and the diagnostic, therapeutic, and laboratory areas. In the ideal metabolic unit there will be a small operating theater that makes a suitable room for processing specimens. Appropriate precautions for sterility and against radioactivity should be imposed. Bacterial or viral infection is commonly a hazard with blood and urine, always with feces. Radioisotopes may occur in any biologic specimen.

The effects of collection, preparation, and storage on compounds to be studied should receive careful attention. Some compounds are inherently unstable and deteriorate quickly or slowly even at the commonest temperature for cold storage, $-20°C$. Some are stable under all conditions, like sodium and other minerals. Glass is still the best all-around container. Some compounds are absorbed into the walls of plastic containers, as is the case with many steroids. Even the liners of caps need attention, Teflon being the best material to minimize contamination, leakage, or loss.

A good validation study requires that blanks, standards, unknowns, and unknowns with added standards be carried through the whole procedure, from collection through storage to final analysis. It also requires a statistical statement on the sensitivity, specificity, reliability, and reproducibility of each method.

Traditionally, certain procedures are supposed to stabilize specimens. Ice baths and refrigerated centrifuges have obvious advantages. Sodium niazide and thymol are most commonly used for bacteriostasis. Urine is acidified with acetic acid to pH 5 or less to protect urea and prevent precipitation of calcium salts. Feces are treated with sulfuric acid to trap the ammonia that might arise from the alkaline reaction that is commonly found in them. The high-speed blender is universal in metabolic work, and ultrasonic dispersion is liked by those who have used it. For stabilizing a suspension of feces against layering out, we use agar in a final concentration of about two percent weight/volume. Agar has a low blank for most substances except carbohydrate.

As a fecal marker we prefer FD & C Blue #1 Dye.* Two 000 gelatine capsules of the dye and a tablespoon of methylcellulose give a sharp marking. Carmine sometimes is hard to see but, more importantly, some batches are contaminated with *Salmonella cubana*, which can give dysentery.

Specimens of urine and feces are best collected under conditions sociably acceptable to patients, which means privacy above everything else. We have a private toilet for this purpose. A stainless steel suspension consisting of straps hangs in the bowl, and a weighed glass pie plate is placed on this. Defecation and urination can then be done, as they commonly are, at the same sitting, kept separate, and quantitatively collected.

THE METABOLIC LABORATORY
The Calculation of Metabolic Balance

The term *balance* has come to have three meanings in the metabolic literature. Only the first can be classified as rigorous. It is the equation of Sanctorius:

$$balance = M_{in} - M_{out} \tag{1}$$

* Brilliant Blue, obtainable from Bates Chemicals, Harleco, or Fisher.

where M is the mass of a substance which is neither anabolized nor catabolized, and the subscripts *in* and *out* refer to the sum of all avenues of intake and output. The common avenues of intake are ingestion, injection, and inhalation. The normal avenues of output are urination, defecation, perspiration and transpiration, exhalation, and bloodletting. Unusual or pathologic pathways are vomiting, salivation, lacrimation, and fistulae, especially after cholecystectomy. A good example of the correct use of equation 1 is in the domain of mineral balance, in which the law of conservation of mass is implicit with respect to sodium.

The second meaning of *balance* can be made rigorous only if endogenous events can be measured. It takes the form

$$\text{balance} = (M_{exog} + M_{endog})_{in} - (M_{exog} + M_{endog})_{out} \qquad (2)$$

Here, the subscripts *in* and *out* refer to the total body system, not to the avenues of intake and output. Endogenous events (endog) are added to the exogenous avenues of equation 1. An example of this meaning of *balance* is *water balance*. A mere computation of H_2O_{in} as fluid water (liquid or in food) is not enough. Water of oxidation also enters the total body system. Likewise a summing of H_2O_{out} as fluid or evaporated water (urine + feces + dermal + pulmonary) is not enough. Water may be sequestrated as water of crystalization or water of hydration and thus leave the system of fluid body water. Sequestrated water cannot be measured by present techniques and so is customarily neglected. Equation 2 implies the law of conservation of mass with respect to H_2O only if the total system of H_2O, H, and O is known.

The concept of *turnover* was developed from equations 1 and 2. If the balance from time 0 to time 1 is known for a nonmetabolized substance, and if the amount of the substance present in the body can be measured for time 0, and is M_0,

$$\text{turnover rate} = \text{balance}/M_0 \qquad (3)$$

or

$$dM/dt = \text{balance}/M_0 \qquad (3a)$$

For a metabolizable substance the concept is strictly valid only for steady state conditions, where anabolism is equal to catabolism.

The third and least rigorous use of *balance* is in relation to equilibrium, not to a difference between input and output. The most widely recognized use of this meaning is *acid-base balance*, which is applied to the buffer pair in the mass law equation:

$$[H^+] = k[HA]/[A^-] \qquad (4)$$

where the brackets identify chemical concentrations of hydrogen ion, undissociated buffer, and dissociated buffer cation. Balance here is almost synonymous with homeostasis: the hydrogen ion concentration is regulated within narrow limits by a buffer system, played upon by exogenous and endogenous events.

Three aspects of renal function are commonly studied by balance techniques under equation 1, 2, or 3. These are nitrogen balance, water balance, and acid-base balance.

Nitrogen Balance

Nitrogen balance is frequently computed erroneously as follows:

$$N \text{ balance} = N_{food} - (N_{urine} + N_{feces}) \tag{5}$$

The error lies in a neglect of the skin as a source of loss of N. In the first place, there is a steady loss of desquamated epithelial cells and hair. Although this varies from day to day in relation to the natural cycle of dermal growth, a figure of 0.3 gm N per day seems reasonable. In the second place, sweat contains urea, ammonia, and amino acids in concentrations at least as high as those in blood plasma. In uremia, actual crystals of urea are sometimes seen on the skin, giving a "uremic frost." Concentrations of total N as high as 200 mg N per 100 ml sweat have been recorded. Also in fever and in exercise the rate of sweating can become surprisingly high. In cross-country runners we have seen losses of 4 liters per hour. Under these extreme conditions, healthy men were losing up to 1.2 gm N in 1 hour.

It seems clear that all studies of N balance should consider dermal loss. Loss of metabolic NH_3 from the lungs has been reported also, but not in large amounts, anywhere near as much as the urea and ammonia in sweat. The correct equation for N balance then becomes

$$N \text{ balance} = N_{ing} - (N_u + N_{fec} + N_{sweat} + N_{derm}) \tag{6}$$

where *ing* means ingested, *u* urine, *fec* feces, *sweat* sweat, and *derm* dermal.

Water Balance

Water balance is truly difficult to measure accurately. Clinically it is often and erroneously calculated as follows:

$$H_2O \text{ balance} = H_2O_{ing} + H_2O_{iv} - H_2O_u \tag{7}$$

where *ing* means ingested, *iv* intravenous, and *u* urine.

Two main errors of omission occur in equation 7. The water of oxidation is omitted from the intake. The output fails to take into account water lost from the skin by perspiration and transpiration and water lost from the lung by evaporation. Water lost in perspiration is variable, depending on thermal load, work load, and body temperature. Water lost in transpiration (insensible loss) amounts to as much as 30 gm per hour. Water lost from the lungs (H_2O_{pulm}) is directly proportional to the difference in absolute humidity of the inspired air and expired air, times the pulmonary ventilation (PV):

$$H_2O_{pulm} = (absolute\ humidity_{exp} - absolute\ humidity_{insp}) \times PV \quad (8)$$

where *pulm* means pulmonary, *exp* expired, and *insp* inspired.

In active persons in dry air the evaporative water loss often exceeds the urinary volume fivefold. The correct version of Equation 7 is

$$H_2O\ balance$$
$$= (H_2O_{ing} + H_2O_{iv} + H_2O_{met}) - (H_2O_u + H_2O_{derm} + H_2O_{pulm}) \quad (6)$$

where *ing* means ingested, *iv* intravenous, *met* metabolic, *u* urine, *derm* dermal, and *pulm* pulmonary.

It may be that for persons at rest H_2O_{met} will balance out $H_2O_{derm} + H_2O_{pulm}$, but that is by no means certain. It would be better to recognize these items and make guesses on their magnitude.

The Peters-Passmore equation permits the water balance to be calculated without any measurements of fluid water intake or output. Their equation is

$$H_2O\ balance = (W_2 - W_1) + (Dry\ W_{out} - Dry\ W_{in})$$
$$+ (gm\ CO_2 - gm\ O_2) + (H_2O_{met}) \quad (10)$$

where W_1 and W_2 = body weights at the beginning and end of a period
$\quad$ O_2 and CO_2 = mass of those gases for that period
$\quad$ Dry W_{in} = dry solids ingested and injected
$\quad$ Dry W_{out} = dry solids in urine, feces, and other sources of loss, particularly skin

and H_2O_{met} is assumed or calculated from the metabolic rate.

This powerful equation is derived from the considerations that the total change in body weight is due to the difference between gas, liquid, and solid gained and lost and that the water balance includes fluid water, water preformed in food, and metabolic water added to the system (body water) minus water lost from all avenues, bowel, kidney, skin, and lung.

From the standpoint of renal function, it is not realistic to talk of water balance separately from osmotic balance. The general equation for osmolar concentration in serum is

$$[Osm]_s = total\ osmols_s/V_s \quad (11)$$

where $[Osm]_s$ refers to the osmolar concentration of the serum (or plasma) and V_s to the volume of the serum (or plasma).

This states that the osmotic concentration in the plasma is calculable if one knows the total osmolar content of the serum or plasma and its volume. A physiologic axiom is that there must be osmotic equilibrium between cells and intercellular fluid and between intercellular fluid and plasma. In a normal, healthy steady state this is achieved by the interplay between water and osmols, the kidney acting as the main homeostatic regulator under hypothalamic-pituitary control, the set point being an $[Osm]_s$ of around 290 mOsm per kilogram H_2O. Primary excess of osmols entails retention of water; deficiency of osmols entails an obligatory loss of water. Primary excess of water leads to retention of osmols; water deficiency leads to loss of osmols. In pathologic states, such as renal failure of some types, the normal, healthy steady state cannot be maintained, and edema follows. In this context the body does not distinguish between non-ionized solutes like urea and ionized solutes like sodium and chloride.

Acid-Base Balance

Acid-base balance has received more attention perhaps than any other aspect of kidney function. One reason is that concepts and techniques were worked out in usable form early in the twentieth century. The modern glass electrode dates back to Clark, and the current nomograms to Sørensen, Henderson, and Hasselbalch, without modification of theory.

One result of the early perfection of concepts and techniques for blood and plasma has been to "lock in," so to speak, the bicarbonate–carbonic acid buffer system as the most important for biologic systems. Yet, in fact, in respect of the total body water, and considering that there has to be electrostatic equivalence in systems with a common interface, the bicarbonate–carbonic acid system is less important than the dibasic phosphate–monobasic phosphate, the protein, the amino acid, and the organic acid systems. Intracellular water, quantitatively speaking, is more important than extracellular.

Good methods for measuring the intracellular control of acid-base balance are needed to reduce this discrepancy. In this respect, urine may be more representative of the body as a whole than is blood.

Peculiarities of nomenclature have become standard in the fields of acid-base balance and osmotic balance. Practically all solutes are commonly expressed in terms of concentrations in the body fluids, in equivalents for electrolytes, and in moles for nonelectrolytes. The Sørensen convention of pH has its uses in physical chemistry, but for most biologic purposes the nonconverted concentration, conveniently in nanoequivalents per liter, would be just as suitable and certainly less confusing. The pH is our only number that expresses an increase by a decrease. In the osmotic field, the custom is to express the osmotic concentration in terms of osmols per kilogram of water. Yet many workers use the term *osmolal* without correcting for the space taken up by substances other than water, especially protein. Properly, they should use the term *osmolar*. A second peculiarity of this way of expressing osmotic concentrations is that unless an empiric activity coefficient is introduced for the effects of concentrations greater than infinite dilution, the values diverge from theory more and more as the concentration rises. We never think of expressing concentrations of sodium and potassium on a molal basis, yet tempers become frayed when we treat osmols like mols. For virtually all medical purposes, the biologic fluids can be regarded as infinitely dilute, and the argument disappears.

In addition to the classic alkaloses and acidoses, two other conditions may come into prominence. The first of these is intracellular alkalosis or acidosis without a corresponding change, or at least with a much reduced change, in the plasma. One model for this is the intracellular acidosis of tissues simultaneously hypoxic and cold. The hypoxia leads to accumulation of organic acids in the cell; the cold, if severe enough, can inhibit the diffusion of the organic acids out of the cell. Thus the normal distribution of acids between cells and interstitial fluid is inhibited.

A second previously neglected acid-base disturbance has been described best in patients with diabetes mellitus. Under some as yet obscure circumstances they may develop a severe acidosis, with accumulation of lactic acid but not the usual keto acids. Presumably the metabolism of their muscles has become anaerobic rather than aerobic.

Body Composition

The development of a practical, sensitive, metabolic bed-scale has facilitated the monitoring of fluid balance as well as studies of body composition in health and disease.

Different models have been used for different purposes. The commonest is the simplest, based on organ weights:

$$M_{total} = \Sigma (M_{liver} + M_{skeleton} + M_{muscle} + \ldots) \tag{12}$$

This direct approach is useful post mortem, when the subjects' organ weights as directly measured, and expressed as a percentage of total body weight, can be compared with a normal standard.

For some chemical purposes it is useful to regard the body as the sum of three phases at $37°C$:

$$M_{total} = M_{gas} + M_{liquid} + M_{solid} \tag{13}$$

where M = mass.

The gases are commonly O_2, CO_2, and N_2, the liquid H_2O (rarely C_2H_5OH or other alcohols), and the solids are the rest—protein, fat, carbohydrate, minerals, and trace substances, both inorganic and organic. One application of this approach is the Peters-Passmore equation for water balance (eq. 10).

If one assumes that the gases are a negligible fraction of the body weight, equation 12 simplifies to the commonest equation for body composition, the two-compartment model:

$$M_{total} = M_{H_2O} + {}_{solid} \tag{14}$$

where M refers to mass.

If one assumes that fat is distinguishable from the rest of the solid mass, equation 14 transforms into a three-compartment model:

$$M_{total} = M_{H_2O} + M_{fat} + M_{fat\text{-}free\ solid} \tag{15}$$

For practical purposes, if two of the three independent variables are known, the third can be calculated. M_{H_2O} can be measured by D^2_2O or T^3_2O dilution, M_{fat} from the density of the body as calculated from water displacement or underwater weighing:

$$\text{Density} = M_{total}/V_{body} \qquad (16)$$

where V refers to volume. $M_{fat\text{-}free\ solid}$ can be measured from the isotope K^{40} total body count and the (assumed) constant percentage of K^{39} in the fat-free lean body mass.

$$\text{Mass}_{fat\text{-}free\ solids} = (f_1 K^{40}\ \text{counts}) \times (f_2\ \text{of LBM/K}) \qquad (17)$$

where f_1 and f_2 are factors derived from calibration with phantoms.

Moore has popularized the term *active cell mass*. This is attractive conceptually, but there is no acceptable way to measure it.

In the three-compartment model, the water component can be subdivided further. Traditionally it is given two main divisions: (1) the extracellular water, composed of water in the plasma, interstitial water lymph, connective tissue, cartilage, and bone, and of transcellular water (mostly from exocrine glands such as the salivary, gastrointestinal, and pancreatic glands, and the liver); and (2) the intracellular water. As a percentage of total body water, the intracellular accounts for some 55 percent and the extracellular for some 45 percent, of which plasma contributes about 8 percent, interstitial water about 20 percent, sequestrated water about 14 percent, and transcellular water about 3 percent. As a percentage of the total lean body mass, the total body water contributes 70 percent. None of these compartments, even the total body water, is easily or certainly measurable by any of the dilution techniques now available. The difficulties lie in the failure of substances to distribute evenly, to stay in their appropriate compartments, and to avoid sequestration, metabolism, or excretion. In addition, some, like antipyrine and sodium thiosulfate, give rise to unpleasant, even dangerous, reactions in a small percentage of patients.

The difficulties in measuring body composition in patients with cardiorenal disease are substantial. The assumptions as to the normal ratios of water to dry lean body mass and the K/N ratio of lean body mass may not hold. Also, in patients with a tendency toward edema, mixing of tracers may not be complete for a very long time.

If one is interested not in absolute values but in the changes of body composition during the course of a regimen, as in weight reduction, then calculations may be made from balance studies, according to the method of Albright. In a patient in a steady state at the beginning and end of a study, one can account for any change in weight from metabolic data. The change in protoplasmic mass is calculated from the N balance, the change in extracellular fluid from sodium or chloride balance, and the change in intracellular fluid from potassium balance. Any discrepancy between the observed change in weight and that calculated from the sum of the three weights computed is attributed to fat.

For practical purposes, the traditional use of body weight as the best simple index of body composition is justified. Edematous fluid shows up on the scales. In our studies we have been struck by a very close correlation between body weight and body volume. Within a homogenous population of young men in military training the body volume of men of a given weight is remarkably constant; at the same time, the larger men have the lower density. There is a good linear relation between volume and weight and therefore between density and weight. The implication is that the body composition within such a population is remarkably constant within a group of the same weight. Observations such as these tend to justify the traditional concept of "ideal" or "best" weight for age and height.

Clearance Studies

The clearance ratio formula has become a central dogma in nephrology:

$$C = UV/P \qquad (18)$$

where $C =$ clearance and is a virtual number, with dimensions in volume per minute

$U =$ the chemical concentration of a substance in the urine

$V =$ urine volume per minute

$P =$ the plasma concentration of the substance.

P is almost never expressed as corrected for plasma water, and it is assumed to be constant for the collection period, or at least representative of that period.

The clearance concept has led to many advances in the study of kidney function, such as the quantitative expression of glomerular filtration rate, renal plasma flow, free water clearance, and so forth. However, for com-

Table 8-1. Raw Data for Clearance Computations

Item	Symbol	Units	Derivation
Time	Δt	min	$T_2 - T_1$
Volume	Vol	ml	Measurement
Rate of urine flow	V	ml/min	Vol/Δt
Concentration of substance Z in urine	U_z	μEq/ml or mg/ml	Measurement
Concentration of substance Z in plasma or serum	P_z	μEq/ml or mg/ml	Measurement
Renal clearance of substance Z	C_z	ml plasma/min	$\dfrac{U_z V}{P_z}$

putational purposes these second-order concepts are algebraically redundant, as the only primary numbers are U, V, and P. In programming we have used two tables. The first (Table 8-1) expresses the raw data and the other (Table 8-2) gives various expressions derived from them. Clearly, when working with the derived items in column 1 of Table 2, the program will express them in terms of the six items in column 1 of Table 1.

Table 8-2. Expressions Computed from Primary Data of Table 1

Item	Symbol	Units	Derivation
Glomerular filtration rate	GFR	ml plasma/min	$\dfrac{U_{inulin}}{P_{inulin}} \times V$
Filtered load of substance Z	F_Z	μEq/min or mg/min	$GFR \times P_Z$
Tubular reabsorption of substance Z	Tr_Z	μEq/min or mg/min	$GFR \times P_Z - U_Z \times V$
Tubular secretion of substance Z	Ts_Z	μEq/min or mg/min	$U_Z \times V - GFR \times P_Z$
Fraction of substance Z bound to protein	fpr	decimal fraction	Measurement by dialysis
Tubular secretion when substance Z is partially bound to protein	Ts_Z	μEq/min or mg/min	$U_Z \times V - GFR \times P_Z \times fpr_Z$
Tubular maximum reabsorption of substance Z	Tm_Z	μEq/min or mg/min	$U_Z V$ when tubular secretion becomes constant with increasing P_Z
Effective renal plasma flow	ERPF	ml/min	C_{PAH}, or $P_{PAH} V / P_{PAH}$
Hematocrit	HCT	ml RBC/ml blood	Measurement
Effective renal blood flow	ERBF	ml/min	$RPF/(1 - HCT)$
Filtration fraction	FF	decimal fraction	$\dfrac{U_{inulin}}{P_{inulin}} \times \dfrac{P_{PAH}}{U_{PAH}}$
Osmotic clearance	C_{osm}	ml plasma/min	$\dfrac{U_{osm}}{P_{osm}} \times V$
Free water clearance	C_{H_2O}	ml H_2O/min	$V - C_{osm}$, or $V\left(1 - \dfrac{U_{osm}}{P_{osm}}\right)$
Negative free water clearance	Tc_{H_2O}	ml H_2O/min	$C_{osm} - V$, or $V\left(\dfrac{U_{osm}}{P_{osm}} - 1\right)$

As in all events related to kidney function, the immediate previous history of the patient may have a profound influence on the results. This is true of diet, activity, and drugs. For instance a high-protein diet raises the creatinine excretion and a low-protein diet does the reverse. Moderate exercise (walking) may raise the endogenous creatinine clearance, whereas strenuous exercise (running) may lower it. One problem has vexed nephrologists for as long as clearance has been studied—what to do about a low flow of urine. The square root of low volumes has been used empirically to handle this problem. We regard the difficulty as a very real one in dealing with normal, healthy, active people. A typical, normal urine flow is around one milliliter per minute. Should one impose a diuresis, or should one accept the low value as normal and go from there?

IV

The Nosology of Renal Disease

9 An Etiologic Classification of Renal Disease

Hereditary disorders
    Anatomic defects and diffuse parenchymatous involvement
        Fabry's disease
        Familial amyloidosis (familial Mediterranean fever)
        Familial nephronophthisis (medullary cystic disease)
        Familial nephrotic syndrome
        Hereditary chronic nephritis
        Medullary sponge kidney
        Microcystic disease
        Polycystic renal disease
        Others
    Tubular nephropathies
        Primary disorders
            Proximal
                Acidosis, renal proximal tubular
                Cystinuria
                Familial renal diabetes
                Glycinuria
                Hypercalciuria
                Others
            Distal
                Acidosis, renal distal tubular
                Diabetes insipidus, renal
                Others
    Disorders secondary to inborn error of metabolism
            Alkaptonuria
            Cystinosis
            Galactosemia
            Hepatolenticular degeneration (Wilson's disease)
            Pentosuria
            Porphyrinuria
            Phenylketonuria
            Tyrosinosis
            Others

Multiple abnormalities of tubular function, uncertain etiology
    Fanconi syndrome, infantile and adult
    Hartnup disease
    Oculocerebrorenal (Lowe's) syndrome
    Others
  Hereditary disorders leading to nephrolithiasis or nephrocalcinosis
    Acidosis, renal tubular
    Cystinuria
    Glycinuria
    Hypercalciuria
    Idiopathic hypercalcemia
    Oxalosis
    Others

Congenital disorders
  Abnormalities in amount of renal tissue
    Deficient renal parenchyma
      Renal agenesis (unilateral or bilateral)
      Simple hypoplasia (unilateral, bilateral, lobular, etc.)
      Oligonephronic hypoplasia (bilateral)
      Others
    Excess renal parenchyma: supernumerary kidney
  Anatomic anomalies
    Anomalies of kidney position, form, or orientation
      Renal ectopia
      Renal fusion
      Renal-adrenal fusion
      Renal rotation
      Others
    Anomalies of renal pelvis
      Bifurcation (ramifying renal pelvis)
      Double pelves
      Extrarenal pelvis
      Pericalyceal cysts
      Pyelocalyceal cysts
      Others
    Anomalies of renal vessels
      Anomalous insertion of origin of renal arteries
      Anomalous renal arteries
      Multiple renal arteries
      Others
  Perinephric anomalies: perinephric pseudocysts
  Dysplastic anomalies (unilateral or bilateral)
    Total dysplasia (aplasia)

Without cysts
With cysts
Segmental dysplasia, with hypoplasia (Ask-Upmark kidney)
Focal dysplasia
Dysplasia associated with congenital obstruction
Others
Cystic conditions
Localized
Cortical cysts (microcystic disease)
Medullary cysts (medullary cystic disease or nephronophthisis)
Medullary sponge kidney
Others
Generalized
Polycystic renal disease
Adult
Infantile
Juvenile, associated with biliary duct fibroadenomatosis
Others
Other types of cysts
Simple (single, multiple, bilateral, unilateral)
Multilocular (unilateral or bilateral)
Peripyelic
Pyelogenic
Teratodermoid
Endometrial (Müllerian)
Other
Congenital diseases of unknown origin
Congenital glomerulosclerosis
Congenital hydronephrosis
Congenital nephrotic syndrome with microcystic disease
Nephronophthisis

Trauma
Mechanical penetrating trauma
Biopsy
Foreign bodies
Gunshot wound
Operative interference
Sharp instruments
Mechanical nonpenetrating trauma
Blunt instrument
Crush
Rupture during childbirth
Shock wave concussion

Ultrasonic waves
Others
Radiation trauma
Chromophosphate
Gold
Mercury
Plutonium
Strontium
Thorium
Others
Thermal trauma
Hyperthermia
Hypothermia
Miscellaneous trauma
Atrophy due to pressure
Cyst following trauma
Foreign body in kidney
Foreign body in pelvis
Perirenal hematoma
Retroperitoneal hemorrhage
Others

Infections
Bacteria
Brucella
E. coli
Mycobacterium tuberculosis
Proteus
Staphylococcus
Streptococcus
Miscellaneous gram-positive organisms
Miscellaneous gram-negative organisms
Metazoa
Cysticercus cellulosae (metacestode of *Taenia solium*)
Echinococcus
Schistosoma haematobium
Schistosoma japonicum
Schistosoma mansoni
Trichinella spiralis
Others
Mycotic organisms
Achromyces bovis
Cryptococcus neoformans
Histoplasma albicans

  Toxoplasma
  Others
 Protozoa
  Leishmania
  Plasmodium falciparum
  Plasmodium malariae
  Plasmodium ovale
  Plasmodium vivax
  Others
 Rickettsia organisms
  Coxiella burnettii (Q fever)
  R. orientalis (scrub typhus)
  R. prowazekii (typhus)
  R. rickettsii (Rocky Mountain spotted fever)
  Others
 Spirochaeteles
  Leptospira autumnale
  Leptospira canicola
  Leptospira icterohaemorrhagiae
  Treponema pallidum
  Others
 Viruses
  Chicken pox
  Cytomegalic inclusion disease
  Green monkey virus
  Hemorrhagic fever
  Infectious mononucleosis
  Measles
  Nephropathia epidemica
  Synpharyngitis
  Yellow fever
  Others

Biochemical or chemical injury
 Endocrine disorders
  Adrenal cortex
  Adrenal medulla
  Bartter's disease
  Hyperparathyroidism
   Primary
   Secondary
   Tertiary
  Ovary
  Pituitary, anterior
  Pituitary, posterior

Testicle
Thyroid
Others

Metabolic disorders
  Acidosis, respiratory
  Alkalosis, respiratory
  Cystinosis
  Diabetes
  Galactosemia
  Hemochromatosis
  Hypercalcemia
  Hyperuricemic nephropathy
  Kaliopenia
  Lipoidoses
  Porphyria
  Sarcoidosis
Nutritional disorders
  Imbalance
  Nutrilite deficiency
  Nutrilite excess
  Overnutrition
  Undernutrition
  Others
Abnormal deposition (storage disease)
  Amino acid storage
  Amyloid deposition
    Primary
    Secondary
  Copper storage
  Glycogen storage
  Iron storage
  Lipid storage
  Others
Toxins or poisons
  Biologic toxins
    Bacterial products (endotoxins)
    Hemolytic products; blood in the gut
    Excess hormones
    Plasma protein products
    Tissue breakdown products
    Others
  Metallic toxins
    Arsenic
    Bismuth

Chromium
Cobalt
Gold
Lead
Manganese
Others
  Nonmetallic toxins
    Amine oxidase inhibitors
    Anesthetic agents
    Antibiotics
    Iron dextran
    Phenacetin
    Osmotic diuretics
    Salicylates
    Sulfonamides
    Others
  Poisons
    Animal venom
    Agents of biologic warfare
    Cantharides
    Carbon tetrachloride and other halogenated hydrocarbons
    Mercuric salts
    Phosphorus
    Plant poisons
    Uranium salts
    Others

Circulatory disturbance
  Anoxia and hypoxia due to various disorders
    Anemia
    Cyanotic heart disease
    Hemorrhage
    High altitude
    Others
  Renal effects of disturbed circulation
    Hematuria of unknown origin
    Infarct
    Ischemia
    Juxtamedullary hypertrophy
    Necrosis
    Urine formation disturbance
  Hemodynamic renal involvement
    Cardiac failure
    Congestion, passive
    Diminished blood flow

Hypertension
Perinephritis
Polycythemia
Raised venous pressure
Shock
Sickling
Others
  Abnormalities of main renal vessels
Compression
Dilatation
Embolism
Inflammation
Ligation
Obstruction
Operative communication
Spontaneous communication
Stenosis
Thrombosis
Others
  Abnormalities of intrarenal vessels
Aneurysmal dilatation
Arteriosclerosis
Arteriovenous fistula
Compression
Fibrinoid change
Inflammation
Scarring
Thrombosis
Bland
Infected
Others

Immunologic disorders
  Conditions associated with infectious agents
Anaphylactoid (Schönlein-Henoch) purpura
Nephritis associated with subacute bacterial endocarditis
Poststreptococcal nephritis
Recurrent hematuria with nephritis
Synpharyngitic nephritis
Others
  Hypersensitivity
Allergic granulomatosis
Animal products (serum sickness)
Animal venoms
Antibiotics

Chemicals (insecticides)
Drugs (sulfonamides)
Foods (perch)
Hormones (pitressin)
Insect venoms
Plant products (pollens)
Plants (sumac)
Others
Conditions associated with urinary excretory defects
Disturbances of conduit system
In the lumen
In the wall
Outside the wall
Disturbances resulting from intrarenal defects
Aminoaciduria
Ammonium response defect
Phosphaturia
Potassium retention or loss
Sodium retention or loss
Others
Disturbances of water excretion
Anuria
Diuresis
Induced
Spontaneous
Hyposthenuria
Isosthenuria
Nocturia
Oliguria
Polyuria
Others

Disorders associated with inflammatory disorders of connective tissue
Amyloidosis
Lupus nephritis
Macroglobinemia
Polyarteritis and other vasculitis
Rheumatoid arthritis
Thrombotic thrombocytopenic purpura and other microangiopathies
(Hemolytic uremic disease)
Scleroderma
Acute
Chronic
Wegener's granulomatosis
Others

Renal disease associated with unknown mechanism
  Nephritis

Not determined or other disorders
  Preeclampsia and eclampsia
  Renal hematuria of unknown origin
  Spontaneous retroperitoneal hemorrhage

Self-induced disorders
  Compulsive water drinking
  Self-induced hematuria (Baron Münchausen syndrome)
  Self-induced glycosuria
  Self-induced proteinuria
  Self-induced (purgative-induced) potassium deficiency

Neoplastic disorders with respect to tissue of origin
  Invasive form
    Adrenal glands
    Liver
    Pancreas
    Retroperitoneal space
    Stomach
    Others
  Lymphoma and myeloproliferative disease
    Benign hematopoietic foci
    Hodgkin's disease
    Leukemia, lymphatic
    Leukemia, myelogenous
    Lymphosarcoma
    Myeloma
    Others
  Mesenchymal neoplasms
    Benign
      Adenoma
      Capillary hemangioma
      Cavernous hemangioma
      Fibroma
      Leiomyoma
      Lipoma
      Transitional cell papilloma
      Others (angiomyolipoma, hamartomas, teratomas, etc.)
    Malignant
      Renal cell carcinoma (hypernephroma)
      Wilms' tumor

Others: mucinous cystadenocarcinoma of renal pelvis, squamous
cell carcinoma of renal pelvis, transitional cell carcinoma of renal
pelvis
Metastatic neoplasms
Carcinoma
Carcinoid
Endometriosis of kidney
Sarcoma
Others

CARDINAL SYNDROMES OF RENAL DISEASE

Acute nephritis
Aldosteronism
Bartter's syndrome
Dialysis disequilibrium
Endotoxin shock
Fanconi syndrome
Glomerulonephritis, rapidly progressive
Hypertension syndrome, malignant
Michel's syndrome
Milk-alkali syndrome
Nephritis, salt-wasting
Nephrotic syndrome
Oculocerebrorenal syndrome
Preeclampsia and eclampsia
Renal failure, acute anuric or oliguric
Renal failure, acute polyuric
Renal insufficiency, chronic
Stillweger's syndrome
Transplant rejection crisis
Uremia
Vasopressin, inappropriate secretion of

A Morphologic Classification of Renal Disease

The Subcommittee on the Morphologic Classification of Renal Diseases, with the aid of several consultants, has prepared a classification of renal diseases which it hopes will be useful to clinicians as well as pathologists.

It might be reasonably argued that in some cases the classification extends beyond the confines of strict morphology, making use of clinical features or etiologic factors. For example, poststreptococcal glomerulonephritis is classified among the diffuse and generalized types of glomerulonephritis. This is correct for the acute but not for the chronic phase of the disease, which is usually focal. But to classify chronic poststreptococcal glomerulonephritis among those types of glomerulonephritis that are characteristically focal in the acute and more typical phase of the disease would be misleading. Similarly, the glomerular changes associated with cyanotic heart disease, classified among the miscellaneous glomerular lesions, are characterized by mild mesangial hypercellularity. However, it would be an error to classify this condition among the proliferative and exudative types of glomerulonephritis.

Considerable difficulty was encountered in classifying those diseases such as gout and amyloidosis, that may have equally serious effects on different segments of the nephron. No attempt was made to modify the classification according to types of functional disturbances associated with each disease. However, some "functional defects" were listed for the sake of completeness and because definite morphologic changes may be present in some of these diseases. Finally, eponyms were eliminated except in those conditions for which no satisfactory morphologic terminology was available.

MORPHOLOGIC (PATHOLOGIC) CLASSIFICATION OF RENAL DISEASES

Congenital anomalies
    Abnormalities in amount of renal tissue
        Deficiency
            Agenesis (unilateral or bilateral)
            Simple hypoplasia (unilateral or bilateral)
            Oligonephronic hypoplasia (bilateral)
            Others

Excess: supernumerary kidney
Anatomic Anomalies
  Anomalies of kidney position, form, or orientation
    Renal ectopia
    Renal fusion
    Renal-adrenal fusion
    Renal rotation
    Others
  Anomalies of renal pelvis
    Bifurcation (ramifying renal pelvis)
    Double pelves
    Extrarenal pelvis
    Pericalyceal cysts
    Pyelocalyceal cysts
    Others
  Anomalies of renal vessels
    Anomalous insertion of origin of renal arteries
    Anomalous renal arteries
    Multiple renal arteries
    Others
  Perinephric anomalies: perinephric pseudocysts
  Dysplastic anomalies
    Total dysplasia (aplasia)
      With cysts
      Without cysts
    Segmental dysplasia, with hypoplasia (Ask-Upmark kidney)
    Focal dysplasia
    Dysplasia associated with congenital obstruction
    Others
Cystic Conditions
  Localized
    Cortical cysts (microcystic disease)
    Medullary cysts (medullary cystic disease or nephronophthisis)
    Medullary sponge kidney
    Others
  Generalized
    Polycystic renal disease
      Adult
      Infantile
      Juvenile (associated with biliary duct fibroadenomatosis)
  Other types of cysts
    Simple (single, multiple, unilateral, bilateral)
    Multilocular (unilateral or bilateral)
    Peripyelic
    Pyelogenic

Teratodermoid
Endometrial (müllerian)
Others
Congenital diseases of unknown origin
Congenital glomerulosclerosis
Congenital hydronephrosis
Congenital nephrotic syndrome with microcystic disease
Nephronophthisis
Acquired induced abnormalities
Absence, surgical (complete, incomplete, unilateral, bilateral)
Atrophy
Hydronephrosis
Homograft
Hypertrophy, compensatory
Trauma
Others

Glomerular disease, predominantly
Diffuse glomerulonephritis
Proliferative (intracapillary and extracapillary)
Exudative
Generalized
Acute and chronic (sclerosing)
Not associated with systemic disease
Intracapillary, predominantly: poststreptococcal
Extracapillary, predominantly: rapidly progressive glomerulonephritis
Mesangioproliferative with circumferential mesangial extensions or
centrilobular sclerotic nodules
Other
Focal glomerulonephritis
Proliferative
Exudative (with or without necrotizing features)
Focal
Acute and chronic
Healing
Segmental scars
Associated with systemic disease
Anaphylactoid purpura
Polyarteritis nodosa
Pulmonary hemorrhagic syndromes (lung purpura)
Subacute bacterial endocarditis
Systemic lupus erythematosus
Wegener's granulomatosis
Others

Not associated with systemic disease
Idiopathic glomerulonephritis
Others
Mild glomerular reaction
Associated with functional defects
Postural proteinuria
Secondary to infectious disease
Rheumatoid arthritis
Others
Diffuse membranous glomerulonephropathy (membranous glomerulone-
phritis): associated with infections or drugs
Lipoid nephrosis (minimal change, foot process disease)
Diabetic glomerulosclerosis
Renal amyloidosis
Preeclamptic and eclamptic nephropathy
Microangiopathies (coagulopathies with or without hemolytic anemia)
Associated with adenocarcinoma
Allograft rejection
Hemolytic uremic syndrome
Associated with malignant hypertension (see under Arterial and
arteriolar diseases)
Schwartzman phenomenon (endotoxin shock)
Thrombotic thrombocytopenic purpura (TTP)
Viper venom
Others
Congenital nephrotic syndrome
Miscellaneous glomerular lesions
Associated with polycythemic states
Congenital heart disease
Cor pulmonale
High altitude
Polycythemia vera
Glomerular storage diseases
Fabry's disease
Metachromatic leukodystrophy
Tuberous sclerosis
Glomerulosclerosis associated with hepatic disease
Hypothyroidism
Hyperlasia of epithelium of the glomerular capsule

Tubular disease, predominantly
Dysproteinemias
Macroglobinemia
Multiple myeloma

Gouty nephropathy
  Primary
  Secondary
Nephrocalcinosis and nephrolithiasis
Obstructive nephropathies: hydronephrosis
Tubular degeneration
  Hydropic change (sucrose, mannitol, dextran, electrolyte disturbance,
    glycogen storage, Armanni-Ebstein lesion, toxic chemicals)
  Fatty changes (anemia, hyperlipemia, ethylene glycol, phosphorus)
  Hyaline droplets
  Inclusions
    Heavy metals: lead, bismuth, others
    Pigments: hemoglobin, myoglobin, bilirubin, others
Tubular functional defects
  Copper storage disease
  Cystinuria
  Diabetes insipidus, renal
  Fanconi syndrome and cystinosis
  Glycinuria
  Hartnup disease
  Maple sugar urine disease
  Oculocerebrorenal syndrome
  Pseudohyperparathyroidism
  Renal glycosuria
Tubular necrosis, focal or generalized
  Acute phase
  Late phase (residual damage, healing, healed)

Interstitial disease, predominantly
  Hereditary nephritis
  Infective interstitial nephritis (pyelonephritis)
    Acute
      Suppurative: bacterial, mycotic
      Nonsuppurative: bacterial, spirochetal, malarial, schistosomal,
        rickettsial, viral, including epidemic hemorrhagic fever
      Granulomatous: tubercular, mycotic, other
    Chronic
  Noninfective interstitial nephritis
    Acute
      Hypersensitivity: infectious agents, drugs, others
      Sarcoidosis
      Balkan nephritis
      Others
    Chronic
  Radiation nephritis

Miscellaneous
    Extramedullary hematopoiesis
    Papillary necrosis
    Rejection of transplanted kidney
    Sickle cell changes

Arterial and arteriolar diseases
  Juxtaglomerular
    Hypertrophy
      Bartter's syndrome
      Hyponatremic hypertrophy
      Ischemic hypertrophy
    Others
  Extraparenchymal (main renal arteries and major branches with or without hypertension)
    Atherosclerosis
    Mural disease
      Adventitial fibrosis
      Fibromuscular hyperplasia
    Others
      Arterovenous fistula
      Aneurysm
      Extrinsic compression
  Parenchymal
    Arterial nephrosclerosis
    Arterial and arteriolar nephrosclerosis (essential or benign hypertension)
    Arterial intimal fibroelastosis and arteriolar necrosis
      Malignant hypertension
      Scleroderma (progressice systemic sclerosis)
    Atherosclerosis
    Arteritis (polyarteritis nodosa, anaphylactoid purpura, etc.)
    Diabetic arteriolar disease (see Glomerular disease, predominantly)
    Embolism
    Infarction
    Microangiopathies
      Hemolyticuremic syndrome
      Thrombotic thrombocytopenic purpura
      Schwartzman phenomenon (see Glomerular disease, predominantly)
      Others
  Thrombosis

Disease of veins and venules
  Increased venous pressure
    Chronic heart failure

Constrictive pericarditis
Tricuspid stenosis
Inferior vena cava obstruction
Phlebitis
Renal vein thrombosis (primary and secondary)
Adult
Infantile

Lymphatic abnormalities

Nerve abnormalities

Neoplasms
Mesenchymal
Adenoma
Benign
Capillary hemangioma
Cavernous hemangioma
Fibroma
Leiomyoma
Lipoma
Transitional cell papilloma
Others (angiomyolipoma, hamartomas, teratomas)
Malignant
Renal cell carcinoma (hypernephroma)
Wilms' tumor
Others
Mucinous cystadenocarcinoma of renal pelvis
Squamous cell carcinoma of renal pelvis
Transitional cell carcinoma of renal pelvis
Metastatic
Carcinoma
Carcinoid
Endometriosis
Sarcoma
Others

V

Criteria for Evaluation of Impairment in Renal Disease

11   Evaluation of the Severity of Established Renal Disease

In the absence of uniform criteria for the description of patients with chronic renal disease, it is difficult to assess the severity of a patient's illness, to determine his need for a specific therapy, and to evaluate therapeutic effectiveness, unless a detailed clinical resume is available. The Renal Section of the Council on Circulation of the American Heart Association has attempted to develop criteria to assist in the more uniform description of the patient with chronic renal disease. It is hoped that these criteria, besides serving as a shorthand index of severity of disease in individual patients, will be of particular value in series of cases appearing in the medical literature. Instead of such gradings as "severe renal impairment," "moderate uremia," "partially rehabilitated," and "mildly symptomatic," which are frequently used for reasons of space, a precise and more meaningful description can be given using the indexes outlined here.

In full realization that a lengthy tabulation may not be used by the busy clinician, we have kept the criteria as simple and brief as possible. Nonetheless, because of the frequent disparity between a patient's clinical manifestations of disease, the absolute reduction in his renal function, and his performance capabilities, it has been felt necessary to include all three of these categories to describe more accurately the severity of disease and its effect upon the patient.

CRITERIA

Classification of Signs and Symptoms by Severity

This classification is designed to describe the severity of the clinical manifestations of renal disease which are displayed by the patient. The patient should be placed in the highest class whose criteria are fulfilled.

Class I: Requires (a) plus one or more of (b) through (f):

      a. No symptoms directly referable to renal disease

---

* Council on the Kidney in Cardiovascular Disease, American Heart Association, 1971. © 1971, 1972 by the American Heart Association.

b. Fixed proteinuria (> 200 mg/24 hours)

c. Repeatedly abnormal urine sediment or bacteriuria in properly obtained urine specimens

d. Demonstrable radiographic abnormality of the upper GU tract

e. Hypertension attributable to past or active renal disease

f. Biopsy-proven parenchymal renal disease

Class II: Any two or more of the following:

a. Symptomatic because of symptoms *directly* referable to the kidney (e.g., hypoproteinemic edema, dysuria, flank pain, renal colic, nocturia)

b. Radiographic evidence of osteodystrophy

c. Stable anemia attributable to renal disease

d. Metabolic acidosis attributable to renal disease

e. Severe hypertension (diastolic BP > 110 mm Hg)

Class III: Any two or more of the following:

a. Symptomatic osteodystrophy

b. Symptomatic peripheral neuropathy

c. Nausea and vomiting without primary GI cause

d. Limited ability to conserve or excrete usual dietary load of sodium and water; tending to sodium depletion, dehydration, or congestive heart failure

e. Impaired mentation attributable to renal disease

Class IV: Any two or more of the following:

a. Uremic pericarditis

b. Uremic bleeding diathesis

c. Asterixis and severely impaired mentation, with or without convulsion

d. Hypocalcemic tetany

Class V: Coma

Classification of Renal Functional Impairment

Exact classification (primary criterion) should be based on measurement of the glomerular filtration rate (GFR) (commonly approximated by the creatinine clearance) when possible, since the plasma creatinine concentration may vary in the presence of muscular wasting and decreased creatinine production. When clearance values are unavailable, the plasma creatinine concentration (secondary criterion) may be used, but the subscript "c" should be added to the classification, e.g., Class D_c.

	Primary	**Secondary**
Class A:	GFR normal	Serum creatinine normal
Class B:	GFR 50–80% of predicted normal	Serum creatinine normal to 2.4 mg percent
Class C:	GFR 20–50% of predicted normal	Serum creatinine 2.5–4.9 mg percent
Class D:	GFR 10–20% of predicted normal	Serum creatinine 5.0–7.9 mg percent
Class E:	GFR 5–10% of predicted normal	Serum creatinine 8–12 mg percent
Class F:	GFR <5% of predicted normal	Serum creatinine >12 mg percent

Performance Classification

A description of what the patient thinks he is able to do and not what the physician thinks he should be able to do.

Class 1: Capable of performing all his *usual* types of physical activity.

Class 2: Unable to perform the most strenuous of *usual* types of physical activity for that particular patient, e.g., sports activity, fast walking, running, shoveling, lawn mowing.

Class 3: Unable to perform all his usual *daily* physical activities on more than a part-time basis, e.g., household duties, employment, driving an automobile, playing with children.

Class 4: Severe limitation of usual physical activity. May need assistance for some facets of self-care, e.g., shaving. Mentation may or may not be impaired. May be confined to bed.

Class 5: Semicoma or coma.

USE OF THESE CRITERIA

Patients should be placed in *one* class from *each* of the three major categories: (1) Severity of Signs and Symptoms; (2) Severity of Renal Functional Impairment; (3) Level of Performance. In each major category, the user should select the highest class whose criteria are fulfilled.

For example, a patient would be graded as II-C-1 if signs and symptoms fit Class II under Severity of Signs and Symptoms, if the creatinine clearance is 30 percent of predicted normal, and if all usual types of physical activity can be carried out. If the patient is unable to carry out his or her usual types of most strenuous physical activity, the classification would be II-C-2. If the patient develops only one Class III criterion under Severity of Signs and Symptoms (e.g., nausea and vomiting), then he or she would be left in Class II. Six months later, as osteodystrophy appears, the necessary two criteria for inclusion in Class III would be fulfilled. If, at the same time, the creatinine clearance is 4 percent of predicted normal and physical activities are limited severely, the patient would be classified as grade III-F-4.

12 Evaluation of Permanent Impairment of the Urinary System

Evaluation or rating of permanent disability has long been recognized as an important and complex subject. In the past much confusion has resulted from inadequate understanding by physicians and others of (1) the scope of medical responsibility in the evaluation of permanent disability and (2) the difference between *permanent disability* and *permanent impairment*.

It is vitally important for every physician to be aware of his proper role in the evaluation of permanent disability under any private or public program for the disabled. It is equally important for him to have the necessary authoritative material to assist him in competently fulfilling his particular responsibility—the evaluation of permanent impairment. It is the purpose of this and other reports of the Committee on Rating of Mental and Physical Impairment to correct a past confusion of terms and to provide a series of practical guides to the evaluation of various types of permanent impairments.

The following is an explanation of terms generally used in programs for the disabled.

1. *Permanent Impairment.* This is a purely medical condition. Permanent impairment is any anatomic or functional abnormality or loss after maximal medical rehabilitation has been achieved, which abnormality or loss the physician considers stable or nonprogressive at the time evaluation is made. It is always a basic consideration in the evaluation of permanent disability.

2. *Permanent Disability.* This is not a purely medical condition. A patient is "permanently disabled" or "under a permanent disability" when his actual or presumed ability to engage in gainful activity is reduced or absent because of *impairment* which, in turn, may or may not be combined with other factors. A permanent condition is found to exist if no fundamental or marked change can be expected in the future.

3. *Evaluation (Rating) of Permanent Impairment.* This is a function that physicians alone are competent to perform. Evaluation of permanent

---

* Reproduced with minor modifications from *Guides to the Evaluation of Permanent Impairment.* American Medical Association Committee on Rating of Mental and Physical Impairment, 1971. Pp. iii, iv, 123–127.

impairment defines the scope of medical responsibility and therefore represents the physician's role in the evaluation of permanent disability. Evaluation of permanent impairment is an appraisal of the nature and extent of the patient's illness or injury as it affects his personal efficiency in one or more of the activities of daily living. These activities are self-care, communication, normal living postures, ambulation, elevation, traveling, and nonspecialized hand activities.

4. *Evaluation (Rating) of Permanent Disability.* In the last analysis, this is an administrative and not solely a medical responsibility and function. Evaluation of permanent disability is an appraisal of the patient's present and future ability to engage in gainful activity as it is affected by such diverse factors as age, sex, education, and economic and social environment, in addition to the definite medical factor—permanent impairment. The first group of factors has proved extremely difficult to measure. For this reason, permanent impairment is in fact the sole or real criterion of permanent disability far more often than is readily acknowledged. However, in actual practice the final determination of permanent disability is an administrative decision as to the patient's entitlement.

Competent evaluation of permanent impairment requires adequate and complete medical examination, accurate objective measurement of function, and the avoidance of subjective impressions and of such factors as age, sex, or employability.

The Committee on Rating of Mental and Physical Impairment believes that permanent impairment cannot vary because of the circumstances of its occurrence or the geographic location of the patient at the time. Furthermore, unlike disability, permanent impairment can be measured with a reasonable degree of accuracy and uniformity, as it is evidenced by loss of structural integrity, loss of functional capacity, or persistent pain that is substantiated by clinical findings.

The Committee is familiar with the various formulas developed in the past for use in evaluation of permanent disability. These formulas are usually administrative devices which equate specific medical criteria to specific percentages of permanent partial or total disability (loss of working or earning capacity). From the medical standpoint the medical criteria may undeniably represent various anatomic or functional impairments. However, it is unrealistic to presume that all of these impairments, especially those of a minor nature, will necessarily at some time result in disability. Although a number of valuable contributions have been made in the past, the Committee has found no comprehensive practical system of the type necessary for the evaluation of permanent impairment by individual body systems or of the whole man. For this reason, the Committee undertook to prepare a series of Guides. All of the guides were developed after careful study of the literature and views of recognized authorities.

Each guide contains recommended percentage values related to the criteria provided. The use of numerical values is preferred because of difficulty in communication and variability in interpretation of such terms as "slight," "marked," and "moderate." Numerical values provide a practical means of expressing and calculating the extent of permanent impairment and encourage accurate, equitable, and uniform evaluation. Methods of calculating impairment are uniform, are explained in detail with examples, and require a minimum of computation. Generally, when a single impairment is involved, the percentage value may be read directly from the text or transposed to a relative value of a unit of the body or of the whole man by referring to appropriate tables.

When two or more impairments are involved, however, the value of each impairment must be ascertained and transposed to a common denominator, such as the whole man. Thereafter, these values must be combined rather than added. A Combined Values Chart is provided by which any combination of impairments may be easily assessed. The method generally used to combine various impairments is based on the principle that each impairment acts not on the whole part but on the portion which remains after the preceding impairment has acted. For purposes of computation, the source and chronology of the impairment values are immaterial.

After the values of all impairments involved have been computed and transposed to a common denominator, the final impairment value, whether the result of single or of combined impairments, should be expressed in terms of the nearest 5 percent.

THE URINARY SYSTEM

This guide provides criteria for evaluating the effects that permanent impairment of the urinary system has on the ability of an individual to perform the activities of daily living.

In this guide the discussion of these systems is in terms of (1) upper urinary tract, with a section on urinary diversions, (2) bladder, and (3) urethra.

METHOD OF EVALUATION. As with the other body systems, no estimation of permanent impairment should be attempted until maximal medical and surgical treatment has been carried out and a reasonable period has elapsed, so that the optimal effect of the treatment may be obtained.

Competent evaluation presupposes that the necessary facilities for clinical and laboratory examinations are available to the physician. Evaluation of impairment is usually possible through the exercise of sound clinical judgment which is based on a detailed history, a thorough physical examination, and the judicious use of necessary laboratory procedures. The text contains a number of useful techniques for evaluating impairment of the reproductive and urinary systems. It is not intended to imply by such enumeration that all the techniques listed are necessary for proper evaluation nor that only the techniques listed are to be considered.

REPORTS. When making oral or written reports, the physician should give a full account of his findings and observations before he gives any statement of conclusions. He should explain and substantiate his conclusions about the patient's impairment. He should also indicate the date on which the findings and conclusions were determined.

Upper Urinary Tract

The parenchyma of the kidneys produces urine, which is conducted by the renal calyces, pelves, and ureters to the urinary bladder. The kidney is an important homeostatic regulatory organ. The manner in which renal and conduit abnormalities may affect the whole man can range from clinically undetectable homeostatic changes to marked specific and generalized manifestations of deterioration of nephron reserve and urine transport impediment.

SYMPTOMS AND SIGNS OF IMPAIRMENT OF FUNCTIONS OF THE UPPER URINARY TRACT. These may include changes in micturition; edema; impairment of physical stamina; loss of weight and appetite; anemia; uremia; loin, abdominal, or costovertebral angle pain; chills and fever; hypertension and its complications; abnormalities in the appearance of the urine or its sediment; and biochemical changes in the blood. It is to be noted that renal disease may often be revealed only on the basis of laboratory investigation.

OBJECTIVE TECHNIQUES USEFUL IN EVALUATING FUNCTION OF THE UPPER URINARY TRACT. Two clinically useful determinations of renal function—the renal clearance of endogenous creatinine and the 15-minute intravenous phenolsulfonphthalein test (PSP)—can ordinarily serve as guidelines for evaluating function of the upper urinary tract.

Measurement of renal clearance of endogenous creatinine (glomerular filtration rate) gives a quantitative estimate of the total functioning nephron population. The reliability of clearance tests of renal function is improved by longer periods of urine collection; therefore, measurement of the 24-hour endogenous creatinine clearance should be used. The normal ranges of creatinine clearance are 130 to 200 liters/24 hr (90 to 139 ml/min) in men, and 115 to 180 liters/24 hr (80 to 125 ml/min) in women.

The 15-minute intravenous PSP test, although affected by stasis in conduit transport of urine, is a clinically useful determination of the general adequacy of renal tubular transport mechanisms. For the test to be valid, the patient must be adequately hydrated and precisely 1 cc of solution containing 6.0 mg of PSP must be injected intravenously, preferably by tuberculin syringe. The normal dye excretion is 25 percent or more in urine in 15 minutes.

If there are any discrepancies in these two tests, e.g., if the glomerular filtration rate is out of proportion to the PSP test (tubular-glomerular imbalance), then it may be desirable to perform additional investigations, such as metabolic studies, serum and urine biochemical determinations, osmolality measurements, concentration-dilution tests, urine analysis, cultures, radiographic investigation, isotope renograms and scans.

Assessment of parenchymal disfigurement and/or conduit abnormality, which by virtue of clinical manifestations impair the function of the whole man, may require such diagnostic procedures as endoscopy with total and separate function studies, biopsy, arteriography and uroradiographic evaluation.

Criteria for Evaluating Impairment of the Upper Urinary Tract

In most instances of stable loss of upper urinary tract function, diminution in creatinine clearance is commensurate with depression of PSP excretion. If a discrepancy exists between these two tests, then additional diagnostic studies should be performed to determine which test is most representative of the loss of upper urinary tract function, and the results of that test used in determining the degree of impairment.

It is to be noted that an individual with a solitary kidney, from a physiologic point of view, may have no actual impairment of renal function; nevertheless, there exists an absence or loss of the normal safety factor which may be of potential significance in subsequently evaluating the disability depending on the cause of the solitary kidney. The individual with a solitary kidney, regardless of cause, should be rated as having 10 percent impairment of the whole man because he has had a structural loss of an essential organ. This value is to be *combined* with any other permanent impairment (including any impairment in the remaining kidney) pertinent to the case under consideration.

CLASS 1—IMPAIRMENT OF WHOLE MAN—0%–10%. A patient belongs in Class 1 when (1) diminution of upper urinary tract function as evidenced by creatinine clearance of 75 to 90 liters/24 hr (52 to 62.5 ml/min) and PSP excretion of 15% to 20% in 15 minutes is present; OR (2) intermittent symptoms and signs of upper urinary tract dysfunction not requiring continuous treatment or surveillance are present.

Example 1: A 22-year-old man when he was 12 years of age developed backache, fever, hematuria, headache, and hypertension during an epidemic of β-hemolytic streptococcal tonsillitis. He was edematous and oliguric, and his renal functions were depressed. The urine contained numerous red blood cells and red blood cell casts, and he passed 2.4 gm protein per 24 hours. The creatinine clearance was 72 liters/24 hr (50 ml/min).

After a stormy illness and a long convalescence, he improved and was well except for microscopic hematuria, which persisted for months but finally cleared. Six months after the illness, the creatinine clearance was 130 liters/24 hr (90 ml/min). Current follow-up studies reveal a healthy man with no evidence of renal disease by biopsy and a creatinine clearance of 158 liters/24 hr (110 ml/min).

Diagnosis: Healthy kidneys, complete recovery from poststreptococcal acute glomerulonephritis.

Impairment: 0% impairment of the whole man.

Example 2: A 40-year-old man had an acute episode of renal colic. He later passed a small stone. He had had two prior episodes of colic with spontaneous passage of stone. Urograms were interpreted as normal; no evidence of metabolic disease is present. Urine, creatinine clearance, and PSP determinations are within normal limits.

Diagnosis: Recurrent ureteral calculi.

Impairment: 5% impairment of the whole man.

CLASS 2—IMPAIRMENT OF WHOLE MAN—15%–30%. A patient belongs in Class 2 when (1) diminution of upper urinary tract function as evidenced by creatinine clearance of 60 to 75 liters/24 hr (42 to 52 ml/min) and PSP excretion of 10% to 15% in 15 minutes is present; OR (2) although creatinine clearance is greater than 75 liters/24 hr (52 ml/min) and PSP excretion is more than 15% in 15 minutes, symptoms and signs of upper urinary tract disease or dysfunction necessitate continuous surveillance and frequent treatment.

Example 1: A 45-year-old man with a history of nephritis as a child was subjected to emergency appendectomy and drainage of an appendiceal abscess. Despite an adequate urinary output during the postoperative period, the serum creatinine rose to 2.8 mg/100 cc. Convalescence was prolonged; his anemia subsided gradually and physical stamina returned slowly. Now, six months postoperatively, the patient feels well and is able to engage in most of his usual activities of daily living. The urine shows a trace of protein (0.75 gm/24 hr). Excretory urograms delineate no architectural abnormality, but the creatinine clearances range from 60 to 70 liters/24 hr (42 to 49 ml/min), and the PSP excretion ranges between 15% and 20% in 15 minutes.

Diagnosis: Asymptomatic persistent proteinuria.

Impairment: 15% impairment of the whole man.

Example 2: A 50-year-old woman was successfully operated on for parathyroid adenoma. She continues to have periodic attacks of pyelonephritis occasioned by residual calculi in both kidneys. She sporadically passes stones. The infrequent clinical attacks of pyelonephritis respond to antibiotics. The symptoms of her ineradicable urinary infection are controlled by continuous medication. The creatinine clearance is stable at approximately 65 liters/24 hr (45 ml/min) and the PSP excretion at 10% in 15 minutes. The bilateral pyelocalyceal deformities and the size of the kidneys, as delineated by excretory urography, have not changed appreciably in a three-year period.

Diagnosis: Renal calculi and bilateral chronic pyelonephritis.

Impairment: 30% due to upper urinary tract impairment which is to be combined with an appropriate value for parathyroid impairment to determine the impairment of the whole man.

Example 3: A 52-year-old man had surgical reconstruction of his left lower ureter because of severe damage to its function from retroperitoneal fibrosis. Despite architectural and apparent functional normalcy of the kidney on the side of the ureteral repair, vesicoureteral reflux can be demonstrated, and repetitive attacks of pyelonephritis have occurred whenever antibacterial medication has been discontinued. The creatinine clearance is 100 liters/24 hr (69 ml/min), and the PSP excretion is 25% in 15 minutes. Since the involved kidney is normal in appearance and has shown no deterioration of function, no further surgical intervention is contemplated.

Diagnosis: Active unilateral chronic pyelonephritis secondary to vesicoureteral reflux.

Impairment: 15% impairment of the whole man.

Example 4: A 36-year-old man, during an insurance examination, was found to have proteinuria. He had been rejected by the army at age 18 because of a similar finding.

The creatinine clearance was 86 liters/24 hr (60 ml/min). A renal biopsy was performed. Through special stains and by electron microscopic examination, a very mild diffuse and generalized membranous glomerulonephritis was noted.

Yearly follow-up studies over six years have revealed no change in the level of proteinuria. The creatinine clearance has fluctuated around 72 liters/24 hr (50 ml/min).

Diagnosis: Chronic membranous nephritis.

Impairment: 25% impairment of the whole man.

CLASS 3—IMPAIRMENT OF WHOLE MAN—35%–60%. A patient belongs in Class 3 when (1) diminution of upper urinary tract function, as evidenced by creatinine clearance of 40 to 60 liters/24 hr (28 to 42 ml/min) and PSP excretion of 5% to 10% in 15 minutes, is present; OR (2) although creatinine clearance is 60 to 75 liters/24 hr (42 to 52 ml/min) and PSP excretion is 10% to 15% in 15 minutes, symptoms and signs of upper urinary tract disease or dysfunction are incompletely controlled by surgical or continuous medical treatment.

Example 1: A 52-year-old woman complained of chronic fatigue. On examination she was found to have elevation of the serum creatinine and a moderate anemia. A clear-cut history of nephritis was not obtainable. A renal biopsy demonstrated diffuse proliferative glomerulonephritis. A high-dose excretory urogram delineated contracted kidneys but normal pyelocalyceal architecture. Results of urine culture were negative; creatinine clearance was 50 liters/24 hr (35 ml/min), and PSP excretion was 10% in 15 minutes.

Diagnosis: Chronic glomerulonephritis with contracted kidneys.

Impairment: 60% due to upper urinary tract impairment, which is to be combined with an appropriate value for the anemia to determine the impairment of the whole man.

Example 2: A 48-year-old man was found to have residual calculi in the minor calyces of both kidneys. He has had multiple endoscopic and open surgical procedures for stone removal. There is marked diminution in the size of one kidney, and there are bilateral pyelographic architectural changes incident to previous surgical procedures and recurrent pyelonephritis. Despite continuous antibacterial medication, the urine remains infected, and periodic episodes of chills, fever, and back pain occur. Creatinine clearance is 65 liters/24 hr (45 ml/min), and PSP excretion is 10% in 15 minutes.

Diagnosis; Renal calculi with bilateral recurrent pyelonephritis.

Impairment: 50% impairment of the whole man.

Example 3: A 52-year-old man was found to have bilateral congenital ureteropelvic junction obstruction, marked hydronephrosis, and bilateral renal calculi. The urine was infected and renal function was depressed. After removal of the calculi and bilateral pyeloplasty, renal function improved and stabilized, but architectural abnormalities have persisted. The creatinine clearance is 70 liters/24 hr (49 ml/min), and the PSP excretion is 15% in 15 minutes. Despite arrest of the functional and anatomic deterioration, occasional episodes of severe pyelonephritis continue to occur.

Diagnosis: Irreparable hydronephrotic changes secondary to congenital ureteropelvic junction obstruction; recurrent pyelonephritis.

Impairment: 35% impairment of the whole man.

Example 4: A 48-year-old man was injured in an automobile accident and developed hematuria. Radiologic studies revealed that the left kidney was damaged. The blood pressure was 150/90 mm Hg. No other abnormalities were noted. He was kept at bedrest in a hospital for a week and then discharged.

Six months later he began to complain of severe headaches. The blood pressure was found to be 240/160 mm Hg, and malignant hypertensive retinopathy was noted.

Investigation revealed a creatinine clearance of 40 liters/24 hr (28 ml/min) and clear-cut evidence of left renovascular hypertension was found. The left kidney was removed. Biopsies from the right kidney revealed malignant hypertensive change. Hilstologic studies of the left kidney revealed ischemia and juxtaglomerular hypertrophy.

Immediately after the operation, the blood pressure fell to 170/110 mm Hg and, during the next six months, leveled off at 155/95 mm Hg. The eyegrounds regressed to Grade 11 (Keith-Wagner) and creatinine clearance rose slowly and has leveled off at 58 liters/24 hr (40 ml/min).

Diagnosis: Left nephrectomy for malignant hypertension due to post-traumatic renovascular ischemia of the left kidney; arteriolonephrosclerosis of the right kidney; and hypertensive vascular disease.

Impairment: 55% due to arteriolonephrosclerosis and 10% due to nephrectomy, which combine to 60% impairment of the whole man, which should be combined with an appropriate value for the cardiovascular impairment.

CLASS 4—IMPAIRMENT OF WHOLE MAN—65%–90%. A patient belongs in Class 4 when (1) diminution of upper urinary tract function as evidenced by creatinine clearance below 40 liters/24 hr (28 ml/min) and PSP excretion below 5% in 15 minutes is present; OR (2) although creatinine clearance is 40 to 60 liters/24 hr (28 to 42 ml/min) and PSP excretion is 5% to 10% in 15 minutes, symptoms and signs of upper urinary tract disease or dysfunction persist despite surgical or continuous medical treatment.

Example 1. A 44-year-old man with a family history of polycystic renal disease experienced loin pain and noted gross hematuria. Endoscopy and retrograde urograms revealed bilateral deformities characteristic of polycystic kidneys. During the past two years the serum creatinine has risen from 8 to 10 mg/100 cc. Until this time the patient had been working regularly and had been relatively asymptomatic. He is maintained on a diet restricted in protein. The creatinine clearance is 35 liters/24 hr (24 ml/min), and the PSP excretion is less than 5% in 15 minutes.

Diagnosis: Bilateral polycystic renal disease; advanced renal insufficiency.

Impairment: 70% impairment of the whole man.

Example 2. A 56-year-old man with bilateral nephrostomies occasioned by obliterative fibrotic ureteral disease of unknown etiology has had removal of renal calculi. An attempt to reconstitute normal conduit function through surgery was unsuccessful. Although the urinary infection is ineradicable, the only complaints are hematuria when the nephrostomy tubes are changed and occasional episodes of pyelonephritis. He continues to engage in most of his usual activities of daily living. The creatinine clearance is approximately 50 liters/

24 hr (35 ml/min), and the PSP excretion is between 5% and 10% in 15 minutes.

Diagnosis: Pyeloureteral disease requiring bilateral nephrostomy diversion.

Impairment: 65% due to pyeloureteral disease and 15% due to bilateral nephrostomies, which combine to 70% impairment of the whole man.

Example 3. A 52-year-old woman, seven years after anterior pelvic exenteration and uretero-ileostomy for carcinoma of the cervix, has no evidence of recurrent cancer. She has had calculi removed from both kidneys and experiences periodic episodes of pyelonephritis even on continual medication. Radiographic changes of pyelonephritis are present. The creatinine clearance is approximately 60 liters/24 hr (24 ml/min), and PSP excretion is about 10% in 15 minutes.

Diagnosis: Uretero-ileostomy urinary diversion and chronic bilateral pyelonephritis.

Impairment: 65% due to bilateral pyelonephritis, 10% due to ureteroileostomy, and 55% due to pelvic exenteration (excision of bladder, lower ureters, uterus, cervix, vagina, fallopian tubes, and ovaries), which combine to 85% impairment of the whole man.

Example 4. A young woman became anuric following severe abruptio placentae. A percutaneous renal biopsy was performed. Renal cortical necrosis was diagnosed and periodic courses of peritoneal dialyses were instituted. After 49 days of anuria and then oliguria, the urine output increased; and on the 60th day the serum creatinine, which was 21.9 mg/100 cc on that day, began to fall without the aid of peritoneal dialysis. Now, four months later, she can perform most of the activities of daily living, despite severely compromised renal function; the creatinine clearance has leveled off at 11.5 liters/24 hr (8 ml/min).

Diagnosis: Renal cortical necrosis; chronic renal failure, severe.

Impairment: 90% impairment of the whole man.

This classification without examples is shown in Table 1.

Urinary Diversion

Permanent, surgically created forms of urinary diversion are usually provided to compensate for anatomic loss and to allow for egress of urine. They are evaluated as a part of, and in conjunction with, the assessment of that portion of the urinary tract which is involved.

Irrespective of how well these diversions function in the preservation of renal integrity and the disposition of urine, the following values for the diversions should be combined with those determined under the criteria previously given for the portion of the urinary tract involved:

	Impairment of Whole Man, %
Uretero-intestinal diversions	10
Cutaneous ureterostomy without intubation	10
Nephrostomy or intubated ureterostomy	15

Bladder

The bladder is a voluntary controllable reservoir for urine which normally permits the patient to retain urine for several hours.

SYMPTOMS AND SIGNS OF IMPAIRMENT OF FUNCTION OF THE BLADDER.
These may include urinary frequency, painful voiding (dysuria), urgency, incontinence, involuntary retention of urine, hematuria, pyuria, crystalluria, passage of urinary calculi, and a suprapubic mass.

OBJECTIVE TECHNIQUES USEFUL IN EVALUATING FUNCTION OF THE BLADDER.
These include, but are not limited to, cystoscopy, cystography, voiding cystourethrography, cystometry, urofluorometry, urinalysis, and urine cultures.

Criteria for Evaluating Permanent Impairment of the Bladder

In evaluating permanent impairment of the bladder, the status of the upper urinary tract must also be considered. The appropriate impairment values for both should be combined in determining the extent of impairment of the whole man.

CLASS 1—IMPAIRMENT OF WHOLE MAN—0%–10%. A patient belongs in Class 1 when there are symptoms and signs of bladder disorder requiring intermittent treatment, but without intervening malfunction.

Example. A 41-year-old woman had been treated with radium 20 years previously for uterine fibroids. Recently, episodes of urinary bleeding occasioned by postradiation telangiectasia of the bladder have required emergency hospitalization and vessel fulguration under anesthesia. The episodes have varied in frequency from one to two weeks to six months. Between attacks, findings from blood and urine studies are normal. After each episode she is able to resume her usual activities within seven days.
Diagnosis: Postradiation telangiectasia of the bladder.
Impairment; 10% impairment of the whole man.

CLASS 2—IMPAIRMENT OF WHOLE MAN—15%–20%. A patient belongs in Class 2 when (1) there are symptoms and/or signs of bladder disorder requiring continuous treatment; OR (2) there is good bladder reflex activity BUT no voluntary control.

Example 1. A 47-year-old man developed such progressive urinary frequency that he was voiding at intervals of every 10 to 15 minutes day and night. The diagnosis of interstitial cystitis was established, but the usual treatment, bladder dilatation with various agents, was ineffective. The upper urinary tract was normal and uninfected. After a ureterosigmoidostomy he was able to resume his usual activities.
Diagnosis: Contracted fixed bladder requiring urinary diversion.
Impairment: 15% due to contracted fixed bladder and 10% due to ureterosigmoidostomy, which combine to 25% impairment of the whole man.

NOTE: The removal of the bladder for any reason and a resultant urinary diversion should be assigned a similar rating of impairment.

Example 2. A 42-year-old man with chronic renal infection, resistant to antibiotic therapy, developed a severe cystitis which required him to empty his bladder at intervals of less than 30 minutes and necessitated the use of a urine collection device. Though his general physical condition was excellent, the urine contained numerous white blood cells and a few red blood cells.

Table 1. Classes of Upper Urinary Tract Impairment*

Class 1 Impairment 0%–10%	Class 2 Impairment 15%–30%	Class 3 Impairment 35%–60%	Class 4 Impairment 65%–90%
Diminution of upper urinary tract function as evidenced by creatinine clearance of 75 to 90 liters/24 hr (52 to 62.5 ml/min) and PSP excretion of 15% to 20% in 15 minutes is present.	Diminution of upper urinary tract function as evidenced by creatinine clearance of 60 to 75 liters/24 hr (42 to 52 ml/min) and PSP excretion of 10% to 15% in 15 minutes is present.	Diminution of upper urinary tract function as evidenced by creatinine clearance of 40 to 60 liters/24 hr (28 to 42 ml/min) and PSP excretion of 5% to 10% in 15 minutes is present.	Diminution of upper tract function as evidenced by creatinine clearance below 40 liters/24 hr (28 ml/min) and PSP excretion below 5% in 15 minutes is present.
OR	OR	OR	OR
Intermittent symptoms and signs of upper urinary tract dysfunction not requiring continuous treatment or surveillance are present.	Although creatinine clearance is greater than 75 liters/24 hr (52 ml/min) and PSP excretion is more than 15% in 15 minutes, symptoms and signs of upper urinary tract disease or dysfunction necessitate continuous surveillance and frequent treatment.	Although creatinine clearance is 60 to 75 liters/24 hrs (42 to 52 ml/min) and PSP excretion is 10% to 15% in 15 minutes, symptoms and signs of upper urinary tract disease or dysfunction are incompletely controlled by surgical or continuous medical treatment.	Although creatinine clearance is 40 to 60 liters/24 hr (28 to 42 ml/min) and PSP excretion is 5% to 10% in 15 minutes, symptoms and signs of upper urinary tract disease or dysfunction persist despite surgical or continuous medical treatment.

* NOTE: The individual with a solitary kidney, regardless of cause, should be rated as having 10% impairment of the whole man. This value is to be combined with any other permanent impairment (including any impairment in the remaining kidney) pertinent to the case under consideration. The normal ranges of creatinine clearance are: Males: 130 to 200 liters/24 hr (90 to 139 ml/min). Females: 115 to 180 liters/24 hr (80 to 125 ml/min). The normal PSP excretion is 25% or more in urine in 15 minutes.

He refused the recommended surgical urinary diversion. As a result, he cannot retain his urine for a sufficient length of time to permit him to perform many of the activities of daily living.

Diagnosis: Chronic cystitis.

Impairment: 20% due to cystitis which is to be combined with an appropriate value for the upper urinary tract disorder to determine the impairment of the whole man.

CLASS 3—IMPAIRMENT OF WHOLE MAN—25%–35%. A patient belongs in Class 3 when the bladder has poor reflex activity (intermittent dribbling) and no voluntary control.

CLASS 4—IMPAIRMENT OF WHOLE MAN—40%–60%. A patient belongs in Class 4 when there is no reflex or voluntary control of the bladder (continuous dribbling).

Urethra

In the female the urethra is a urinary conduit containing a voluntary urethral sphincter. In the male the urethra is a conduit for urine and seminal ejaculations, and possesses a voluntary urethral sphincter and propulsive musculature.

SYMPTOMS AND SIGNS OF IMPAIRMENT OF FUNCTION OF THE URETHRA. These include dysuria, diminished urinary stream, urinary retention, incontinence, extraneous or ectopic openings, periurethral mass or masses, and diminished urethral caliber.

OBJECTIVE TECHNIQUES USEFUL IN EVALUATING FUNCTION OF THE URETHRA. These include, but are not limited to, urethroscopy, urethrography, cystourethrography, endoscopy, urethrometry, and cystometrography.

Criteria for Evaluating Permanent Impairment of the Urethra

When evaluating permanent impairment of the urethra, the status of the upper urinary tract and bladder must also be considered. The appropriate values for all should be combined in determining the extent of impairment in the whole man.

CLASS 1—IMPAIRMENT OF WHOLE MAN—0%–5%. A patient belongs in Class 1 when symptoms and signs of urethral disorder are present which require intermittent therapy for control.

Example. As the result of an injury, a 27-year-old man has a urethral stricture which requires dilatation every few weeks. Between dilatations he is entirely free of symptoms and has difficulty only when the urethra gradually constricts, at which time he notices ever-increasing difficulty in voiding. There is no associated upper urinary tract infection.

Diagnosis: Traumatic urethral stricture.

Impairment: 5% impairment of the whole man.

CLASS 2—IMPAIRMENT OF WHOLE MAN—10%–20%. A patient belongs in Class 2 when there are symptoms and signs of urethral disorder which cannot be effectively controlled by treatment.

Example 1. A 23-year-old man experienced considerable laceration of the ventral surface of the penis which created a surgically uncorrectable fistula. He was able to perform most of the activities of daily living, but could not void normally. He could ejaculate with sexual awareness, but the fistula was so situated that impregnation was impossible.

Diagnosis: Urethral fistula.

Impairment: 15% due to urethral fistula and 10% due to impaired sexual function, which combine to 25% impairment of the whole man.

Example 2. After an automobile accident, a 31-year-old man experienced a urethral stricture which necessitated weekly or biweekly urethral dilatations. Because of the magnitude of the injury to the urethra, corrective surgery was ineffective. Repeated urinary tract infections secondary to urethral dilatations continue to occur, and pyelonephritis has developed. The creatinine clearance is 65 liters/24 hr (45 ml/min), and PSP excretion is 10% in 15 minutes.

Diagnosis: Traumatic urethral stricture with chronic pyelonephritis.

Impairment: 20% due to urethral stricture and 25% due to upper urinary tract damage, which combine to 40% impairment of the whole man.

Example 3. A 21-year-old factory worker was crushed between a lift and a wall. His bony pelvis was fractured, his urethra was totally severed at the apex of the prostate, and his perineum was severely lacerated. Immediate reconstructive urethral surgery was unsuccessful, and one year after the accident a urinary diversion procedure was necessary (ureterosigmoidostomy), which resulted in hydronephrosis of the right kidney with repeated urinary tract infections. This diversion was subsequently converted to a conduit, and renal infection occurred only sporadically thereafter. He is now totally impotent. The pelvic fracture healed without evidence of musculoskeletal impairment, but, because of his occasional urinary tract infections, he periodically is unable to perform some of the activities of daily living. Creatinine clearance is 70 liters/24 hr (49 ml/min).

Diagnosis: Severed urethra, hydronephrosis with recurring urinary tract infections, impotency.

Impairment: 20% due to severed urethra, 30% due to upper urinary tract impairment, 10% due to uretero-ileostomy, and 30% due to loss of sexual function, which combine to 65% impairment of the whole man.

Index

Diagnostic criteria—*Continued*
   polycystic renal disease, 185
   preeclampsia and eclampsia, 185–187
   primary aldosteronism, 303–304
   pyelonephritis, 187
     acute nonobstruction, 187
     asymptomatic, 187
   radiation nephritis, 188–189
   radiologic examinations, 257–293. *See
     also* Radiologic techniques
   renal arterial disease, 304
   renal failure, 189
     acute anuric or oliguric, 189
     acute tubular necrosis, 189
   renal insufficiency, 189–190
     acute nonobstructive, 189
     acute polyuric, 189–190
   renal osteodystrophy, 190
   renal rickets, 190
   renal schistosomiasis, 190–192
   renovascular hypertension, 191–193
   Schönlein-Henoch purpura, 193–194
   sponge kidney, medullary, 194
   tuberculosis, renal, 194–195
   urinary tract infections, 223–232
   uropathy, obstructive, 195
Dialysance, 87
Dialysate, 113
Dialysis, kidney, 113
   peritoneal, 113
Dialysis disequilibrium syndrome, 153–154
Diffusion, 87
   nonionic, 87–88
Dilatation, renal arteries, 106
   aneurysmal, 106
   poststenotic, 106
Dip slide technique, 226
   screening tests, 225
Disability, evaluation of permanent, 349
Disappearance curve, 101
Disequilibrium pH, 84
Diuresis, 88
   induced, 88
   osmotic, 88
   spontaneous, 88
   water, 88
Diuretics, 88
Doll kidney, 127
Drip infusion technique, 162
Dromedary hump, 162
Droplets, 54–55
   hyaline, 54
   lipid, 54–55
   lipofuscin granule, 55
   protein, 55
Ducts, 7–8
   anatomy, 7–8
   collecting ducts, 7–8
   connecting segments, 7
   duct of Bellini, 8
   mesonephric ducts, 8
   papillary, 8, 33
   pronephric, 8
   wolffian, 33
Dunbar's crescent, 162
Dwarf kidney, 127
Dysplasia, renal, 113–114, 116
   anomalies, 324–325
   hypoplasia with, 127
Dysproteinemia, 114
Dysuria, 88

Eclampsia, 156–157
Ectopia, renal, 114
   crossed, 114
   simple, 114
Edema, 50, 51, 55–56
   endothelial cell, 55
   epithelial cell (podocyte), 55
   interstitial, 55
   tubular, 55
Efferent arterioles, 8, 25, 35
   medullary, 35
Embolism, renal arteries, 106
Embryoma, 151
Encephalopathy, hypertensive, 114
Endocarditis, subacute bacterial, associated with nephritis, 114
   diagnostic criteria, 173–174
Endocrine disorders, 327–328
Endocytic apparatus, 8, 31
Endopeptidases, 82
Endothelial cells, 5–6
   edema, 55
Endothelium, 22
   capillary wall of glomerulus, 4
Endotoxin shock, 154
   diagnostic criteria, 174
Enhancement, 41
Enuresis, 88, 114
Eosinophils, 67
Epidemic hemorrhagic fever, 114
Epinephrine
   metabolic pathways of norepinephrine and, 300
   in renal venography, 293
Epithelial cells (podocytes), 4–6
   edema, 55
   inclusions, 66
Epithelium, visceral, 24
Erythropoietin, 88
Essential hypertension, 125
Ethylene glycol nephrotoxicity, 115
Etiologic classification of renal disease, 323–333
   abnormal deposition (storage disease), 328
   biochemical or chemical injury, 327
     endocrine disorders, 327–328

Hemorrhagic fever, epidemic, 114
Hemorrhagic pulmonary renal syndrome, 132, 178
Hemosiderosis, 121
Henle, loop of, 10, 19
Hepatic fibrosis and renal lesions, 121–122
Hepatolenticular degeneration, 110, 248
Hepatomas, 77
Hereditary disorders, 323–324
  anatomic defects and diffuse parenchymatous involvement, 323
  chronic nephritis, 249
  leading to nephrolithiasis or nephrocalcinosis, 324
  multiple abnormalities of tubular function, 324
  tubular nephropathies, 323
Heterologous, 41–42
Heterophagy, 10
Heymann's nephrosis, 42
High altitude hypoxia, 128
Hilus, glomerular, 9, 17
Histocompatibility, 42
History of patient, 310, 320
HL-A unit, 42
Hodgkin's disease, renal involvement in, 122
Homologous, 42
Hospitals, metabolic ward, 309–311
Howard test, 192
Hyalin, 62
Hyaline casts, 53
  in urinary sediment, 213, 214
Hyaline deposits, 58
Hyaline droplets, 54
Hyaline lesions, 62–64
Hyaline thrombi, 77
Hydrogen secretion, 91
Hydronephrosis, 122
Hydropic change, 55
Hypercalcemia, 122
  conjunctival metastatic calcification and, 247–248
  ophthalmic diagnosis, 249
Hypercalciuria, 122
Hypercellularity (hyperplasia), 64–65
  extracapillary, 64
  glomerular, 64
  intracapillary or endocapillary, 65
  tubular, 64
Hypergranulation, juxtaglomerular cells, 65
Hyperkalemia, 122–123
Hyperlipidemia, 123
Hypernatremia, 123
Hyperparathyroidism and impaired renal function, 123
Hyperphosphatemia, 123
Hyperplasia, 64–65

fibromuscular, 116
juxtaglomerular hyperplasia with hyperaldosteronism, 153
Hypersensitivity, 123
  disorders, 330–331
Hypertension, 123–125
  arterial, 123
  benign or malignant arteriolonephrosclerosis, 124, 155
  diastolic, 123
    with renal involvement, 123
  heart disease and, 120
  laboratory aids in treatable causes of, 299–307
    determinations of aldosterone and plasma renin activity, 304–307
    pheochromocytoma, 299–302
    primary aldosteronism, 302–304
    renal arterial disease, 304
  malignant, 123, 125
    hypertension syndrome, 155
  postpartum, 125
  primary, 125
  renal, 125
  renoprival, 125
  renovascular, 125
    diagnostic criteria, 191–193
  retinopathy, 249–251
  secondary, 125
  systolic, 123
  vascular disease, 150
Hyperthermia and renal trauma, 125–126
Hypertrophy, 65–66
  degranulation and, 66
Hyperuricemic nephropathy, 126
Hypervitaminosis D, 126
Hypokalemia, 126, 153
Hypokalemic alkalosis and normal blood pressure, 153
Hypokalemic nephropathy, 126
  acute, 126
  chronic, 126
  self-induced, 126
Hyponatremia, 126
Hypophosphatemia, 127
Hypoplasia, renal, 127
  with dysplasia, 127
  lobular, 127
  oligonephronic, 127
  pluricystic, 127
  segmental, 127
  simple, 127
Hyposthenuria, 91
Hypothermia, renal trauma due to, 127–128
Hypoxia, 128, 329
  anemic, 128
  associated with chronic hypoxic lung disease, 128

Kimmelstiel-Wilson (nodular) lesion, 131
Korean fever, 115

L-forms, detection of, 227–232
Laboratory procedures
  amino acid, determination of, 245–246
  ammonia, determination of, 243–245
  antibiogram studies, 226–227
  biochemistry of renal diseases, 233–246
    creatinine, determination of, 240–242
    identification of bacteria organisms, 226–232
      detection of bacterial variants, 227–232
  metabolic ward and laboratory, 309–320
  nephron dissection, 294–298
    acid maceration, 295–296
    autoradiography of isolated nephron, 297
    collagenase maceration, 296
    measurement of, 297
    microdissection techniques, 296–297
    permanent record and photographs, 298
    selection of material, 295
  pheochromocytoma, 299–302
    clinical features, 299–300
    diagnosis, 300–302
      catecholamine assays, 301
      chemical tests, 300–302
      metanephrine assays, 301
      pharmacologic tests, 302
      vanillylmandelic acid assays, 301–302
    pathology, 299–300
  radioimmunoassay procedure for aldosterone and plasma renin activity, 307
  radiologic techniques, 257–293. *See also* Radiologic techniques
  treatable causes of hypertension, 299–307
    aldosterone and plasma renin activity, 304–307
    pheochromocytoma, 299–302
    primary aldosteronism, 302–304
    renal arterial disease, 204
  urea determination
    by urease and Berthelot reaction, 236–238
  urea nitrogen determination
    by diacetylmonoxime, 239–240
    by urease and nesslerization, 238–239
  urinalysis, 199–200
  urinary sediment, 200–224
    caution and care, 201
    collecting and handling, 200
    constituents. *See* Urinary sediment
      contamination by vaginal discharge, 220
    urinary tract infections, 224–232
      identification of organisms, 226–232
Lacis cells, 6, 26, 27
Lacis celluloconjunctif cells, 6, 13
Lamina densa, 4
Lamina fenestrata, 4
Lamina rara externa, 4
Lamina rara interna, 4
Laminagraphy, 164
Lead toxicity, 131
Leiomyomas, 78
Leptospira icterohaemorrhagiae, canicola, autumnalis, bataviae, 131
Leptospiral nephritis, 131
  diagnostic criteria, 176
Lesions, 69–70
  hyaline, 62–64
  pelvic and calyceal, 72
  segmental glomerular, 75–77
Leukemia, renal involvement in, 132
Leukocyte accumulation, 70–71
  glomerular, 70–71
  tubular, 71
Leukocyte (polymorph) casts, 53
  and white blood cell casts in urinary sediment, 212–213
Ligation, renal artery, 107
Light cells, 6, 25
Lipid droplets, 54–55
Lipofuscin granule, 55
Lipoid nephrosis, 132
  diagnostic criteria, 176–177
Lipomas, 78
Lobe, 10, 17
Lobule, 10, 18
  glomerular, 10, 19
  renal, 10, 17
Loop of Henle, 10, 19
  thick limb, 10, 19
  thin limb, 10, 19
Lowe's syndrome, 156
Lung purpura, 40
  with nephritis, 132, 177–179
    diagnostic criteria, 177–179
Lupus nephritis, 61, 62, 148
  diagnostic criteria, 179–182
Lymphangiography, 161, 291
Lymphatic capillary dilatation, 71
Lymphatic circulation, kidney, 92–93
Lymphatics, renal, 10
Lymphoma and myeloproliferative disease, 332
Lymphosarcoma, 132–133
Lysosomes, 10, 31, 65

Macula densa, 25, 26
Malacoplakia, 133
Malaria, renal involvement in, 133

Mannitol clearance, 85
Maple sugar urine disease, 133
Marchiafava-Micheli syndrome, 121
Masugi nephritis, 40
Medial fibroplasia, 116
Medulla, 11
Medullary cystic kidney, 169, 170
    diagnostic criteria, 169–171
Medullary interstitial cells, 6
Medullary lipomatosis, 71
Medullary ray, 11, 28
Medullary sponge kidney, 194, 262
Medullary zones, 11, 17, 19
Membranoid material, 71
    basement membrane abnormalities, 47
Membranoproliferative lesions, 71
Membranous glomerulonephritis, 70
Membranous nephropathy, 133
    diagnostic criteria, 179, 182–183
Membranous transformation, 71
Mercury toxicity, 133–134
    diagnostic criteria, 184
Mesangial cells, 6–7, 18–20, 22, 24
Mesangial deposits, 59, 62
Mesangial matrix, 11, 18
Mesangial stalk, 11, 19
Mesangiolysis, 71
Mesangium, 11, 20, 21, 24
Mesenchymal neoplasms, 332–333
Mesonephros, 11
Metabolic balance
    acid-base balance, 312–313, 315–316
    body composition and, 316–318
    calculation of, 311–316
    clearance studies, 318–320
    concept of turnover, 312
    definition, 311–312
    equations, 312–313
    monitoring of fluid balance, 316–317
    nitrogen balance, 313
    water balance, 312–315
        Peters-Passmore equation, 314
Metabolic disorders, 323, 328
Metabolic laboratory, 311–312
    body composition, 316–318
    calculation of metabolic balance, 311–
        316
        acid-base balance, 315–316
        nitrogen balance, 313
        water balance, 313–315
    clearance studies, 318–320
Metabolic ward, 309–311
    collection and processing of specimens,
        310–311
    nutrition, 310
    patients' environment, 310
    physical activity, 310
Metanephrines, 301
Metanephrogenic blastema, 11
Metanephros, 12

Metastatic neoplasms, 333
Methylguanidine, 236
Michel's syndrome, 155
Microangiopathy with thrombocytopenia,
    71, 148
Microbody, peroxisome, 12
Microculture technique, for urine cul-
    ture, 226
Microcystic disease, 134
Microdissection technique, 294–298
    acid maceration, 295–296
    selection of material, 295
Microperfusion, 93
Micropuncture, 93
Microscopic studies, urinary sediment,
    201–202
Microvillus, 12, 30, 57, 73
Micturition, 93, 147
Milk-alkali syndrome, 155
Miniature kidney, 127
Minimal change disease, 132
Minimal lesion disease, 132
Monge's disease, 128
Morphologic classification of renal dis-
    eases, 335–342
    arterial and arteriolar diseases, 340
    congenital anomalies, 335
    cystic conditions, 336–337
    glomerular disease, 337–338
        diffuse glomerulonephritis, 337
        focal glomerulonephritis, 337
        microangiopathies, 338
    interstitial disease, 339
    neoplasms, 341
        malignant, 341
        mesenchymal, 341
        metastatic, 341
    tubular disease, 338–339
    veins and venules, disease of, 340–341
Moschcowitz's syndrome, 148
Multilobar kidney, 12, 17
Multilocular renal cyst, 136
Münchausen, Baron, syndrome, 121
Mycoplasma, detection of, 227
Myeloma, renal involvement in, 134
Myeloproliferative diseases, 332
Myoepithelial cells, 7
Myoglobinuria, 134

Neck, tubular, 12, 21
Necrosis
    coagulation, 72
    glomerular, 72
    papillary, 113, 137, 168
        intravenous pyelograms, 265
Necrotizing angiitis, 139
Necrotizing arteritis, 139
Neoplastic disorders, 332–333, 341
    invasive form, 332

Splay, 98–99
Split renal function tests, 99
Sponge kidney, medullary, 147
    diagnostic criteria, 194
    radiologic technique, 262–263
Staghorn calculus, 164, 258
Stamey test, artery lesions, 192
Steblay nephritis (autoimmune glomeru-
        lonephritis), 43
Stenosis, renal artery, 107
Stillweger's syndrome, 158
Stop-flow analysis, 99
Storage disease (abnormal deposition),
        328
Strangury, 147
Streak method, semiquantitative, 226, 228
Stress incontinence, 128
Subendothelial deposits, 59, 61
Subepithelial deposits, 59, 60
Sublimate poisoning, 133
Sulfonamide toxicity, 147
Swan-neck tubular lesions, 75–76
Swelling
    glomerular cells, 76
    tubular cloudy, 76
Syndromes, cardinal, of renal disease, 333
Syndromes glossary, 153–159
Syphilis, congenital, with nephrotic syn-
        drome, 148
Systemic lupus erythematosus, 148, 180–
        182

Takayashu's syndrome, 139
Tetany, 100
Thick ascending limb, 10, 13
Thick descending limb, 10, 19
Threshold, 100
Thrombosis, 76–77
    renal artery, 107
    renal vein, 144
Thrombotic thrombocytopenic purpura
        (TTP), 148
Tissue, renal, abnormalities in amount of,
        324
Titratable acid, 100
Tolerance, 43
Tomography, 164
Toxemia of pregnancy. *See* Preeclampsia
        and eclampsia
Toxicity, 328–329
    mercury, 133–134
        diagnostic criteria, 184
    salicylate, 145
    sulfonamide, 147
Toxins or poisons, 328–329
Transit time, 100
Transplant rejection crises, 158–159
    acute transplant rejection, 158
    chronic transplant rejection, 158

hyperacute transplant rejection, 158–
        159
Transplanted kidneys, intravenous pyelo-
        gram of, 266
Transport, 100–101
    active, 100
    competitive, 100
    maximum, 96
Trauma
    mechanical nonpenetrating, 325
    mechanical penetrating, 325–326
    radiation, 326
    thermal, 326
Treponema pallidum, 148–149
Tuberculoid granulomata, 68–69
Tuberculosis
    epididymal, 149
    prostatic, 149
    renal, 149
        diagnostic criteria, 194
    retrograde pyelogram showing, 276
Tubular atrophy, 45–48
Tubular basement membrane abnormali-
        ties, 47
Tubular cells
    inclusions, 65
    regeneration, 73
Tubular edema, 55–56
Tubular leukocyte accumulation, 71
Tubular necrosis, 72
Tubular nephropathies, 323
Tubule, renal, 10, 28
    anatomy, 14–15, 29–32
    convoluted portion (*pars convoluta*),
        15, 19, 31
    distal segment, 15
    intermediate portions (*pars maculata;
        macula densa*), 15
    pars recta of proximal tubule, 28
    proximal convoluted segment, 14, 21,
        29–32
    proximal segment, 14
    secretions, 97
    straight portion (*pars recta*), 14–15, 19
    thick ascending limb, 10, 15, 19
    thick descending limb, 10, 14, 19
    thin segment, 10, 15, 33
    uniniferous, 14
Tubulorrhexis, 72, 77
Tuft, glomerular, 16
Tumors
    adrenal, 77
    clear cell, 109
    extrarenal malignant and invasive, 77–
        78, 149
    metastatic, 78, 149
    pathology, 77–78
    renal arteriograms, 282–286
    renal and benign, 78, 149
    Wilms' tumor, 136, 151